DOCTORS AND THE LAW

Medical Jurisprudence in Nineteenth-Century America

JAMES C. MOHR

D0017770

The Johns Hopkins University Press
Baltimore and London

Originally published in a hardcover edition by Oxford University Press.
Johns Hopkins Paperbacks edition, 1996
05 04 03 02 01 00 99 98 97 96   5 4 3 2 1

The Johns Hopkins University Press
2715 North Charles Street
Baltimore, Maryland 21218-4319
The Johns Hopkins Press Ltd., London

A catalog record for this book is available from the British Library.

ISBN 0-8018-5398-2 (pbk.)

Library of Congress Cataloging-in-Publication Data
Mohr, James C.
    Doctors and the law : medical jurisprudence in nineteenth-century America / James C. Mohr.
       p.   cm.
    Originally published : New York : Oxford University Press, 1993.
    ISBN 0-8018-5398-2 (pbk. : alk. paper)
    1. Medical jurisprudence—United States—History—19th century. I. Title.
    [DNLM: 1. History of Medicine, 19th Cent.—United States. 2. Jurisprudence—history.   WZ70 AA1
M6d 1993a]
RA1022.U6M64   1996
614'.1'097309034—dc20
DNLM/DLC
for Library of Congress   95-48061

DOCTORS AND THE LAW

To Elizabeth

Acknowledgments

Historians owe enormous debts of gratitude to librarians and archivists, without whom we simply could not do our work. I had the privilege of benefiting from the services of a great many librarians and archivists during the years of research that went into this book, and I would like to acknowledge their collective efforts here, even though I cannot list them individually. It has been a genuine pleasure to interact with so many professionals who are so good at what they do, who offer the right suggestions, who stay beyond normal closing times for an out-of-town scholar, who find lost material, who arrange to make and mail xeroxes, and generally advance the task of historical research.

Chief among the repositories I used was the National Library of Medicine in Bethesda, Maryland. The Historical Branch of that library holds an unmatched collection for the nineteenth century. If librarians ever establish a hall of fame, I would nominate Dorothy Hanks, head of historical reference services at the NLM during the key years of my research, as their first inductee. The staff of the Library of Congress in Washington, D.C., also proved accommodating, particularly in the Rare Books and Manuscripts Division and in the Law Division. Librarians at the University of Maryland, Baltimore County, were unceasingly supportive, especially in the patient location of interlibrary loans. I was also fortunate to enjoy the generous services of other Baltimore-area libraries and librarians, including those at the Health Sciences Library and the Marshall Law Library of the University of Maryland at Baltimore, the Baltimore Law Library, the library and archives of the Medical and Chirurgical Faculty of Maryland, the Peabody Library, and the Welch Medical Library of the Johns Hopkins University.

I found valuable evidence in Philadelphia at the College of Physicians of Philadelphia and at the University Archives of the University of Pennsylvania; in New Haven at the Sterling Library, the Yale Law Library, and the Yale University Archives; and in Boston at the Countway Library of the Harvard Medical School. In New York City the Rare Books and Manuscripts Division of the New York Public Library proved both helpful and important, as did the Rare Book Room of the New York Academy of Medicine Library. The staff of the New York State Library at Albany generously expedited access to rich resources there. Reference librarians at the American Medical Association headquarters in Chicago kindly copied records for me and sent them east.

Abroad I encountered equally dedicated and helpful librarians and archivists. In Paris the Institut Médecine Légale, thanks to Professors Léon Dérobert, André Hardengue, George Heymans, and Michele Rudler, opened its holdings to me and put a special reference assistant at my disposal. The manuscript division of the Archives Nationales granted special access to the Orfila papers. In London, my inquiries at the Wellcome Institute for the History of Medicine yielded unexpected leads at the Institute for Advanced Legal Study at the University of London. P. B. Freshwater, Lesley De-Jean, and Dorothy Wardle of the Special Collections division of the Edinburgh University Library pulled rare notebooks from their vaults and had them waiting in the Manuscripts and Rare Books Room to be read. The Royal College of Physicians of Edinburgh and the National Library of Scotland also offered useful materials related to my inquiries.

Sustained financial support is also crucial to historians, especially those engaged in relatively large, long-term projects like this one. Heading the list of my benefactors on this front is the John Simon Guggenheim Foundation, which appointed me a fellow for the academic year 1983–84. That award allowed me to launch this lengthy undertaking in the first place. I am also extremely grateful to the University of Maryland, Baltimore County, which steadily underwrote aspects of this research in the form of special library purchases, graduate assistants, and research expenses.

Several audiences have listened to papers and asked questions that helped me focus or rethink various aspects of this work. An early version of Chapter Two was presented at a National Library of Medicine Staff Seminar, under the direction of James Cassedy. Portions of Chapter Four were presented in a seminar at the Johns Hopkins Institute of the History of Medicine, under the direction of Gert Brieger. Portions of Chapter Five were presented in a seminar at the University of Wisconsin, Department of the History of Science, under the direction of Judith Leavitt and Ronald Numbers, and as a public lecture at the University of Wisconsin Law School, under the direction of Hendrik Hartog. Portions of Chapter Eight were presented as a lecture and discussion session in the Law and Medicine series at the College of Physicians of Philadelphia, under the direction of Janet Tighe, and to a class at the Yale Law School, under the direction of Michael Les Benedict. A slightly altered version of Chapter Eight appeared as "The Emergence of Medical Malpractice in America," in the *Transactions & Studies of the College of Physicians of Philadelphia*, ser. 5, vol. 14, no. 1 (March 1992): 1–21; and a slightly altered version of Chapter Nine appeared as "The Trial of John Hendrickson, Jr.: Medical Jurisprudence at Mid-Century," in *New York History*, vol. 70, no. 1 (January 1989): 23–53.

Many fellow scholars have helped me wrestle with this subject over the years. A few are acknowledged in specific notes. Some will recognize an idea here or a reference there, which they were kind enough to share. Others will see lines of analysis or inquiry to which they alerted me. Harder to notice are items that do not appear in the book: mistakes or misconceptions that colleagues have caught or corrected in conversation or in draft. I wish sincerely that I could thank by name the scores of people who have been so forthcoming in these and other ways, but the list would be too long. Suffice it to say that I remember in some detail a great many kindnesses and contributions, and I am tremendously grateful. Three people read the manuscript closely, and I would like to thank them personally: James H. Cassedy, William G. Rothstein, and Robert K. Webb. They are first-rate scholars, insightful critics, and excellent editorial readers, as well as good friends.

Finally, I would like to acknowledge the understanding and patience of my family. My children, Timothy and Stephanie, tolerated the ever-present subject of medical jurisprudence in our household with remarkable grace through periods of their lives when lots of children are not especially graceful about their parents' interests. My wife, to whom this book is dedicated, has been a tireless companion, perceptive reader, and marvelous helpmate. She remains all three and much more.

Eugene, Oregon   J.C.M.
November 1992

Contents

xii   *Contents*

Introduction

Most modern Americans take for granted the relationship that now exists between the medical profession and the nation's legal processes, especially since the essential elements of that relationship have been firmly in place for most of the twentieth century. But the essential elements of that relationship were neither in place nor somehow preordained when the nation was founded. Instead, they are the direct legacy of professional developments that took place during the nineteenth century. This book is the story of those developments and of the evolution of the present relationship between American physicians and American legal processes: a history of medical jurisprudence from the early national period, when the ultimate structural principles of medical jurisprudence in the United States were yet to be determined, through the end of the nineteenth century, when the basic structure of modern medical jurisprudence in the United States was essentially fixed.

Medical jurisprudence may be defined in at least two principal ways. First and most important, medical jurisprudence is the interaction between those who possess medical knowledge and those who exercise legal authority. Since that interaction must take place in some fashion, the ideal system of medical jurisprudence would be as fair, as effective, and as sensitive to the general well-being of society as it possibly could be. Second and more specifically, medical jurisprudence may also be defined as the separate professional field whose focus is the interaction between those who possess medical knowledge and those who exercise legal authority, a sort of facilitating or mediating field between medicine and law. Although modern Americans may consider this second definition somewhat hypothetical, medical jurisprudence as a separate professional field had existed on the European continent for centuries prior to the American Revolution. For at least fifty years following that Revolution, leading physicians in the United States hoped to establish a prominent role for the field in their new republic.

This study looks at the history of medical jurisprudence in both of its principal definitions. Though the double meaning risks some confusions, to be sure, the reciprocal relationship between the two definitions of medical jurisprudence makes consideration of them together both historically necessary and analytically essential. Without some understanding of the way American physicians actually interacted with the nation's legal processes, and how those interactions changed over time, it would be difficult, if not impossible, to understand why physicians interested in those interactions were flourishing or fading at any given time within their own medical profession.

Although the subject of medical jurisprudence by any definition might seem at first rather arcane and narrow, it certainly is not. The history of medical jurisprudence in the United States through the end of the nineteenth century involves large and significant issues of enduring interest, including the role of legal medicine in the evolution of the medical profession in the United States, the impact of physicians on general social policy, the quality and character of justice in American courts, and the shifting relationship between the medical profession and the state. Also involved are key issues in the history of medical education, the care and treatment of the mentally deficient, the origins of modern medical malpractice, and what might be called the civic consciousness of doctors, who would become in the twentieth century one of the nation's most powerful professional groups.

The study of medical jurisprudence also brings back into the historical spotlight individuals of towering importance in their own time, whose names are barely recognized even by specialists today, and dramatic trials of great symbolism and social significance, which riveted the attention of Americans at various points in the nineteenth century and helped shape popular attitudes toward medical jurisprudence. Those forgotten figures deserve recognition, and those trials remain just as dramatic today as they were when they were being conducted. Even the smaller byways associated with legal medicine prove inherently fascinating, and the history of medical jurisprudence offers an intriguing perspective on the overall development of American society through the beginning of the twentieth century, a perspective which emphasizes the place and role of the professions in the shaping of American life.

Nor is the early history of American medical jurisprudence by any means a static subject. Even though the current relationship between American physicians and the nation's legal processes has been essentially in place since the first decade of the twentieth century, that relationship evolved only after a series of dramatic developments during the nineteenth century. At least through the 1840s, for example, leading American physicians believed that the future of their profession lay in civic-minded interaction with the nation's courts, legislatures, and lawyers; by the end of the century the vast majority of American physicians had withdrawn from most legal processes, and relations between doctors and lawyers were, to say the least, strained. Through the first half of the nineteenth century, American medical schools gave medical jurisprudence a prominent place in their professional curriculum; by 1900 the field had essentially disappeared from professional schools. Medico-legal problems stimulated exciting research through the first half of the nineteenth century and created for the United States at least one professional of international standing; by 1900 few people conducted serious medico-legal research in the United States. Leading physicians tried during the nineteenth century first to create a system of medico-legal officers in the United States and then, failing that, at least to ensure professional compensation for physicians acting as medico-legal experts in the public interest. By the end of the century, however, they acquiesced in a politico-professional compromise that created prototypes in New England of the twentieth-century medical examiner, a very different officer from the one earlier physicians had anticipated as an important agent in the long-term well-being of the nation.

Many of the developments analyzed in this book seem in retrospect even more striking still. In 1800 medical experts had no particular standing in American courtrooms; by 1900 the system now taken for granted was fully functional, complete with a pool of contradictory opinions for hire on any given subject. Through the first half of the nineteenth century the medico-legal aspects of insanity provided the field of medical jurisprudence with some of its most progressive material; during the second half of the nineteenth century the medico-legal aspects of insanity became the nightmare they have remained through the twentieth century. In 1800, astonishing as it might seem to anyone involved in legal medicine today, actions for medical malpractice were virtually unknown in the United States; by 1900 medical malpractice had assumed its modern place in American professional relations.

These, then, are the sorts of developments discussed in this book, the developments that largely determined the evolution of the present relationship between the American medical profession and the nation's legal processes. They are developments played out against larger shifts in American history from the founding of the republic through the end of the nineteenth century, and they are developments that continue to have a remarkably direct effect upon United States citizens even as the nation enters the twenty-first century.

DOCTORS AND THE LAW

CHAPTER ONE

Medical Jurisprudence
in the New Republic

The United States emerged from the American Revolution with its previously imposed English approach to medical jurisprudence virtually unaltered. But to many prominent physicians, who were trying to help shape both the future of American society and the place of their profession within it, that old English approach appeared dysfunctional. Under traditional English law and civil procedure, public authorities could, if they wished, solicit the opinion of medical practitioners on any given subject under a number of circumstances; but the public authorities were not obliged to do so, even when the matter under consideration seemed obviously to involve medical questions. In those instances when they did want medical opinions, coroners and justices had the power to subpoena physicians and require them to conduct any appropriate examinations, including post-mortem analyses. Doctors were generally not paid for those publicly mandated investigations and generally tried to avoid such coerced service. When compelled to lend a hand, or even when they were anxious to help, most American physicians were too poorly trained in systematic methods and forensic applications to be significantly useful in any event. Coroners and justices, in turn, who did have to pay the peripheral expenses of medical examinations, even though they did not have to compensate the individual physicians for conducting them, usually preferred to take a given situation on its circumstantial appearances rather than spend time, trouble, and public money probing beneath the surface.[1]

To make matters worse, when physicians were directly involved in legal processes as expert witnesses, whether impressed by the state or retained by private parties, they almost always testified not as neutral seekers of the whole truth, but as advocates for one side or the other in overtly adversarial settings. Sometimes those settings were political forums, as in the case of disputes before a town council (imagine, for example, the hard feelings engendered in a small village where one group of citizens wanted the business of another group of citizens shut down for the sake of public health), or legislative hearings (as in the case of proposed quarantines, which had huge implications for trade); more often the settings were civil or criminal courtrooms, where intense personal battles of various sorts were fought to bitter and often divisive conclusions. As a consequence, physicians not infrequently found themselves before the public as a group of people who were intellectually fragmented and only occasionally useful in the cause of justice or the protection of the general welfare. Though such characterizations may have been closer to the truth than many physicians cared to admit, they regarded their relationship to legal processes as frustrating, professionally counter-productive, and in need of reformation.

The best-informed American physicians realized that the English system they had inherited was by no means the only way to approach medico-legal questions. Many of the governments of continental Europe, for example, had long retained specific individuals, trained as experts in medical jurisprudence, whose job was to guarantee, at least in theory, that relations between medicine and law would be as close and effective as possible. Pope Gregory IX had officially recognized the role of physicians in certain types of trials in 1234, and the Italian city-state of Bologna had an officially sworn medico-legal officer as early as 1249. A number of other city-states followed suit, and by the end of the thirteenth century state-sanctioned legal medicine had spread through Provence to Aragon and the Iberian peninsula. Rulers in northern and central Europe also began to see the advantages of giving official authority to medical experts in many sorts of legal proceedings, especially since the rulers themselves retained power over their appointed physicians. While the interests of the state were not always identical to the interests of the folk, as became painfully obvious when some of the early medico-legal experts were enlisted as court torturers, somewhat systematic medical jurisprudence gained an institutional base and an official status in most of Europe. The best-known milestone in the development of the Continental tradition had been the so-called Carolingian Code promulgated by the German emperor Charles V in 1533. That Code authorized government spending to train medico-legal experts, stipulated that paid officers with formal status would be responsible for applying the advances of medical science to the law and its processes, and provided a rationale for appropriations designed to advance both forensic medicine and public health.[2]

By the 1790s, American physicians were also aware of growing uneasiness with the British approach to medical jurisprudence even in Great Britain itself, especially among the Scots. At the University of Edinburgh, which then housed the most prestigious, progressive, and practically-oriented medical school in the English-speaking world, the faculty expressed grave concern about the low quality of medical jurisprudence in the United Kingdom. Drawing upon his own extensive knowledge of the Continental traditions, Andrew Duncan, Sr., professor of the institutes (i.e. the basic underlying principles) of medicine, began to offer formal lectures on medical jurisprudence in 1791, the first of their kind in English.[3] His initial efforts to upgrade the civic consciousness and forensic skills of Britain's future physicians were simply tacked on at the end of his regular courses. Soon, however, Duncan began to teach separate classes designed to boost the popular awareness and social significance of medical jurisprudence. He opened these classes to the general public and encouraged lawyers and local officials in particular to attend. Because American physicians continued to regard Edinburgh as the medical school of choice and emulation in the United Kingdom, they also paid attention to Duncan's initiatives.[4]

Like many other influential physicians on both sides of the Atlantic, Duncan believed that medical experts should play a more systematic and effective role in the formation and implementation of social policy, particularly in areas related to what would now be labeled criminal justice and public health. Physicians should be working more and more closely both with the policymakers who made the laws and with the lawyers who worked out their practical implications. As the decade progressed, Duncan devoted an increasing proportion of his course work to public health concerns. By 1797 he was asserting both to his students and to the citizens of Edinburgh that it was "incumbent on a medical Practitioner to suggest the Causes of particular Diseases to Magistrates," and by 1800 Duncan's public lectures addressed at length such subjects as air circulation, sanitation, noxious odors and gases, fresh food and water, quarantines, hospitals, the treatment of the insane, and a special interest of his, cemetery regulations, in addition to such traditional topics as toxicology, the causes of death, and the conduct of a post-mortem examination.[5]

Duncan's efforts paid direct personal dividends. In 1807 the government in London authorized creation of a formal chair in medical jurisprudence at Edinburgh. The new chair was opposed by a majority of the existing faculty, who did not want to thin the ranks of their own paying students by adding more courses to the curriculum, and by the opposition in Parliament, including George Canning, who considered the move an audacious example of unnecessary spending. But the strong support of the Edinburgh townspeople, who had been won over by Duncan's visions of a higher quality of justice and better public health, helped bolster the government's resolve. Duncan thereupon maneuvered successfully to have his son, Andrew Duncan, Jr., appointed to the new chair. This activity at Edinburgh seemed to ensure that more systematic attention would be paid in future to the subject of medical jurisprudence in the United Kingdom. Formally appointed scholars would now be able, at least in theory, to spend their time investigating the various questions associated with medical jurisprudence and impressing the importance of medico-legal issues upon forthcoming generations of British doctors.

The subsequent history of the new jurisprudential chairs in British medical schools proved anticlimactic in the short run. Because students paid for their education course by course, and because a course in medical jurisprudence was not required for graduation with an M.D. degree, relatively few students laid out extra money to hear lectures on the subject, either at Edinburgh or elsewhere around the United Kingdom where similar chairs were subsequently authorized. Since a faculty member's teaching income depended directly upon the number of students who paid to take his courses, chairs in medical jurisprudence gained a reputation as being cheap posts, professorships without much direct compensation. Most of the doctors who accepted these appointments during the early decades of their existence did so as a way of getting a foot in the faculty door. But their goal was to move as quickly as they could to a more lucrative chair. Few of the early professors actually did serious work in medical jurisprudence; it was more important to them to keep up in the fields to which they ultimately aspired. The younger Duncan himself transferred to Edinburgh's chair of materia medica (a required course) in 1820, and his successor in medical jurisprudence, William Pulteney Alison, served only until 1822, when he seized a chance to become professor of the institutes of medicine (another required course). During the 1820s there was widespread agitation to eliminate the medical jurisprudential chairs, but the government eventually rescued their occupants by making medical jurisprudence a required course in 1833. It is surely no coincidence that British medical educators began to produce serious work in the field only after that year.[6]

Physicians in the United States at the beginning of the nineteenth century could not have foreseen the less-than-immediate impact of the Edinburgh reforms. But like the Scots, the Americans were increasingly uncomfortable with the way the old English system was operating in practice. Looking ahead toward the future place of their profession in the emerging republic, they began to reconsider the relation of medicine to law. The times seemed perfect for reform, and the United States seemed to epitomize an exciting spirit of institutional experimentation. Medical jurisprudence, a subject little studied and poorly practiced through the colonial period and the Revolution, appeared ready for major readjustment.

The United States had two chief centers of medical activity and medical education by 1800. One was at Philadelphia, where the oldest and most prestigious medical school in the country was located, and the other was at New York City, where a relatively high number of European-trained physicians worked and taught. During the first decade of the nineteenth century influential professional leaders in both cities launched efforts to improve American medical jurisprudence. In Philadelphia, the *Medical Museum* first brought the cause to the attention of the city's professionals. In 1808 that journal published a manifesto written ten years earlier by Andrew Duncan, Sr., entitled "A Short View of the Extent and Importance of Medical Jurisprudence, Considered as a Branch of Education." The essay had originally been presented privately to the Patrons of the University of Edinburgh, then made public in 1806, when Henry Erskine, Lord Advocate for Scotland, submitted it to the cabinet in Westminster in support of the government's proposal to create professorial chairs in the subject.[7] Erskine, a leading lawyer and moderate reformer, saw the improvement of legal medicine as part of the larger effort he was involved in at the time "for the better regulation of the courts of justice in Scotland."[8]

In his essay Duncan had divided medico-legal interactions into two fundamental categories: "judicial medicine," by which he meant the application of medical knowledge to court cases; and "medical police," by which he meant the orderly regulation of public health.[9] Duncan went on to review the importance of both branches, to trace the history of medical jurisprudence on the Continent, and to assert the tremendous need he perceived for the systematic teaching of medical jurisprudence in the British world. Duncan also outlined the chief topics he considered essential to any course in medical jurisprudence. John Redman Coxe, editor of the *Museum*, underscored his endorsement of Duncan's position by announcing that efforts at improvement were already under way in New York City and by publishing in the same issue of the journal an article on urban public health by the American physician Elijah Griffiths. Entitled "An essay on the means necessary to be employed for correcting and rendering wholesome the atmosphere of large cities," the article advocated municipal sewers and legal restrictions on the industrial pollutants emitted from such "domestic manufactories" as soap-making plants, distilleries, refineries, and slaughterhouses.[10]

A number of Philadelphia's most prominent doctors soon came forward to champion the new cause of improving medical jurisprudence. Foremost among them was the redoubtable Benjamin Rush. While a student in England in the 1760s, Rush had known William Hunter, one of the few British physicians who tried to undertake systematic research on medicolegal issues prior to the end of the eighteenth century.[11] Rush's subsequent career as a public figure in the United States during and after the Revolution heightened his appreciation of the subject, for he was forced to think seriously about the various roles that his own profession might play in the new republic. Rush was a signer of the Declaration of Independence, a delegate to the Pennsylvania ratification convention, and a treasurer of the United States mint at Philadelphia as well as a practicing doctor and a medical school professor. Even the professionals who cordially disliked the intrigues, postures, and controversial therapeutics of this physician-politician had to take seriously anything to which he turned his attention.[12]

In 1810 Rush decided to make a public gesture in behalf of better relations between medicine and law in the United States. In June of that year he wrote his son, who was then himself studying in England, that he intended to highlight some aspect of medical jurisprudence in his next introductory lecture at the University of Pennsylvania. Since introductory lectures were public showpieces, and because his lecture would certainly be published, Rush's choice of material represented a conscious decision to use his renown to try to stimulate the study of medical jurisprudence in America. Dismayed that so little was available on the subject, Rush found himself wishing that he had "a copy of young Dr. Duncan's lectures upon medical jurisprudence" to help him prepare one of his own. Notwithstanding the paucity of material, however, Rush made his long-term goal explicit: "At a future day that science [medical jurisprudence] I hope will be taught in the University of Pennsylvania."[13]

Rush eventually chose to speak on the problem of mental competence because he thought that subject would allow him to demonstrate the "usefulness" of medical jurisprudence.[14] While it is tempting for scholars of the late twentieth century, who are still struggling with the slippery concept of legal sanity, to see in this decision another example of Benjamin Rush's legendary tendency to expound idiosyncratic opinions, he was, for once, not being perverse. For reasons that will be assessed later, Rush seems to have had a better insight than many subsequent writers into the ways in which the issue of legal insanity, as distinguished from insanity itself, affected ordinary Americans.

"To animate you to apply to the study of medical jurisprudence," Rush exhorted his students,

> I beg you will recollect the extent of the services you will thereby be enabled to render to individuals and the public. Fraud and violence may be detected and punished; unmerited infamy and death may be prevented; the widow and the orphan may be saved from ruin; virgin purity and innocence may be vindicated; conjugal harmony and happiness may be restored; unjust and oppressive demands upon the services of your fellow citizens may be obviated; and the sources of public misery in epidemic diseases may be removed, by your testimony in a court of justice. Nor is this all. By cultivating this science I am now recommending, you may extend its benefits beyond our courts of justice, to the legislatures of our country, and thereby become the means of obtaining laws formed upon modern discoveries and opinions in physiology.[15]

That was a powerful prescription. Rush clearly envisioned medical jurisprudence as a tool for greatly expanding the social role of his own profession. As he phrased it himself, "they entertain very limited views of medicine who suppose its objects and duties are confined exclusively to the knowledge and cure of diseases."[16] And significantly, he apparently never anticipated, either in his private letters on the subject or in his public exhortations, that the expansion he envisioned might provoke conflict with other professional groups. If anything, Rush believed the reverse: stronger medico-legal skills among physicians would be welcomed by professionals and the general public alike. Though his sentiment now seems hopelessly naive, Rush in all good faith urged his students to obtain a strong grounding in the medical jurisprudence of insanity so they might "relieve judges and jurors from the painful necessity of acting in a discretionary manner."[17] Enthusiastic about the possibility of upgrading medical jurisprudence in the United States, Rush wrote to Thomas Jefferson right after his introductory lecture on the subject was published, urging the former President to pay particular attention to it.[18]

Rush died in the spring of 1813, but the cause of medical jurisprudence in Philadelphia was taken up by two of the city's other prominent physician-scientists, Charles Caldwell and Thomas Cooper. The former, who had gone from being Rush's favorite pupil to being one of Rush's most bitter enemies and then back again to close colleague, began to offer public lectures on the subject of medical jurisprudence. The lectures were open to any interested Philadelphians willing to purchase a subscription to hear them. For educated citizens, open courses like these were one of the principal intellectual reasons to live in a city that had a college or a professional school, and for aspiring medical practitioners, extramural courses in such subjects as human anatomy played a crucial role in practical training.[19] Caldwell offered his medical jurisprudence lectures on a public subscription basis because his faculty appointment was in the University of Pennsylvania's collegiate department rather than the medical school and because he hoped to attract Philadelphia's leading lawyers and already practicing physicians in addition to students still in training. Caldwell claimed in his autobiography that his goals were at least partially met, for several of the elite lawyers of the city took his course.[20] Though the effort failed as a business venture, he maintained throughout his influential career a strong personal commitment to the field.[21]

Caldwell's colleague Thomas Cooper tried to bolster the study of medical jurisprudence in the United States by collecting, annotating, and publishing the first major compilation of the subject to appear under an American imprint. Though little known today, Cooper was one of the most fascinating and multi-talented men of his own generation; a sort of aristocratic, intellectual, and professional version of Thomas Paine. Cooper had been born and educated in England, where he studied both the classics and the sciences before becoming a barrister. A confirmed rationalist and radical, however, he emigrated to the United States in 1793 along with two of the sons of his friend Joseph Priestley. Cooper's example helped resolve the elder Priestley later to make the same migration, and the two settled near each other in Pennsylvania. Cooper became a Jeffersonian judge in Pennsylvania, a professor at Carlisle College (now Dickinson), and a confidant of Thomas Jefferson himself, before accepting a chair in chemistry and mineralogy at the University of Pennsylvania.[22] There, while serving as Caldwell's colleague, Cooper brought out his *Tracts on Medical Jurisprudence*.[23]

In his *Tracts* Cooper reprinted the four English-language essays on medical jurisprudence that he considered most useful: Samuel Farr's "Elements of Medical Jurisprudence . . . To Which Are Added, Directions for Preserving the Public Health" (which had been published in England in 1787 and was closely based upon a Swiss text that appeared in 1767); William Dease's "Remarks on Medical Jurisprudence; Intended for the General Information of Juries and Young Surgeons" (Dease was himself a surgeon); George Edward Male's "An Epitome of Juridical or Forensic Medicine, for the use of Medical Men, Coroners, and Barristers" (Male was a student of Duncan and his work clearly reflected his mentor's views); and John Haslam's "Medical Jurisprudence, as it relates to Insanity, according to the Law of England" (the most recent statement on the subject, this piece had appeared in 1817). To this core Cooper added a preface, extensive annotations, a digest of the law of insanity in the United States, several snippets that threw light upon American court practice in medically related cases, and a paper that Cooper had read to the American Philosophical Society on the chemical methods of detecting arsenic.

Of greatest interest to modern analysts were Cooper's annotations, since they revealed the sorts of things this champion of a new order wanted to change. As befitted this outspoken defender of scientific inquiry and individual freedom, the chief theme of those notes was Cooper's belief that medical jurisprudence should first and foremost concern itself with protecting defendants against wrongful conviction. Cooper highlighted several well-known instances where the English system had failed to do that, and he exhorted his fellow professionals to see that the American system did not perpetuate similar flaws. Experts should testify when called into court, juries should defer to professional judgment, and circumstantial evidence should never be sufficient to convict in capital cases. Regardless of a defendant's past history, public standing, general behavior, or possible motives, it was up to experts in medical jurisprudence to prove that the accused had committed the specific act alleged, a suspected poisoning, for example, or what looked like an intentional drowning. In the absence of scientific proof, the defendant should go free.[24] Persecuted in England for his radical views, convicted and fined under the notorious Sedition Act in the United States in 1800, and removed as a judge by political partisans who considered him too arbitrary, Cooper saw in the field of medical jurisprudence a potential bastion of individual rights.[25]

Cooper realized, partly on the basis of his own experience as a judge, that medical jurisprudence did not always operate in the idealistic fashion he prescribed. Consequently, he was at some pains to make explicit what he thought necessary. First on his agenda was upgraded, systematic training in forensic science for America's physicians. He was appalled at the scanty knowledge of basic chemistry among American physicians, even those frequently called to conduct chemical tests for use in courtrooms. He railed openly at "the gross ignorance in Chemistry and Pharmacy of physicians educated" at his own institution, the University of Pennsylvania, though it was "by far the most fashionable place of resort for medical education in the United States."[26] That was why he included his own paper on toxicology in his Tracts; he viewed it as the latest research by a prominent professor of chemistry.[27]

Second, the public would have to spend more money on the training of medico-legal experts, provide them institutional settings where they could conduct ongoing research, and afford them the high social status that experts in such a crucially important field deserved. Here Cooper's political radicalism coexisted uneasily with his traditional professional elitism. He considered the medical expert the defender of the ordinary citizen against powers greater than himself, yet the medical expert must also be an archetypical "gentleman," to use Cooper's own word, in order to be effective. Cooper consistently favored training in the classical languages, certification procedures in related sciences, and relatively high age requirements for those who wished to practice medicine, in large part because they would be entrusted with jurisprudential responsibilities.[28]

Third, the American legal system itself would have to be adjusted to accommodate better medical jurisprudence. Post-mortem examinations would have to be conducted by experts, who would take careful notes and work in the presence of a competent jury. The experts should be appointed by the jury "specially . . . for the purpose," as distinguished from using physicians brought in after the fact by one party or the other to search for evidence useful to those who engaged them. In this same vein, Cooper praised the Napoleonic Code, which he quoted from its 1813 Paris edition, on a number of subjects. In his view the French had come closest to melding effectively the old Continental tradition of medical jurisprudence in the service of the state with the Americans' post-Revolutionary sensitivity to individual rights. The Code was "so full of good sense" that he was confident "readers will be glad to peruse" its provisions.[29] Obviously, Cooper hoped that American medico-legal practice would move in the same direction as the French, a hope that would grow steadily stronger among American physicians after 1820.

For all its value, Cooper's contribution to medical jurisprudence had serious weaknesses, one of which was an obvious oversight. Perhaps because the author wanted to appear more in the vanguard of a new field than he already was, or perhaps because of the intense rivalry between the two medical centers in Philadelphia and New York, Cooper failed to mention activities under way in the latter city. That was not only ungracious, but historically short-sighted. By the time Cooper published his *Tracts* in Philadelphia in 1819, New York physicians had pushed the study of medical jurisprudence further than their counterparts in Philadelphia. They had also offered the first formal lectures in the United States on the subject, established the nation's first professorial chair in the field, and trained the man who would later become the greatest American authority in the field.

The first formal lectures on medical jurisprudence had been offered by James Stringham. Stringham grew up in New York City during the Revolutionary era. His parents managed to maintain their considerable wealth through that tumultuous period, and sent him to Columbia. There he studied the classics, anticipated a career in the ministry, and obtained his B.A. degree in 1793. But Stringham was plagued by what appears in retrospect to have been a form of congenital heart disease. He abandoned his postgraduate theological studies in the mid-90s and became interested in medicine; he was, after all, almost constantly being doctored. Stringham, under the guidance of Samuel Bard and David Hosack, mastered all of the material then taught by what was called the Faculty of Physic in New York City. To complete his medical education in the fashion appropriate to an able, wealthy, and well-educated gentleman, he went to Edinburgh. Awarded an M.D. from that university in 1799, he returned to his native city and accepted a professorship of chemistry at Columbia.[30]

Stringham took seriously his responsibilities to promote science in the

United States "at a period when comparatively few could be found engaged in so good a cause," as one of his faculty colleagues somewhat sardonically noted.[31] While in Edinburgh, Stringham had attended the elder Duncan's lectures on medical jurisprudence and decided voluntarily to prepare a similar series for American audiences. Like Duncan, Stringham inaugurated his series as an addendum to his regular courses. Student response proved favorable, and in the words of James Thacher writing twenty years later, "The utility of the science [of medical jurisprudence] was cheerfully acknowledged by all."[32] Thacher's use of "cheerfully" was telling rather than quaint, for New York medical education was then an intensely competitive and highly politicized business. To put it mildly, anyone who tried to gain personal advantage in any way, including the introduction of a popular new subject, would expect opposition. That Stringham's medical jurisprudence encountered none of substance testified to the professor's popularity and the subject's appeal. By 1808 Columbia recognized the potential drawing power of the nation's only systematic instruction in medical jurisprudence and in its advertisements touted Stringham's courses formally as "Chemistry and Legal Medicine."[33]

Stringham continued as Columbia's professor of chemistry and what might be considered adjunct lecturer in medical jurisprudence through 1813, when a major reorganization of medical education in New York forced him to shift his position. David Hosack had been engineering a merger between the College of Physicians and Surgeons of New York, a de facto proprietary school of which he was a principal, on the one hand, and the medical branch of Columbia, which Hosack hoped to eliminate, on the other. Though some of the members of the Columbia faculty, including Stringham, resisted Hosack's attempt to hug them to death, the merger finally took place. Hosack, who would remain throughout his stormy and contentious career a consistent advocate of medical jurisprudence, arranged for a formal chair in the subject at the newly enlarged College of Physicians and Surgeons, then offered it to Stringham, partly as a way to win Stringham's approval of the merger. Rather than battle on, Stringham accepted his old mentor's offer, and in this Byzantine fashion the United States gained its first formal professorship of medical jurisprudence.[34]

While Stringham certainly constructed his course in medical jurisprudence around the notes he had himself taken in Edinburgh, he added the insights of his own reading in the classics and, more important, the latest research emanating from France. Stringham's attention to French activity was perhaps to be expected, and certainly important to the development of medical jurisprudence in the United States. As a professor of chemistry, he was doubtless aware of the advances being made in that field in France, and his predecessor in Columbia's chair of chemistry, Samuel L. Mitchill, had introduced the new French chemical nomenclature into the United States.[35]

Stringham's attention to French developments, which paralleled Cooper's strong endorsement of the medico-legal aspects of the Napoleonic Code, helped establish from the beginning a tendency in the field of American medical jurisprudence to admire and to keep abreast of French medical jurisprudence. The political and intellectual climate of Jeffersonian America no doubt encouraged scholars in all fields to take French ideas and French institutions more seriously than had the English during the colonial era. President Jefferson was a francophile; the French had not only backed the Americans in their rebellion against the British empire but tried to establish a republic of their own; and the English after 1812 would reappear as military invaders. Over the next several decades American professionals would benefit enormously from their close attention to French developments, because the French during the first half of the nineteenth century went through one of their most impressive periods of creativity in the medical sciences generally and in medical jurisprudence specifically.[36] In the areas of toxicology and insanity, for example, both of which were central concerns of nineteenth-century medical jurisprudence, virtually all historians of medicine concur that the French were doing the most heuristic and valuable work undertaken in the Western world during that period.

Stringham never published the lectures he prepared, though his colleagues encouraged him to do so while he was alive and unsuccessfully importuned his widow to release them after his death. Consequently, scholars must rely on the notes taken by his students, preserved in their lecture-books, and on an outline syllabus of Stringham's course, published in 1814. The latter appeared in a journal edited by Hosack and John W. Francis, the man who took over Stringham's course in medical jurisprudence after Stringham died. The volume was dedicated to James Kent, Chancellor of the State of New York, who presided over New York's equity court system and had to deal regularly with medico-legal questions that often involved large amounts of money.[37]

Stringham had divided his material into twenty topical discussions. The first ten dealt generally with issues related to sex and reproduction: the ages at which various physiological developments took place, the problem of knowing when to risk a Caesarean section, questions related to virginity (including the methods of detecting rape and sodomy), concealed pregnancies, abortion, unusual births (including twinning, birth defects, or "monstrosities," and abnormalities of the sex organs, or "hermaphrodites"), impotence, and sterility. Sections eleven and twelve were devoted to extensive discussion of feigned disease, which usually arose in cases where people sought to avoid public work or military service; and concealed disease, which usually arose in cases where people sought to avoid quarantines or anti-contagion laws. Under the thirteenth heading was a long series of lectures on poisons. As might be expected of a former chemistry professor, this section of Stringham's course was remarkably sophisticated by the standards of his day. Next came instructions on how to proceed in a forensic autopsy, and a substantial discussion of wounds. The sixteenth section of the course was devoted to the issue of infanticide and how to detect it. How to save individuals near death from hanging or drowning, along with the ways to detect hanging and drowning as causes of death, followed. In the eighteenth section Stringham addressed professional behavior and medical etiquette. The final two sections dealt with aspects of public health: "the propriety of permitting certain manufactories in thickly inhabited places," and "the salubrity and insalubrity of particular kinds of water."[38]

Stringham was not a strong or original scholar. Though his eulogists praised him for his publications, those publications were neither numerous nor penetrating.[39] Moreover, Stringham did not last long in the chair that was created for him. The congenital heart ailments that led him to become interested in medicine in the first place continued to dog him. A student taking his class during the 1815–16 school year noted that Stringham could not continue to the end of the term. Leaving his lectures to be read aloud by a physician-friend in New York City, Stringham went to St. Croix, where colleagues felt his heart condition might improve. Unfortunately, it did not, and he died there June 29, 1817.[40]

Stringham deserves credit, nonetheless, for more than simply being the first full-time expositor of medical jurisprudence in the United States. Everyone acquainted with his professional efforts agreed that Stringham was an excellent teacher, and through his erudite lectures and manifest enthusiasm for the subject, he inspired one of the College of Physicians and Surgeons' best students, Theodric Romeyn Beck, to choose a medical jurisprudential topic for his dissertation. That choice proved to be the beginning of a lifelong commitment to the subject, which would by the middle of the nineteenth century make T.R. Beck the best-known expert in medical jurisprudence in the world.

CHAPTER TWO

T. R. Beck and the Elements of Medical Jurisprudence

In 1812 the Regents of the State of New York persuaded the legislature to charter a new medical school to serve upstate citizens in a more convenient way than the distant College of Physicians and Surgeons at New York City was then able to do. Located at Fairfield in Herkimer County, the new school was called the College of Physicians and Surgeons of the Western District of the State of New York.[1] Aware of the rising professional interest in medical jurisprudence, the board of trustees of the new institution wanted that subject taught at their school from the outset. They approached one of James Stringham's former students, Theodric Romeyn Beck, who was then practicing medicine in Albany. Beck accepted their offer and in 1815 joined the faculty as professor of both the institutes of medicine and medical jurisprudence. Because Western's new professor would eventually come to embody American professional interest in medical jurisprudence, and because his writings would earn him an international reputation in the field, his approach to the subject is well worth reviewing.

Beck had been born in Schenectady, New York, in 1791, and was to be the oldest of five brothers.[2] His paternal grandfather and father had both been prominent lawyers. His mother, who raised her sons alone after the death of her husband in 1798, was strongly committed to a family tradition of learning in general and higher education in particular.[3] Her own father and brother were both doctors of divinity and Dutch Reformed pastors; a cousin was president of the state medical society. In 1807, at the age of sixteen, T. R. Beck graduated from Union College, which one of his grandfathers had founded. From there he went first to Albany to serve a brief medical apprenticeship, then to New York City to study medicine formally at the College of Physicians and Surgeons. Although technically a student of David Hosack, Beck was most influenced by James Stringham and his lectures on medical jurisprudence, which Beck found "a source of great gratification" and full of potential "utility."[4] For his dissertation, which he defended successfully in 1811, Beck had sought a topic that would lend

15

itself to medico-legal discussion. He chose insanity, the same topic that Benjamin Rush used to showcase the field in Philadelphia that same year.

Beck's dissertation foreshadowed some of the intellectual characteristics that would later make its author a famous man. Most of its forty pages consisted of a concise survey of the literature then available on the issue of insanity. Beck would remain extremely skillful throughout his career in the art of the precis; he could identify clearly and express well the important ideas of other researchers. The dissertation also revealed Beck's essentially humane attitude toward human problems of all sorts. To the extent his dissertation had a thesis, it was to champion the efficacy of "removing [insane] patients from their residence to some proper asylum; and for this purpose, a calm retreat in the country is to be preferred." There he felt patients could be placed under a "system of human [i.e. humane] vigilance," rather than the "blows, stripes, and chains" tolerated for centuries by medical authorities. As his daughter testified after his death, Beck always retained "the most intense horror of oppression and injustice whether practiced by corporations or individuals."[5] Finally, along with his ability to summarize and his enduring sympathy toward those in trouble, the dissertation demonstrated Beck's fascination with statistics and quantifiable assertions. He appended a survey of asylums in Europe and the United States, for example, complete with tables. Although Beck's dissertation was favorably received by the medical press of the day and may have been a harbinger of things to come, it did not make any particular splash.[6]

The new M.D. returned to Albany to begin the difficult job of trying to establish a paying practice. Through his family's powerful connections, Beck obtained an appointment as physician to the Albany almshouse, a post that provided a degree of public visibility and financial stability. But the job of expanding his practice proved frustrating, and he received little help from his jealous competitors, whom he characterized in a private letter to his close friend and former medical-school classmate, John W. Francis, as "a set of plodding, mean, lowlive [sic] Blockheads, with a few exceptions."[7] Beck's lack of paying patients did offer him the somewhat ironic opportunity of pursuing further his fascination with medical jurisprudence. In October 1811, he noted that he had "read a number of books with reference to Legal Medicine, making extracts to enlarge my store of facts on that subject." He confided to his friend Francis that "I still hold out to myself the idea of one day being enabled to prepare a work on that subject, which may be of some use or value[.] 'Every Man . . . owes something to his profession and to mankind'." He also asked Francis to help him obtain the latest works from France on the subject.[8]

By the autumn of 1812 Beck was sufficiently discouraged with his prospects in Albany that he decided to enlist in the army's "Hospital Department." His motivation was partly patriotic and partly economic. On the one hand, war had been declared with England, and Beck was at this stage of his life and would remain to his death a fervent nationalist and outspoken champion of the new American republic.[9] On the other hand, his practice was "hardly worth more than $350 a year at present & the war will probably prevent its increasing." But he wanted to keep his enlistment a secret until he received some sort of confirmation from the government.[10]

Beck's circumspection saved him considerable embarrassment because the army never responded to the young physician's offer to enlist. He had submitted his credentials to the Quartermaster General at Albany for forwarding to Washington, but somewhere along the line the papers were lost. "So much for visions of patriotism," wrote a bemused Beck to his confidant, adding that at least business was picking up in Albany because of an epidemic. In view of what he considered to be the unscientific puffery and crackpot theories proffered by most of the other local physicians in response to the epidemic, Beck persuaded himself that his services would be "more important & useful at home at the present" than at the front.[11]

Through 1813 Beck continued to read and summarize the most important studies of medical jurisprudence then available, especially those emanating from the Continental tradition. He borrowed and translated Francis's copy of Paolo Zacchia's *Questiones medico-legales.* Though Beck considered the *Questiones* "very heavy & written in the most barbarous Latin," Zacchia's works, which had originally been published during the 1620s, were in Beck's day and are still today considered to have laid the basic foundations of modern Western medical jurisprudence.[12] Most of the problems that Zacchia addressed in the seventeenth century would reappear in Beck's own great work two hundred years later.

More to Beck's taste were François Foderé's 1799 *Les Lois éclairees par les sciences physiques, or Traité de médecine légale et d'hygiène publique,* an example of the exciting new work coming out of France; and back issues of the *Edinburgh Medical and Surgical Review,* whose editor, Andrew Duncan, Jr., tried to keep his readers informed about the latest and most interesting developments in medical jurisprudence.[13] Throughout this period, perhaps precisely because it was so professionally frustrating, Beck clung to his private resolve. He continued to be "engaged in collecting Notes on Legal Medicine" wherever he could find them, he wrote Francis. "My original plan on that subject remains unaltered. I hope one day or other to prepare something for publication."[14]

In 1814 Beck married Harriet Caldwell. Judging from the half-philosophical and half-sophomoric accounts of the romance relayed to Francis, Beck delighted in the company of his new wife. Also to the point, however, was the fact that Harriet's father was one of the wealthiest of the old Albany-based upstate gentry. Beck's marriage eliminated the young scholar-physician's financial uncertainties and freed him to continue to pursue his interests in medical jurisprudence, aided during the winter of 1814–15 by a fresh supply of French texts. His goal was to "finish two subjects of Disquisition this winter, one in Legal Medicine *Feigned Diseases* & one in Medical Police *on the effects of Manufactures on the Public Health,*" which would serve "as specimens" of the sort of larger work he had in mind. As the war drew to a close in the early months of 1815, Beck waxed rhetorical about the limitless potential of the United States, now finally secure from reconquest by England. He clearly envisioned young professionals like himself playing a key role in the realization of that potential.[15]

When Beck accepted the professorship tendered by Western College in 1815, medical teaching was neither a full-time nor a full-salaried occupation. Faculty often served schools far removed from their own homes, residing at the college only while school was in session, typically a couple of months during the winter. For most of the rest of the year they would retain a home base elsewhere, as Beck continued to do in Albany. Through most of the nineteenth century, moreover, faculty members were paid directly by their students, who quite literally bought tickets to each of the courses they took. As in Britain, faculty members thus preferred to teach required courses, for those courses would generate more fees. It is unlikely, however, that any American faculty lived on their lecture fees alone. Most medical educators in the United States prior to the early decades of the twentieth century generated far larger amounts of income by parlaying their scholarly reputations as faculty members and their considerable chunks of free time into handsome private practices. Many also grew wealthy by serving as specialists and consultants to their former pupils, when the latter went out on their own.[16]

Beck was out of step with his contemporary colleagues, for he took the occasion of his faculty appointment, coming as it did upon the heels of his financially favorable marriage, to cut back on his private practice. Beck had alluded to this course of action a year earlier in a letter to his uncle, Dr. Nicholas Romeyn, who had himself apparently lectured on forensic medicine in 1813.[17] "I have begun to look upon medicine in a very different manner from what I formerly did," he wrote. "Although delighted with the study yet I dislike the practice, and I had not acquired sufficiently comprehensive views of its value and great importance as an object of research. I now find it a subject worthy of my mind, and for some time past I have brought all my energies to its examination."[18] Now in a position to devote full time to his scholarly interests, Beck completed his manuscript on feigned diseases by the end of 1815.[19] Even though he realized that his projected study of medical jurisprudence would be "a work . . . of years," and even though he was "not anxious to hurry it," Beck was assuming the position of a full-time academic.[20]

Through 1815 and 1816 Beck continued to chip away at the vast subject of medical jurisprudence. He had to postpone his essay about the effects of manufacturing on public health "for want," as he put it, "of sufficient facts."[21] In an era when many would not have been deterred by such a consideration, that comment testified forcefully to Beck's essentially modern, scientific temperament. He had earlier been frustrated by Rush's inaugural lecture on insanity for the same reason; he thought Rush wasted too much effort "descending to speculation."[22] So Beck turned away from what would now be called environmental concerns to what he labeled "Poi-

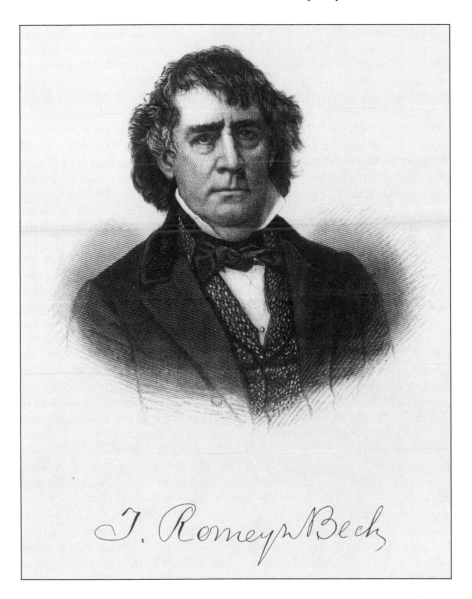

J. Romeyn Beck

sons," a subspecialty of medical jurisprudence where the data seemed more amenable to rational analysis.[23]

In the long run the study of poisons, or forensic toxicology, would prove to be one of the crucial foundations of serious medical jurisprudential work during the remainder of Beck's own lifetime. Chemistry was booming as a field of scientific experimentation, and many of the discoveries being made, as Thomas Cooper had emphasized earlier in his *Tracts*, held medico-legal implications. In 1817 Beck abandoned private practice altogether and accepted the post of principal of the Albany Academy, an eclectic institution that combined elements now parceled out to high schools, colleges, professional schools, and research institutes. There he assigned himself the courses in chemistry and began to teach himself and his students as much as he could about that subject. This arrangement proved fruitful for Beck, who would incorporate a good deal of this knowledge into his later works, and fruitful as well for his students, who must have been receiving some of the best scientific training then available in the United States. One of those students was Joseph Henry, whom Beck, in essence, discovered and trained. Henry had hoped to become an actor, but Beck considered the penurious young man's scientific talents superior to his theatrical skills. To help Henry finance his education Beck awarded him what amounted to a teaching assistantship, and the two of them explored chemistry together before Henry did the work in electromagnetism that made him an important figure in the history of science. Henry left Albany in 1832 for Princeton and headed the Smithsonian Institution from 1846 to 1878, but never did anything again, in the words of his biographer, which "equaled the achievements of his young struggling years in Albany" with Beck.[24]

Through the early 1820s Beck continued to offer his lectures on medical jurisprudence at the Western Medical College as well as supervise the Albany Academy, teaching math and science at the latter as the need arose. This busy schedule, which involved frequent travel under primitive conditions, forced Beck to cut back on his writing. He also spent a good deal of time as a lobbyist in behalf of science and medicine in the state legislature at Albany.[25] "Legal Medicine comes on slowly," he confessed to Francis, but he continued to amass materials and to organize his topical essays.[26]

Throughout the period from 1815 to 1822 Beck corresponded with other physicians, scientists, and researchers, including such prominent figures as Jacob Bigelow at Harvard and Benjamin Silliman at Yale, both of whom were experts in what might be labeled medical chemistry; Sterling Goodenow, an early practitioner of statistical geography; Elisha Harris and John Griscom of New York, both of whom would later become significant pioneers in the fields of vital statistics and public health; and a number of researchers in France, with whom Beck corresponded in French, a language he considered essential to anyone seriously interested in medical jurisprudence.[27] Finally, sometime late in 1822 or early in 1823, Beck completed his manuscript and gave it to a publishing firm in Albany, Webster and Skinner. They issued the work in two volumes, totaling over 900 pages, in the summer of 1823 under the title *Elements of Medical Jurisprudence*; that work would dominate the field for the next thirty years.

In the first volume Beck included an introduction and twelve chapters. The first chapter, on "Feigned Diseases," was the pilot project he had sent to Francis eight years earlier. Chapter Two, "Disqualifying Diseases," dealt with a related subject. Both subjects had long been included in the tradition of medical jurisprudence, since European rulers had wanted to know from an early date which military conscripts were trying to avoid service and which should be excused for their own sake or for the sake of others. The principles adduced in those investigations, however, could be applied to other situations as well. In his discussion of disqualifying diseases, for example, Beck neatly summarized the working regulations then operative in both England and France. The only American material Beck was able to find was a compilation of disqualifying considerations prepared in 1818 by Samuel L. Mitchill, then surgeon-general of the New York state militia, for Beck's long-time friend, Governor DeWitt Clinton.[28] Beck's own comments typified the combination of social practicality and individual sensitivity that suffused his work. Americans could afford to be more flexible and generous than European nations in excusing people from state-imposed services, he believed, but American governments should learn to enforce their regulations with firmness and fairness in peacetime rather than responding only to war.[29]

The bulk of the rest of the Volume 1 dealt with issues related to the general subject of procreation. These too had a long and hallowed history in the development of medical jurisprudence, for the feudal states of Europe rested upon a social structure in which the circumstances of birth mattered a great deal. Chapter Three discussed "Impotence and Sterility," for such questions were often germane in cases of disputed paternity. Chapter Four addressed "Doubtful Sex." Males, after all, inherited; females did not.

There followed chapters on "Rape," "Pregnancy," and "Delivery." On the crime of rape Beck took direct issue with the long-standard European authorities. The latter believed that emission had to be proved, but Beck disagreed. Instead he endorsed Thomas Cooper's opinion that the forcible use of another's body was the real crime. Beck advised his readers that prosecutors in the Albany area had solved the problem by abandoning the charge of rape itself, which was so difficult to prove, and instead pursuing successfully indictments for attempted rape. Beck also quoted with approval an 1819 Illinois act, which explicitly declared "that so much of the law regulating the evidence in case of rape, as makes emission necessary, is hereby repealed."[30] The discussions of pregnancy and delivery were straightforward distillations of standard obstetrical works of the early nineteenth century.

Beck's younger brother John Brodhead Beck wrote Chapter Eight, on infanticide. John had graduated first in his class from Columbia in 1813, and then followed his brother to the College of Physicians and Surgeons. There in 1817 John submitted his dissertation on the subject of infanticide and quickly became an international expert on the subject, perhaps the leading international expert.[31] Under the general heading of infanticide John Beck included both neonatal murder and what would now be called abortion. His views concerning the latter, which he opposed, would eventually have national impact.[32] Like his brother, John Beck continued to revise and expand his material in subsequent editions of the *Elements*, and his chapter on infanticide eventually grew to hundreds of pages. John Beck gained a chair of his own at the College of Physicians and Surgeons in New York City in 1826, where he taught medical jurisprudence himself through mid-century.[33] In 1835 Theodric Romeyn Beck began acknowledging both his brother's contribution to the *Elements* and his brother's standing in the field by listing him as a full co-author.[34]

Chapters Nine, Ten, and Eleven discussed legitimacy, presumption of survivorship, and age and identity. These issues had most frequently arisen in disputes over inheritance. Suppose, for example, that a widow remarried almost immediately upon the death of her husband, then had a child seven or eight months after her second wedding. Could that child be the posthumous heir of its mother's first husband? Could it be the legitimate heir of the new husband, born prematurely? Could it be the illegitimate child of the second husband (or someone else) conceived before the ailing first husband actually died? Since older authorities differed on such fundamental facts as the length of gestation, how were judges to decide such matters in the face of disputed claimants, especially if large estates were at stake?

But large estates were not always at stake, and Beck seems to have been intrigued by the sheer drama often associated with identity problems. His illustrations still make good reading. One of them was the sixteenth-century French case of Martin Guerre, the peasant impostor case recently brought back to light by Natalie Z. Davis.[35] Another example involved a charge of bigamy tried before Judge Livingston in New York City in 1804. The case hinged upon whether a bridegroom before the bar was the same man who had earlier married a different woman under a different name; the earlier bride swore he was, but the jury eventually decided he was not.

Volume One of the *Elements* concluded with the chapter "Mental Alienation." Although the material was taken in large part from Beck's dissertation on that subject, he rearranged it and focused it more sharply because he wanted "to confine [him]self to those points which are particularly noticed in civil and criminal cases": the symptoms that constituted a state of insanity; the problems of identifying feigned and concealed insanity; the legal rules governing insanity in court proceedings; the various types of mental impairment short of insanity; the state of mind necessary to make a legally valid will; and the legal status of the deaf and dumb, who were often lumped with the insane as mentally deficient.[36]

Taken as a whole, the first volume of the *Elements* was Beck's attempt to summarize for Anglo-American readers the issues that had concerned the great medico-legalists of the Continental tradition since the Middle Ages. It placed Beck in a line of writers that went back at least to Zacchias and included such eighteenth-century commentators as B.D. Mauchartus, J.E. Hebenstreit, Gottlieb Ludwig, and J.T.C. Schlegel, all of whom were products of the Germanic, state-sponsored approach to medical jurisprudence.[37] The outpouring of praise and appreciation, not to mention the booming sales and the strong demand for revised editions, demonstrated beyond doubt that Beck had performed a valuable service to physicians and attorneys in bringing these traditional concerns together in a systematic fashion, commenting in English on research published in German and French, and illustrating specific points wherever possible with English and particularly with American court cases. Nonetheless, it was Volume 2 of the *Elements* that revealed the excitement and promise that so many professionals of Beck's generation seemed to sense in the field of medical jurisprudence; there Beck began to apply the new science, especially chemistry, to the sorts of problems encountered in medicine and law.

The first chapter, "Persons Found Dead," began with a useful discussion of the duties of the office of coroner. This mini-lecture was a minor masterpiece of practical preaching and was surely most welcome to those coroners interested in trying to do a better job. In it, Beck laid out his own philosophy of how authorities should deal with cases of sudden or mysterious death. Not surprisingly, he campaigned in favor of letting professional physicians play a more prominent role during inquests than they customarily did. "In many instances," he exhorted local coroners, "the evidence of medical men is required. Sometimes, indeed, the facts are so clear that no professional opinion can be wanted, *but whenever there is the least uncertainty,* such opinions should be taken, and for the most part a dissection must be made."[38]

He then warned physicians to beware of popular rumor. "There is nothing more common among the populace, who crowd around the bodies of persons found dead, than to suspect that they have been murdered," but the physician's job was to keep a clear head, squelch wild theories before they could "gain strength by repetition," and remember that most sudden deaths had perfectly natural explanations.[39] The duty of professionals was to proceed to a systematic autopsy. Some 75 pages of instruction and practical advice followed, in which Beck carefully led physicians through a forensic dissection and explained not only why certain steps should be taken but what to look for when taking them. Special sections highlighted specific types of problems: how to deal with putrefaction, for example, or how to decide whether a person found in water had actually drowned or been placed there after death.

Early in his discussion Beck tried to impress upon his fellow physicians the importance of preparing clearly written reports and giving testimony that was "as simple and plain as possible, avoiding all those terms which are unintelligible to a court and jury."[40] That was good advice in a republic whose common citizens would be judging one another. But it was difficult advice to follow in a society where even the most rudimentary anatomical and scientific terms were unfamiliar to those same common citizens. Moreover, as the subsequent history of medical jurisprudence in the United States would reveal, many physicians never even tried to deliver opinions in a style "simple and plain."

The next chapter addressed problems associated with wounds. How could a physician determine whether a wound was fatal, for example, or what the secondary physiological results of a given wound might be? As was the case throughout the *Elements*, Beck presented comparative context whenever he commented on law, then offered his own conclusions. One of the perennial problems associated with the question of wounds provided a nice illustration of Beck's procedure.

Lawyers, lawmakers, judges, and physicians throughout Europe and the United States had long debated the length of time that could elapse between a wounding and a death and still justify an indictment for murder. In Lombardy, a charge of murder could be brought if the victim died anytime within a year of the wounding; in England and hence in the American colonies through the Revolution, according to William Blackstone's famous *Commentaries* of the 1760s, it was a year and a day. In France, on the other hand, the victim had to expire within forty days to justify a charge of murder against the person who had delivered the wound; and in Prussia, where the official code was silent on the subject, officials did not bring murder indictments in practice unless the victim died within nine days of being wounded. Beck's own New York State copied a stabbing statute enacted during the reign of James I that stipulated six months. Beck concluded that they were all wrong. Because careful forensic methods could "strictly and indisputably" ascertain whether a given wound did or did not result in the death of a given person, all time provisions in law and in practice should be dropped.[41] In effect, though Beck never said so outright, this gave judicial power to the professional experts whom Beck was hoping to instruct. This attitude would also figure prominently in the future history of the field.

All the rest of Volume 2, nearly 300 pages, was devoted to "Poisons." Chapter Four addressed issues associated with poisons generally; Chapters Five, Six, and Seven focused separately on specific aspects of mineral, vegetable, and animal poisons. These last chapters were the most systematically scientific in the book, and they revealed the ways in which Beck hoped to apply modern experimental techniques to the traditional issues of medical jurisprudence. Poisoning, after all, had been a subject of forensic inquiry since antiquity, and it remained into the 1820s, according to contemporary observers in the United States, a crime easily committed, difficult to detect, and widely feared by the general population.

Beck had available to him, however, something that centuries of previous scholars did not have: the rapidly breaking discoveries of modern chemistry, a field then coming into its own. Throughout Europe and the United States, work was going forward that had obvious forensic applications in addition to a host of less obvious implications for public health and legislative policy. At the forefront of this activity stood French researchers, led by Matthieu J.B. Orfila, then the world's best-known authority on poisons and their detection.[42] This brilliant son of a Spanish merchant had been sent to Paris in 1807 at the age of twenty by his professors in Spain, who realized that their best student should pursue his chemical research in collaboration with stronger scholars than they could provide. Essentially adopted by his senior French mentors, then naturalized as a French citizen, Orfila had published in four parts between 1813 and 1815 the work on poisons that brought him a lasting international reputation.[43] That study quickly became the world standard on forensic toxicology and made its author his nation's most sought-after expert whenever a poisoning case went to trial.

Printers in the United States had already brought out two different English translations of Orfila's work on poisons: the first appeared in Philadelphia in 1817, the second in Baltimore in 1819.[44] Since printers were unlikely to venture competing versions of a book for which there was no market, those translations suggested a real interest in the subject among American professionals. In 1817 Orfila issued an important volume on applied medical chemistry.[45] Beck added all of this new French material to findings that he and others were bringing to light in the United States. In his discussion of mineral poisons, for example, he included a commentary on the method of detecting arsenic advanced by Thomas Cooper in the latter's *Tracts* four years earlier. Beck felt obliged to point out that experiments conducted independently by Porter and Silliman at Yale threw doubt upon the applicability of Cooper's procedure.[46]

Beck's book received a simply astonishing reception, which testified not only to the surging interest in medical jurisprudence in the United States but also to the great need for a systematic summary that would be of practical use to a wide range of professionals: judges, attorneys, physicians, and medical school professors. Beck benefited enormously from the fact that the *Elements* responded to that tremendous demand. Physicians now had a reliable guide to follow when called upon to act in legal or forensic situations; lawyers and lawmakers had a handbook to refer to when wrestling with medically related questions; judges and juries had a foundation upon which to test medically related evidence. No one since Zacchias had been able to compile and update so comprehensively and usefully the body of knowledge included under the rubric of medical jurisprudence; no one in the English-speaking world had even come close.

Medical reviewers in the United States hailed Beck's achievement quickly and enthusiastically. The *Philadelphia Journal of the Medical and Physical Sciences*, though often cool toward the efforts of writers associated with their rivals in New York, praised Beck's "plain, manly and unpretending language" and considered the *Elements* the most important evidence yet of the fact that medical jurisprudence, after a long period of neglect in England, had "in comparatively a short time . . . reached a high degree of perfection" in the United States.[47] R.E. Griffith, who was teaching medical jurisprudence at the University of Pennsylvania when the *Elements* appeared, hoped that Beck's book would mark nothing less than "the commencement of a new epoch in the history of American medical science."[48] The *New York Medical and Physical Journal* devoted eighteen pages to a glowing summary of the *Elements'* chief topics.[49] Most importantly, virtually every medical school in the country quickly adopted the *Elements* as the chief text for their proliferating courses on medical jurisprudence.[50]

The initial response of the nation's legal profession is harder to judge historically than the initial response of the medical profession because bar

associations did not yet publish professional journals. But the reaction of
lawyers may be inferred from three other sources. One was the booming
sales of the *Elements* from its first appearance. Many attorneys purchased
the two-volume set, which almost instantly became a standard in private
legal libraries.

A second inference may be drawn from the fact that Beck's book quickly
became the most frequently cited medico-legal text in American court cases.
Lawyers referred to the *Elements* whenever they made medico-legal points,
and their phrasing made obvious the fact that it was considered the national
standard.[51] Given the magnitude of Beck's undertaking, the quality of the
work, the fact that the book was in English, and the practical organization
of the volumes, the *Elements* would probably have achieved great popularity
with lawyers even if Beck had followed traditional British legal precedents
throughout. But, of course, he did not. The fact that Beck was at pains to
cite post-Revolutionary American cases wherever and whenever he could
made the *Elements* especially useful to American attorneys.

A third inference about the reception of the *Elements* in the legal profession comes from the direct testimony of James Kent, Chancellor of the
State of New York and one of North America's most prominent legal authorities. Chancellor Kent was so impressed with the *Elements* that he wrote
Beck personally. "I had not seen any qualified work on the Subject," Kent
observed, "except *The Tracts* published by Dr. Cooper . . . in 1819, & the
allusions to this department of Jurisprudence in Reviews under corresponding Articles [i.e. medico-legally related snippets sent to editors and published in professional journals on an irregular and ad hoc basis]." This was
no idle comment, coming as it did from a man who was both a widely read
legal scholar himself and the chief judge of New York's equity courts, where
cases often involved medico-legal matters. "Be pleased to accept thanks for
the work, & for the great and valuable addition which you have made to
the Jurisprudence & to the Scientific reputation of our Country." Kent hoped
that the *Elements* would become "a Text Book in all our forensic & judicial,
as well as medical, Inquiries on the Subject."[52]

Even more startling than the reception afforded the *Elements* in the
United States was its reception abroad. The most prominent outlet for medical
jurisprudential material in Great Britain, the *Edinburgh Medical and Surgical
Journal*, reviewed the book in glowing terms.[53] Andrew Duncan, Jr., editor
of the *Journal*, pronounced the *Elements* so thorough and so useful "that few
cases can occur in practice on which it will be necessary to seek elsewhere
for farther information."[54] Privately, Duncan wrote Beck that the book

> has astonished me, and makes me ashamed every time I see it. Had I
> the abilities to execute it as you have done such a work ought to have
> come years ago from me, who was appointed to teach the Subject, and
> I had often projected it and as often shrunk from the task as beyond
> my powers and behold the work performed by a gentleman who from
> his being placed at such a distance from the old established centers of
> learning, laboured under infinitely greater disadvantages & performed
> in the most able manner.[55]

George Edward Male, another of the pioneers of British medical jurisprudence, quickly joined the chorus of praise. Like Stringham, Male had
encountered medical jurisprudence as a student at Edinburgh. His own
*Epitome of Juridical or Forensic Medicine for the Use of Medical Men, Coroners,
and Barristers* had been published in 1816, revised and reissued in 1818,
reprinted in the United States in Cooper's compilation of *Tracts*, and cited
by Beck in the *Elements*.[56] In the *Edinburgh Medical and Surgical Journal*, however, Male generously acknowledged the supersession of his own contributions and labeled Beck's *Elements* "one of the best works ever to appear in
this or any other country."[57]

A physician from Liverpool wrote Beck in 1825 to "unite in opinion
with those of my professional brethren on this side of the Atlantic who
have perused it, that [the *Elements*] is unquestionably by far the best work
on the subject which has yet appeared in the English language."[58] Another
Liverpool physician wrote in 1826, "Your Medical Jurisprudence has become very popular in this country, and is considered the best standard of
its kind in all our Courts of Law."[59] Beck's book became so prominent in
Great Britain that Dunlop, a London publisher, issued a new edition of the
Elements in 1825. Beck conscientiously supplied Dunlop with revisions and
fresh examples from court cases that had occurred since the first Albany
printing two years before. Half a century later Alfred Swaine Taylor, by
then England's greatest author on medical jurisprudence, remembered reading the Dunlop edition of Beck's *Elements* in 1825; Taylor was a second-
year medical student at the time and Beck's work so impressed him that he
turned his career to the subject. For the rest of his life Taylor saved the
actual volume that had inspired him.[60] Dunlop's printing did so well in
Britain that Darwell of London brought out a third edition of the *Elements*
in 1829.[61]

Also impressive was the fact that Dunlop's 1825 revised London edition was reprinted in Weimar in 1827 under the title *Elemente der gerichtlichen Medicin*.[62] Given the prestige and long tradition of medical jurisprudential activity in the German-speaking states, that was a rare tribute to
American scholarship. For centuries material on medical jurisprudence had
flowed the other way across the Atlantic. Indeed, Beck's book may have
occupied a more lofty place in the world of European science and letters in
its day than any other American book of the nineteenth century.

While his reputation soared in Europe, Beck continued his own reading and research in Albany. The result was a major new version of the
Elements, which appeared in 1835. Beck estimated that he spent as much
effort on the 1835 revisions as he had spent to produce the 1823 original.
But the product proved well worth his efforts. This magisterial fifth edition
was meant to be as exhaustive and definitive as Beck could make it, and as
up-to-date. Now totaling 1352 pages, it was about half again as large as the
first edition. In this edition of the *Elements* Beck also incorporated another
decade of his brother's research on infanticide and abortion, as well as his
own matured thoughts on the subject of medical evidence. The result was
one of the greatest achievements of early American professional scholarship.

Though virtually unknown today, the 1835 edition of the *Elements*, clearly and elegantly written, internationally respected, and preeminently useful, deserves a place among the triumphs of American science and letters.[63]

In 1838, with the 1835 edition evidently already sold out, a Philadelphia publishing house issued a sixth edition. To this printing Beck contributed an expanded version of his section on "Persons Found Dead," for he continued his special interests in forensic pathology and the role of coroners. Otherwise, the 1838 edition of the *Elements* followed the 1835 version. A seventh edition was printed in London in 1842. The publisher noted in his own preface that the seventh edition was essentially a copy of the sixth, though "various manuscript additions" had been "communicated by the Authors." This third British printing was publicly "enscribed" by the Becks to Robert Christison, then the United Kingdom's most eminent toxicologist.[64]

Eighth and ninth editions followed during the 1840s before another major revision, the tenth edition, appeared at Albany in 1850. By now the *Elements* had grown to some 1825 pages or about 30 percent larger than the fifth edition. Beck had intended simply to reprint previous editions in 1850, but by his own admission could not resist adding several hundred pages of fresh material. It is also significant that the 1850 edition was produced and distributed by Little and Company, "Law Booksellers." Their marketing orientation was clear. Attached to the back cover of every copy of the tenth edition of the *Elements* was Little's catalogue of legal publications, additional strong evidence that the book was being sold as vigorously to attorneys as to physicians.[65]

John B. Beck died of arteriosclerosis in 1851 and T. R. Beck succumbed to the same condition in 1855.[66] So successful was their book, however, that two posthumous editions appeared. In 1860 the Beck family approached C.R. Gilman, who had become professor of medical jurisprudence in the College of Physicians and Surgeons of New York, and urged him to revise and reissue the *Elements* on the basis of notes that T.R. Beck had made between 1850 and 1855. Gilman agreed, cajoled "an association of the friends of Drs. Beck" into helping him, and contracted with Lippincott to publish what became the eleventh edition.[67] Lippincott subsequently published a twelfth and last edition of the *Elements* in 1863, because the eleventh edition sold out completely in two years. Two recently decided cases that dealt with mental alienation were added to the last edition along with some recent work on poisons by Samuel St. John, professor of chemistry at the College of Physicians and Surgeons of New York.[68]

Though extraordinarily successful, T.R. Beck and his *Elements* did not stand alone; though largely forgotten today, they were by no means isolated or singular in the professional consciousness of their own era. Beck and his great book stood instead at the symbolic center of one of the most dynamic and rapidly growing areas of professional activity in the United States between 1820 and 1850. The first and most obvious manifestation of that dynamism and growth appeared in the nation's proliferating medical schools.

CHAPTER THREE

Medical Jurisprudence as a Burgeoning Field in Early American Medical Schools

Professional interest in medical jurisprudence spread throughout the United States during the first half of the nineteenth century, as training in medical jurisprudence came to be considered crucial to the future role of American physicians. Both Charles Caldwell and Thomas Cooper, whose efforts in behalf of medical jurisprudence at the University of Pennsylvania were discussed in the first chapter, left Philadelphia in 1819, and their subsequent careers illustrated the diffusion of the field they helped to pioneer. Caldwell went west to become a founding member of the new medical department of Transylvania University in Lexington, Kentucky, then well-funded and bidding aggressively to become the most prominent seat of higher learning west of the Appalachian Mountains.[1] In 1823 Caldwell published *Outlines of a Course of Lectures on the Institutes of Medicine*, which served as a vehicle for his philosophy of medical training in general and his hopes for Transylvania in particular.

Caldwell believed that the basic institutes, or underlying principles, of scientific medical education fell into four categories: physiology, pathology, therapeutics, and hygiene. In the last he also included "Medical Police." Caldwell noted that "some schools" separated out "the principles of Medical Jurisprudence" as a fifth and separate pillar of proper professional training, which he clearly approved, even though Transylvania had decided to fold medical jurisprudence into hygiene. The salient point was not whether professional training for physicians should be structured as four divisions or five, but that medical jurisprudence, wherever fitted in, had become an established essential of the ideal professional curriculum. Caldwell ended his *Outline* by announcing his intention to bring out "a synopsis of Hygiene and Medical Jurisprudence" as his next major publication.[2] Unfortunately for him, Beck's *Elements* appeared in Albany even as Caldwell's announcement went to press in Lexington; Beck had provided exactly what Caldwell thought the nation's serious professionals needed.

While Caldwell headed west, Cooper went south to the College of South

Carolina (now the University of South Carolina). There he was made professor of chemistry and mineralogy, then almost immediately appointed president as well.[3] Cooper's commitment to improving the interaction of medicine and law became clear in his subsequent roles as chief founder of South Carolina's first insane asylum and as chief editor of the state's statutes. The latter, one of Cooper's last great works, was completed during the late 1830s after his retirement from the college presidency.[4]

Caldwell and Cooper were not alone in preaching the new gospel of medical jurisprudence. "Three years ago," Stringham had told his last group of students at the College of Physicians and Surgeons of New York back in December 1815, "the only Professorship of Legal Medicine in the United States was held in this College—There are now 5 Professorships of Legal Medicine in the United States—which fact—Shows the rising importance of the Subject."[5] Developments in New England illustrated the trend that Stringham had detected, a trend which would continue in American medical schools for three decades.

Where medical schools already existed in New England, curricular changes were introduced to accommodate the inclusion of medical jurisprudence. Reuben Mussey, for example, a Rush student, began teaching medical jurisprudence at Dartmouth in 1814 and continued to do so through 1837.[6] Walter Channing, another Rush student, who had subsequently studied at Edinburgh as well, brought the subject to Harvard in 1815, when he was appointed professor of obstetrics and medical jurisprudence. Channing remained in that chair through mid-century and maintained his mentor's commitment to a positive vision of medical jurisprudence, imploring four decades of Harvard medical students to try to improve legal medicine in the United States.[7]

Where medical schools were founded in New England during the first half of the nineteenth century, medical jurisprudence was generally included as a central subject of instruction from the outset. The case of the Berkshire Medical College, organized at Pittsfield, Massachusetts, in 1821, offers an unusually well-documented example of the commitment to medical jurisprudence so typical of most early American medical schools. And because the National Library of Medicine has preserved a unique collection of lecture notes taken by students in Berkshire's medical jurisprudence classes in 1821, 1822, and 1824, the experience of that college also offers a chance to learn directly from contemporary medical students what they were actually being taught in medical jurisprudence classrooms in the 1820s.[8]

Finding someone to teach the subject proved difficult for this struggling new college. To solve their problem for the October term of 1821, Berkshire's first, the trustees prevailed upon Amos Eaton, then teaching natural science at nearby Williams College, to come to Pittsfield to lecture on medical jurisprudence. Though Eaton had no medical training, he had practiced law for fifteen years before returning to his alma mater to pursue botany, mineralogy, and geology; and he was a man of genuine scholarly abilities.[9] Berkshire's first medical students thus received their introduction to medical jurisprudence not from a physician but from a lawyer-scientist.

Defining the field as "Medical Skill applied in aid of the Judiciary," Eaton offered nine lectures. As might be expected from a mineralogist, the class learned in detail the ways to identify accurately the mineral poisons. But they also learned that even a leading botanist could not identify with certainty the vegetable poisons after they entered the human system. If death resulted from one of the vegetable poisons, Eaton observed, "it must be determined by the symptoms preceding death and by concomitant extenuating circumstances." Eaton went on to cover other causes of death, rape, infanticide, questions of legitimacy, procured abortions, venereal diseases, "nuisances," feigned diseases (including false pregnancies and pretended insanity), "idiotism," insanity, and the legal aspects of obstetrical practice.

Eaton taught his students to take what many modern Americans might consider to be a surprisingly liberal or tolerant interpretation of most subjects. Always give the benefit of the doubt to the person in trouble, he advised, especially in matters affecting women. In cases of rape, for example, defense attorneys had long argued that no woman who became pregnant could claim to have been raped, for she almost certainly must have consented. Judges and juries apparently tended to share that view. But Eaton, emphasizing that pregnancy was not dependent upon female volition, insisted that women could become pregnant as the result of a rape, and thus be even more tragic victims than those who escaped pregnancy.

More striking still was Eaton's discussion of infanticide. When investigating an allegation of infanticide, Eaton told his students, they should always keep mercy uppermost in their minds. If a woman had been deserted or was unmarried or in unusually difficult straits, the doctor should try to give her the benefit of every possible doubt, no matter how implausible her story, even if that meant hypothesizing some theoretical course of events that fitted the circumstances without condemning the mother. In this bold lesson, Eaton could hardly have gone further without openly condoning infanticide in cases involving desperate women.

Eaton also stressed the responsibility of professionals for public health.

It is the duty of every Practitioner of Medicine to search for Every cause of disease there may exist in his neighborhood. Carbunenetted Hydrogen arising from low marshy grounds is undoubtedly the cause of intermittant fevers. . . . Slaughter houses, sinks, etc. ought not to Escape the notice of the Medical Practitioner [.] [I]t is his duty to analize all the waters in the circle of his practice[,] to detect poisons in Liquors sold by merchants[,] to inform his employers of an epidemic when it makes its appearance[,] to quell all false alarms and most of all to expell a quack from his neighborhood when one makes his appearance.

Clearly, Eaton envisioned local physicians operating as quasi-public agents, defending individuals against the powers of the state and protecting the public's health against threats both natural and imposed.

Eaton left Berkshire at the end of his first and only term of part-time teaching there, having been nominated by T. R. Beck's friends Stephen Van Rensselaer and DeWitt Clinton to make a scientific survey of the lands adjoining the Erie Canal. The trustees then turned to a full-time faculty member, John P. Batchelder, whom they asked to offer lectures on medical jurisprudence. Though Batchelder had come to Pittsfield to teach anatomy and surgery, he agreed to pinch-hit in medical jurisprudence for the autumn term of 1822.

Although Batchelder approached the subject as a doctor rather than a lawyer, and although he organized his lectures quite differently from Eaton's, the two men shared strikingly congruent conceptions of what medical jurisprudence was ultimately all about. For Batchelder the field was taught primarily in order to make possible "the application of Medical Knowledge to testimony in Courts of Judicature." He believed that the ends of government were the protection of individuals and the protection of property. Like Eaton, Batchelder also believed that professionals ought to play a civic role by employing their superior knowledge of special subjects to uphold the laws of nature and basic ideals of right and wrong.

Batchelder divided medical jurisprudence into three main headings: the "propagation of our species," the "destruction of our species," and the issue of insanity. Under the first he discussed such questions as the length of pregnancy, the problem of monsters and hermaphrodites, the types of sterility (which often figured in lawsuits for divorce), and the question of virginity. In his discussion of abortion, Batchelder took the same tolerant attitude that Eaton had taken toward women in difficult circumstances. He cautioned his students not to perform abortions, but when investigating one, he urged them to lean to the side of understanding. "If we must Err," he advised, "let it be on the side of charity" toward the accused woman.

Batchelder's lectures on the causes of death were thorough and more balanced than Eaton's. Where Eaton had stressed poisoning almost exclusively, Batchelder also went over the signs of death by various diseases in order to help his students make distinctions. When teaching about insanity, his third chief heading, Batchelder forthrightly admitted the near impossibility of definitive conclusions. "All we know of the mind is from words actions Signs and intentions," he told his students, and those generally would not satisfy lawyers in court.[10]

Though he performed in an altogether creditable fashion, Batchelder, like Eaton before him, abandoned Berkshire's medical jurisprudence course after one term in order to return full-time to his own specialties. If the board of trustees had any misgivings about medical jurisprudence, this would surely have been an occasion to drop the offering from their curriculum. After all, basic survival of the school was still very much at issue, and they would now have to locate another new faculty member to continue the course. That they persisted underscores the place of medical jurisprudence in professional training in the 1820s. The subject was one of roughly half a dozen thought to be essential for physicians in the future. If aspiring medical schools like Berkshire wanted to establish a first-rate reputation, they would have to teach the subject.

Accordingly, the trustees brought in Stephen W. Williams from nearby Deerfield, Massachusetts, to lecture in the fall term of 1823. Williams was a little-known thirty-three-year-old practitioner with a scholarly bent, a genuine interest in the subject, and a willingness to work.[11] The last was important, because he had to prepare his lectures with very little help. "When I was appointed Professor of Medical Jurisprudence in the Berkshire Medical Institution, in the year 1823," he later remembered, "not a single treatise, embracing a full view of the subject, had been published in the English language, of which I could avail myself, except the collection of Cooper, and that I did not receive until I had nearly prepared my lectures for delivery."[12] Williams had, however, heard Stringham lecture at Columbia in 1813, and he wrote to an old classmate to obtain a set of notes from those lectures. Otherwise he did his own research in journals and court records, in American, English, Scottish, and French sources, and even in the Bible. By his own testimony he spent hundreds of hours preparing his first course.[13] But the Williams appointment brought stability and continuity to Berkshire's offerings in medical jurisprudence: he would teach the subject for the next eight years.

Williams defined his subject much as his two predecessors had done, as "the application of medical knowledge in courts of justice."[14] He began by trying to impress upon his students why formal training in medical jurisprudence would be so important to them. Though English courts had traditionally permitted physicians simply to state their views, in the new republic "an opinion will not be received in our courts of justice without the reason for the Physician's opinion." Williams no doubt emphasized the word "reason." That insistence upon the justification of medical opinion had been established in Berkshire's own Massachusetts by Judge Parsons, according to Williams, and the so-called Parsons rule was generally followed elsewhere in American courts. In short, when American physicians got involved with legal matters, they had better understand what they were talking about. Williams then covered each of the topics addressed by his predecessors, despite some obvious weaknesses in his own understanding. He was distinctly less secure than Eaton had been in toxicological chemistry, and he differed with both Eaton and Batchelder on the probability of pregnancy following rape.[15] Yet the fundamental themes remained constant.

Williams believed strongly that physicians should bring their expertise to bear upon the problems of their communities. Every "jury of inquest ought always at least to contain one Physician," and that physician's special expertise should weigh heavily in any result. Williams also believed that doctors could and would have to expand their knowledge of legal processes in order to be effective. "Positive evidence only," wrote a student notetaker, capturing his professor's emphasis, "must—must have positive declaration." Finally, like his predecessors, Williams urged his pupils explicitly, "When in doubt, lean to the side of mercy."[16]

What was happening at Berkshire was happening elsewhere: medical colleges went out of their way to include medical jurisprudence in the curriculum. In Ohio, most of the medical schools that were organized and frequently reorganized prior to mid-century created posts in medical jurisprudence, just as their models in the East and their great rival over the river in Kentucky had done.[17] Typical was the appointment in 1836 of James B. Rogers in the Medical Section of Cincinnati College. Like the Becks, Rogers was a broad-gauged scientist and a strong teacher with good connections (his brother later founded the Massachusetts Institute of Technology), who had also been involved in geological surveys in Virginia and Pennsylvania. Like T.R. Beck, Rogers's chief interest lay in medical chemistry, a subject he would teach at several medical schools during a career that would eventually end at the University of Pennsylvania.[18]

In the upper South, Robley Dunglison, another of the giants of early American medical education, taught medical jurisprudence at the University of Virginia in the 1820s. He had graduated from the University of Erlangen in Germany, where all candidates for the M.D. degree were required to study the Continental traditions of legal medicine, and he was invited to teach medical jurisprudence at Virginia by former president Jefferson. Dunglison subsequently taught at the University of Maryland in the 1830s, before settling in at Philadelphia's Jefferson Medical College in 1836, where he remained for thirty-two years.[19] R.E. Griffith, who had carried on the strong tradition of medical jurisprudence at the University of Pennsylvania after the departure of Caldwell and Cooper, traveled the other way, succeeding Dunglison first in Baltimore and then in Charlottesville.[20] Richard Wilmot Hall continued medical jurisprudence at the University of Maryland into the 1840s.[21]

In the lower South, Lewis DeSaussure Ford, one of the founders of the Medical College of Georgia in 1829, taught medical jurisprudence there for decades. Ford, whose father was a superior court judge in New Jersey, had also studied medical jurisprudence at the College of Physicians and Surgeons of New York, probably under Francis Wharton and John Beck. Like so many of the other early champions of medical jurisprudence, Ford too was nationally prominent in his efforts to raise the professional standards of American medicine; indeed, his circular letter of 1835, which called for a convention of medical school educators to explore the possibility of standardizing medical curricula, is often considered a precursor of efforts a decade later that led to the founding of the American Medical Association.[22]

Additional examples abound, but the overarching point is clear: during the first half of the nineteenth century, medical schools endorsed with remarkable unanimity and tenacity the concept that medical jurisprudence should be an essential aspect of professional training for America's future physicians. Through an upgraded knowledge of medical jurisprudence, doctors could work with lawyers, judges, and legislators to enhance both the public contribution and the social role of professionals in the new nation. William Frederick Norwood, who meticulously surveyed the institutional history of American medical schools prior to the Civil War, observed that many, if not most, of them had faculty chairs in medical jurisprudence by 1840.[23] Chester R. Burns, in a more recent survey of American medical education, identified by name at least forty-eight individuals who taught medical jurisprudence at thirty-seven different medical schools throughout the nation prior to 1860. Burns concluded accurately that "medical jurisprudence received a remarkable amount of attention in nineteenth-century American medical schools from both physicians and lawyers."[24]

Burns was right to add "and lawyers." The mutual interest that doctors and lawyers were assumed to have in the field was shown in the willingness of medical schools, many of which had only a half-dozen faculty positions available, to appoint attorneys to to teach medical jurisprudence. Some of the appointments given to lawyers were stopgaps, to be sure, like Eaton's term at Berkshire, while others were more permanent. Some were certainly made to win the support of locally influential lawyer-politicians, while others were made for sound academic reasons. But they were made.[25]

What may have been the supreme example of this phenomenon occurred at the Albany Medical College. Beck's home city did not have a medical school through the late 1830s. Teaching at the Vermont Academy of Medicine across the Champlain Valley were two born promoters, Alden March and his protégé James H. Armsby.[26] In January 1836 those two came to Albany and offered lectures on anatomy, physiology, and surgery to test the market and drum up enthusiasm for a professional school in the capital of the nation's most powerful and influential state. They were at pains to attract as much public attention as possible, and they deliberately offered their lectures during the months the legislature was in session.[27]

For the next two years, March and Armsby worked to put together an organizational coalition of prominent professionals in Albany to boost their project. One of the people whose support they most wanted was Amos Dean, a leading Albany lawyer. Dean had already organized the Albany Young Men's Association and would later organize a law school for Albany.[28] Through Dean, March and Armsby assembled a politically powerful board of trustees, who eventually won key legislative appropriations for the nascent Albany Medical School.[29] The school opened formally in 1839, with one of its chairs devoted to medical jurisprudence. The required reading for the course, as might be expected, was the Becks' *Elements*, along with some supplemental volumes. The professorship of medical jurisprudence, however, did not go to the world's leading expert in the field, Albany's own T. R. Beck, but to Amos Dean, Esquire.[30]

Dean's appointment was neither ludicrous nor corrupt, for Dean was genuinely interested in medical jurisprudence and later published in the field. Moreover, T. R. Beck, still occupied with the Albany Academy and now constantly busy as a world-renowned author and editor, was not a member of the original faculty of the Albany Medical College.[31] In 1842, Beck agreed to join the faculty; not, surprisingly, as professor of medical jurisprudence but as professor of materia medica and librarian. Dean, the influential lawyer, continued on until after Beck's death as Albany's professor of medical jurisprudence, all the while assigning Beck's *Elements*.[32] Although this case clearly owes more to professional politics in Albany than it does to scholarly logic, it provided a dramatic illustration of the fluid interaction of law and medicine.

The spread of courses in medical jurisprudence also stimulated additional publication in the field. A number of physicians who taught the subject, including Robley Dunglison, the professor whom Jefferson coaxed to the University of Virginia, published their lectures, hoping no doubt to gain at least a small share of the huge market Beck had captured with the *Elements*.[33] Dunglison urged fellow professors to follow the general outlines suggested by an English writer, John Gordon Smith, but recommended the work of Beck, Cooper, Foderé, and Orfila for student reading.[34] Dunglison was well grounded in toxicology and spent a large part of his course introducing American students to "chemical knowledge," the possession of which he considered "the great distinction as to the qualifications of the practitioner for clearing up the obscurities of poisoning by minerals."[35] He then taught the latest tests for mineral poisons and the physiological indications of the non-mineral poisons. In comparison with other writers, Dunglison paid more attention than most to poisoning and infanticide, less to insanity.

Dunglison was also among the first to point out to his students the potentially large role for physicians in the new life insurance business. In an era without actuarial figures, insurance companies paid doctors to estimate the probable survival of would-be policyholders, and Dunglison offered advice on how to do that.[36] This emphasis apparently endured at the University of Virginia, since Henry Howard, professor of medical jurisprudence at Virginia from 1839 through his retirement in 1867, was also known for his lectures on the relationship between doctors and insurance companies. Life insurance was so novel in this era, incidentally, that Professor Howard began his remarks on the subject as late as 1851 by defining exactly what such a policy was. By then physicians were also being hired to verify posthumously the so-called declarations of policyholders concerning their age, health, and physical condition. If any of the declarations were found to have been false or erroneous, the companies did not have to pay off, and large sums were often at stake.[37]

Another of the early professors who published some of his lecture material was Stephen W. Williams, the man who taught medical jurisprudence at Berkshire from 1823 through 1831. Though he believed that Beck's *Elements* was the best book on medical jurisprudence in any language, he thought it was probably too costly and too weighty for many ordinary practitioners of law and of medicine; an opinion that implied a good deal about the status of lawyers and physicians. To help them deal both quickly and easily with the most common basic problems that were likely to arise in the vast majority of cases, in 1835 Williams brought out a *Catechism* of some 200 pages that offered summary answers to many traditional medico-legal questions.[38] While the need for a "popular manual," as R.E. Griffith put it in a review of the Williams book, was certainly great, the *Catechism* itself proved disappointingly weak and ill-informed.[39]

Amos Dean also entered the lists. He published an early version of his material in a limited printing in 1840, then wrote a much more substantial volume in 1850.[40] His book was designed to fit between the short, superficial gloss contained in Williams's *Catechism* and the massive, encyclopedic treatment contained in the *Elements* by mid-century. As Dean himself put it, he had no desire to "supersede" the work of others, including that of his Albany colleague, "but to furnish, in as intelligible and concise a form as possible, the substance of what they contain." As he distilled the principles, he cited appropriate references so that readers could run down "fuller discussions and minuter details" as they wished.[41] Though it took Dean over 600 pages to accomplish his goal, this approach proved effective, and Dean's book appeared frequently on required reading lists in medical jurisprudence classes through the rest of the century.

Also common on course reading lists and in courtroom citations were American editions of several British works, once the British began to produce a more extensive literature of their own after 1830. In 1832 R.E.Griffith brought out an American edition of Michael Ryan's *A Manual of Medical Jurisprudence*. Ryan's book had been published in London the year before and was reviewed favorably by Griffith for American readers. In the American edition, Griffith entirely rewrote the chapter on "the laws relating to the profession, so as to accommodate it to the laws of the several states," and made extensive editorial notes throughout.[42] The firm of Carey, Lea and Blanchard of Philadelphia, which printed Griffith's edition of Ryan, also issued an American edition of *A Practical Treatise on Medical Jurisprudence* by Joseph Chitty in 1835. This too was only a year after its initial printing in England, and like the Ryan book, Chitty's *Treatise* was favorably received by the American champions of medical jurisprudence.[43] Joining Ryan and Chitty as frequently cited British studies were American editions of Robert Stewart Traill's *Outlines of a Course of Lectures on Medical Jurisprudence* (American edition, 1841), Alfred Swain Taylor's *A Manual of Medical Jurisprudence* (American edition by R. E. Griffith, 1845), and Robert Christison's *A Treatise on Poisons in Relation to Medical Jurisprudence, Physiology, and the Practice of Physics* (American edition, 1845).[44]

After 1840 the field of medical jurisprudence began to spawn specialized studies that became rapidly too numerous to list here and increasingly narrow for general courses in medical schools. Scholarly monographs on insanity, pregnancy, poisons, homicide, and the causes of death appeared before mid-century. After mid-century, efforts to summarize the entire field of medical jurisprudence in a single general work began to attract joint authors, typically one from law and one from medicine. The first and eventually most enduring example of this development was *A Treatise on Medical Jurisprudence* by Francis Wharton and Moreton Stillé, which appeared in 1855.[45] Wharton was already a well-established author of legal texts;[46] Stillé a young physician then teaching in Philadelphia. Though Stillé died before the book actually appeared, the professional collaboration in which he had participated was very well received by those interested in medical jurisprudence in the United States.[47] Published the same year T.R. Beck died, this "stereoscopic view" of the subject, as one reviewer put it, came closer than any other book to supplanting the *Elements*.[48] With Alfred Stillé, then Truman Abbe, taking over for Moreton Stillé, and Frank Bowlby eventually taking over for Wharton, the *Treatise* went through several editions and remained in print well into the twentieth century.[49] It appeared frequently on medical and law school reading lists through the second half of the nineteenth century.[50]

To understand a final significant aspect of the spread of medical jurisprudence through the nation's medical schools, a brief glance at the shifting history of medical education is in order. Prior to 1800 the vast majority of people who practiced medicine in North America had no formal training. Few medical schools existed and few students attended them. Most practitioners had uneven practices; they typically offered general advice on the treatment of maladies, set broken bones, compounded crude medicinals, and occasionally attempted something dramatic in the face of emergencies. The great majority of practitioners did not earn their chief livelihoods as doctors. Even for those few who aspired to a full-time practice, the usual route to success ran not through medical school but through an apprenticeship. Would-be physicians learned by watching and doing. Theoretical instruction of a formal sort may have "crowned," to use a verb contemporaries liked, a physician's standing, but theoretical instruction, in the eyes of the general public, did little to make a person a better practical doctor. The United States in 1800 was a nation whose people relied on folk remedies and vague notions about the way the body worked; the doctor was the otherwise ordinary person deemed best at administering the former and interpreting the latter.

Between 1800 and 1850, and at an accelerating rate after 1830, Americans began self-consciously and overtly to abandon the traditional and ultimately class-based attitudes toward professionals and the social place of the professions which they had inherited from the British.[51] De facto circumstances in the new republic had radically opened access to traditionally elite professional undertakings, like medicine and law, and a democratic political philosophy had largely prevented the establishment of privileged professional groups with the legal authority to sanction and monitor those undertakings. The result was an increasingly fluid and competitive marketplace for anyone who wished to provide what had been traditionally professional services to the citizens of the new United States. Under those circumstances, more and more would-be providers of traditionally professional services began to seek formal credentials to present to the public; in the absence of established sanctions, either class-based or legal, a claim to advanced knowledge made them more attractive to the public and, everyone hoped, more effective. Nowhere was this general tendency more evident than in medicine. The imprimatur of a formal degree increased in desirability during the first half of the nineteenth century and so, partly as a consequence, did the prestige of a faculty post. The almost inevitable result was a striking proliferation of medical schools, which in turn fed the cycle of credentialing, a cycle paradoxically generated not by the existence of formal standards and legal sanctions, but by their absence.

The proliferation of American medical schools during the first half of the nineteenth century has been the subject of a great deal of excellent scholarly analysis and debate. While some of those early medical schools tried to maintain high standards, according to the benchmarks of the period, the quality of others, responding as they sometimes did to a lowest-common-denominator phenomenon, could be, to say the least, suspect. A few were out-and-out diploma mills, where an M.D. degree could be virtually purchased. The subsequent elimination of many of these early schools during the first decades of the twentieth century and the transformation of those that survived into the rigorous, scientific, research-oriented, university- and hospital-affiliated medical colleges of the modern era has likewise been the subject of intense scholarly analysis and debate.[52]

For present purposes, however, the quality and character of these early schools was less important than the fact that they were substantially demand-driven institutions. Not only could a student go elsewhere if he (or more rarely she) did not like either what a school was offering or the price at which it was offered, he quite literally paid by the course even if he stayed. The consumer-student could be forced to purchase those courses required by the supplier-faculty for a degree, but might otherwise subscribe or decline to subscribe to specific series of lectures as he chose. There was, moreover, a strong incentive to keep down the number of required courses, lest the students flee to a rival institution that required fewer (which happened repeatedly during the first half of the century), and to keep up the number of optional electives that might on their own merits attract and hold students. Under those circumstances, faculties had powerful incentives to offer practical and practice-oriented courses.[53]

Medical jurisprudence thus spread into American medical schools at a time when the conditions in those schools militated against the imposition of arbitrary or idiosyncratic subjects. The professions in the new republic really did welcome it. "The demand of the public [for upgraded medical jurisprudence]," observed Amos Dean, who was looking back over the first half of the nineteenth century, "is sufficiently evidenced in the multiplication of the means of instruction, that is every where taking place. No medical institution in this country or Europe, could now deem its organization complete, without a department devoted exclusively to an exposition of the facts and principles embraced in Medical Jurisprudence."[54] As late as 1848

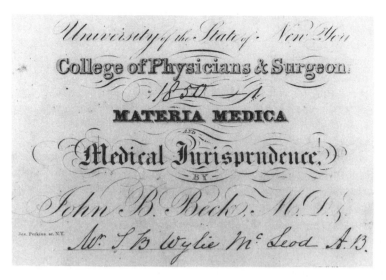

An admission ticket to John B. Beck's course on materia medica and medical jurisprudence at the College of Physicians and Surgeons of New York for the academic
year 1850–51, the last one in which he taught the course. *(Courtesy of the New York
Academy of Medicine)*

the faculty of the recently established Rush Medical College in Chicago
unanimously petitioned their board of trustees to add "a course in Medical
Jurisprudence . . . to those now given in this institution."[55]

Had there been no demand, real or perceived, there would have been
no great spread of the new subject, no matter how appealing it might have
been to a few of the intellectual elites of law and medicine. The rank-and-
file faculty members of early nineteenth-century medical schools, those who
saw themselves shaping the future of the medical profession, believed medical jurisprudence not only inherently important to the future of physicians
but sufficiently attractive to students to be included in the curriculum. Both
considerations had to be present; the second almost uniquely so. Furthermore, the students themselves, at least enough of them to sustain offerings
in the field, were subscribing voluntarily, cash-at-the-door, to hear the field
propounded.

No one could legitimately argue that medical jurisprudence was a fully
established academic field in the United States by mid-century, nor could
anyone demonstrate that the subject was universally taught by well-trained,
professional scientists. Both gaps and gaffes were obvious. Medical jurisprudence was not taught in every medical school. Where it was taught, it
was often tacked onto the duties of a professor whose chief interests might
well lie elsewhere. Catalogues through the 1840s were full of professorships
of "surgery, obstetrics, and medical jurisprudence" (Mussey's chair at Dartmouth), "obstetrics and medical jurisprudence" (Channing's chair at Har-

vard and W. T. Leonard's chair at Washington Medical College of Baltimore), "obstetrics, hygiene, and medical jurisprudence" (Hall's chair at
Maryland), "medical jurisprudence and insanity" (Samuel M. Smith's chair
at Willoughby), "physiology and medical jurisprudence" (H. M. Bullit's
chair at St. Louis University and John C. Dalton, Jr.'s chair at the University of Buffalo); "chemistry and medical jurisprudence" (Rogers's chair at
Cincinnati), or "botany, materia medica, and medical jurisprudence" (John
B. Beck's chair at the College of Physicians and Surgeons of New York).[56]
Courses in medical jurisprudence could vary from a few cursory lectures
read aloud from standard works to a complete and thorough investigation
that included pathological specimens and chemical demonstrations.

Those who taught the subject ranged from brilliant to ridiculous, and
a few who held chairs in medical jurisprudence clearly knew little or nothing about it. When C. E. Pierson was appointed to a newly created chair
in medical jurisprudence at the Medical College of Ohio in 1830, for example, he asked for and received a year's leave to go to New York to learn
something about the subject.[57] Benjamin Rush Rhees, who taught medical
jurisprudence in Philadelphia during the 1820s, was described by his most
famous student as an adequate lecturer but a "superficial man, with few
original ideas and no adequate conception of the importance" of the field he
was responsible for teaching.[58] On the other hand, men like John Beck at
the College of Physicians and Surgeons of New York and Walter Channing
at Harvard were insightful and effective professors who maintained strong
interests in and commitments to research in medical jurisprudence through
their entire careers.

Even conceding the weaknesses and fragilities of the field, however,
the growth of medical jurisprudence in America had been remarkable. A
discipline that did not exist in 1790 had been established in medical schools
as a significant subject of inquiry and instruction by 1850. A substantial
cadre of influential educators, including many who consciously believed they
were shaping the future role of professionals in the United States, had been
attracted to the field.[59] A large and reasonably sophisticated literature, by
the standards of the day, had been produced. Yet the spread of medical
jurisprudence through American medical schools was only one part of a
larger story. Outside the medical schools individuals pressed their own fas-
cinations with the field; journals began to pay attention to medical jurisprudential issues, even to feature them; and researchers found in medico-legal
and public health questions new stimuli for research.

CHAPTER FOUR

Medical Jurisprudence
and American Medicine,
1820–1850

Interest in medical jurisprudence rose among American physicians outside the medical schools as well as inside them during the second quarter of the nineteenth century. Journal articles on jurisprudential issues multiplied dramatically in the medical literature of the period, piquing further interest and broadening the national knowledge base in the field. Medico-legal research done abroad, especially in France, was eagerly received in the United States and disseminated in prominent publications. Individual practitioners saw in medical jurisprudence an emerging field in which to make a mark, and a number of them undertook studies of their own on various aspects of medical jurisprudence. Finally, specific medico-legal questions served as stimuli for investigations that produced inadvertent, though significant, results in other fields of medicine. New lines of professional development seemed to be opening up; new knowledge was being uncovered; a new field seemed about to emerge.

A separate book would be required to document and summarize the appearance and proliferation of articles about medical jurisprudence in the journals published for American physicians between 1820 and 1850. The phenomenon was unmistakable, widespread, and pervasive. Almost all of the journals that started up during that period paid some attention to the field from the outset. Journals that already existed before the great surge of interest in medical jurisprudence added that subject to the others they regularly covered. Two examples of this broad development should suffice: the first was a New York-based journal that existed for less than a decade; the second, published in Philadelphia, became one of the nation's most influential medical magazines.

For historians looking back more than a century and a half, the journal that best captured the first wave of excitement and potential that early nineteenth-century professionals saw in medical jurisprudence was the *New-York Medical and Physical Journal*. Established in 1822 by John B. Beck, in association with John W. Francis and Jacob Dyckman, this publication lasted seven years before changing management and going under.[1] That short life span was not unusual; many medical publications appeared and disappeared during the first half of the nineteenth century. What was unusual was the quality of the material published and the intriguing subjects explored. Though several of the initiatives suggested by the *NYMPJ* would lie buried for decades, the work that appeared there epitomized medical jurisprudence in the 1820s.

The first volume of the journal, published in three issues during 1822, signaled both the eclectic approach and the basic interests of the editors. T. R. Beck, whose presence just behind the editorial managers was obvious from the beginning, published a historical discussion of the legal status of physicians in the colony and state of New York. Though he was still comparatively unknown in 1822 and readers would have had no reason to take his views on the subject any more seriously than anyone else's, Beck argued forcefully for strengthening the mutual obligations and responsibilities that he saw historically existing between doctors and the government. That theme would become explicit in the *Elements* and remain a dominant principle in Beck's fundamental understanding of the ways in which medical jurisprudence could be improved. Beck noted, for example, that the state of New York in 1809 had dropped a long-standing exemption for physicians from military service. But he believed that the exemption should be reinstated because physicians, especially if they all became better-grounded in medicolegal skills, would be routinely serving the state in ways that ordinary citizens could not.[2]

The first volume also included an article by John B. Beck entitled "An Examination of the Medico-Legal Question, whether, in Cases of Infanticide, the Floating of the Lungs in Water can be depended on as a certain test of the Child's Having Been Born Alive."[3] In this impressive piece, John Beck, who had done extensive research on the subject and who probably knew more about it than any other person in the country, rehearsed with clarity and skill the long-standing debate over what was called the hydrostatic test, a debate that went back to Latin texts and famous English court cases. Though Beck acknowledged that decomposition could produce gases in the lungs of an infant who had never breathed, and therefore make a case of stillbirth look like a case of infanticide, he believed physicians might still employ the test under most conditions, provided they did not draw unwarranted conclusions. Even though John Beck was the leading anti-infanticide and anti-abortion advocate of the day, the implication here, as in most other early medical jurisprudential writings in the United States, was in favor of giving actual and potential defendants, in this case the accused mother, the benefit of the doubt.

A third subject addressed in the first volume of the *NYMPJ* was poisoning, a subject that would become more and more important in this and other journals around the country. The *NYMPJ* described the use of an early version of the stomach pump to save poison victims, and the editors endorsed a proposal to ban the indiscriminate sale of arsenic except "as an instrument of research, in the chemical laboratory."[4] Long before legislatures began to take such advice seriously, the early advocates of medical jurisprudence thought the public interest would be served by prohibiting "apothecaries and druggists" from carrying dangerous substances. Poisoning, accidental and intentional, posed a genuine threat to Americans, and toxicological chemistry was a area of research that attracted increasing attention among the early champions of better medical jurisprudence.

Through the rest of the decade, the *NYMPJ* continued to present the latest material in the field of medical jurisprudence. In 1823 the journal discussed the medico-legal implications of such subjects as barrenness, impotence, pelvic deformity, pregnancy and its detection, lightning, congenital diseases, venereal diseases (including the time it took for a rash to appear; on this point a recent rape case had been erroneously decided), and, of course, poisons and poisoning. An article in 1824 explored an insanity case that ended up in the New York legislature. In 1825 the journal began to translate and publish for its readers the latest French work in forensic chemistry, and in 1826 the editors began setting aside a regular, separate section for that purpose.

In 1826 T.R. Beck launched the first of a series of "Contributions in Medical Jurisprudence and Police," which would continue through 1828 and which eventually included five outstanding articles. The first focused on the medico-legal aspects of life insurance, at precisely the time when Robley Dunglison was introducing the subject at the University of Virginia. As Beck put it, the "novel" subject of "insurance upon lives," though among "the most important" new topics for the field of medical jurisprudence, was "comparatively unknown in this country, and indeed has but very lately been broached in professional works."[5] Beck had to rely on British and French cases, most of which hinged upon whether policyholders had committed fraud by concealing important medical information when taking out their policies. The second article in the series was Beck's analysis of the 1825 New York state census. The chief burden of the piece was to convince readers that the problems of the deaf, dumb, and insane were much more widespread and hence deserving of more attention at the state level than most citizens commonly supposed.[6] The essay revealed an unusually sophisticated sense of the use and persuasive value of statistical data.

The third article discussed two recent murder trials in which medical testimony had proved crucial. In one, physicians persuaded the court that a blow to the midsection could leave little or no mark but still be powerful enough to cause death. Beck viewed the case as a good example of scientific demonstration prevailing over commonsensical appearances, for the defense had argued that any blow sufficient to cause death would necessarily have to leave plenty of evidence of external violence. In the other, medical witnesses, including John W. Francis, Beck's close friend and a founding editor of the *NYMPJ*, had to distinguish between strangulation and apoplexy in a confusing case where one man strangled another to the point of interrupting his breath and blood flow, but not to the point of death, only to have the victim die later. At the end of the article, Beck made his message overt: confusions like that would continue "until coroners and coroner's juries are more impressed with the importance of their functions—until dissections shall be more minute and complete—and (above all) until the study of legal medicine is made the actual business of at least a portion of the profession, rather than, as it now is, a subject of speculation and hasty examination, by witnesses too suddenly summoned, and too often imperfectly prepared."[7]

Both the fourth and fifth articles in Beck's series addressed key questions from inheritance cases: the length of human gestation, on the one hand, and whether it was possible to demonstrate that an infant who died at or near childbirth had ever been legally alive, on the other. Debate over the length of pregnancy had been touched off throughout the English-speaking medical world by the so-called Gardner Peerage Case, tried in the House of Lords in 1825. In that case, the Lords had recognized as legitimate an heir born after an unusually long pregnancy, and most physicians considered the decision suspect. Beck was clearly among them and argued for the application of a norm of 280 days, adjusted only within reason, not several months, for a possible miscalculation of the menstrual cycle.[8] The final article in the series served to update and review, six years after John Beck's original article on the subject, the signs of live birth.[9] While a debate like that might seem excessively academic, fortunes could hang in the balance. A man might die with a conditional will, for example, in which his children, if he had any, would inherit everything, and if he did not, his estate would go to a close friend. Suppose his posthumous baby dies in childbirth. If the infant ever legally lived, the baby technically inherited, then died intestate, in which case the general intestate rules of the jurisdiction would apply, probably giving the estate to next-of-kin, however distant. The next-of-kin, not to mention the close friend in the original will, suddenly had a real interest in whether the child who died in childbirth had ever been legally alive.

In addition to his formal series, T.R.Beck wrote a major piece on medical testimony in courts, which will be examined later, and another effective essay on insane asylums in the United States, a subject that continued to command his attention.[10] In the latter, he renewed his ongoing exhortation in behalf of systematic state support for asylums and asylum treatment. Beck also contributed scores of letters, snippets, notices, reviews, and translations of foreign material. Published correspondence made clear the fact that T.R.Beck had become the nation's personal clearinghouse for interesting information and inquiries about medical jurisprudence, and Beck used the *NYMPJ* as his chief outlet. But the *NYMPJ* was far from a one-man show.

Along with articles by the founding editors, the journal published material from such advocates of better legal medicine as Alexander H. Stevens, a learned and well-informed physician who kept abreast of the latest French research, and Charles A. Lee, who would remain influential in the field of medical jurisprudence for decades.[11] Nor did the *NYMPJ* shy away from the industrial hygiene aspects of medical jurisprudence. Information appeared on the chemical analyses of local mineral springs in New York state; on the occupational diseases of tailors, carpenters, and bakers in Germany; and on the effects of tobacco on the health of workers employed in the snuff factories of France.[12]

Finally, the *NYMPJ* also published one of the most intriguing public health articles of the decade, which was written by Lewis C. Beck, the youngest of the four Beck brothers, in 1828.[13] Entitled "On the Nature of the Compounds, usually denominated Chlorides of Soda, Lime, &c., With Remarks on Their Uses as Disinfecting Agents," the essay provided easy directions for preparing crude chloride compounds. Following French leads, primarily those suggested by Labarraque, Lewis Beck described how the compounds could be used in industry (especially those that processed animal remains as raw products), and for "the disinfection of corpses, of hospitals, lazarettoes, merchandise in quarantine, and the most filthy receptacles." Lewis described how his brother T. R. Beck used the chemicals in autopsies to eliminate the "highly offensive odour" often involved and to stop further putrefaction of the corpse. Care had to be taken not to contaminate with the chlorides any of the viscera to be examined, but sheets soaked in chloride solutions had the potential of making post-mortem examinations much more tolerable procedures than they had ever been before in the eyes of the ordinary practitioner. For the purposes of spreading serious medical jurisprudence more widely throughout the profession, this was no trivial matter, since autopsies had a well deserved reputation during the nineteenth century as one of the most nauseating procedures a physician could perform. Moreover, Lewis reported, the chlorides appeared to have the ability to retard putrefaction even on living tissue, when "applied to ulcers, &c.," though appropriate strengths and doses had yet to be worked out. And all this could be accomplished "at a trifling expense." Appearing forty-nine years before Lister demonstrated antiseptic surgical techniques, this was an unusually forward-looking and potentially heuristic essay.[14]

Though the *NYMPJ* epitomized the new visibility and positive view of medical jurisprudence that characterized America's professional journals during the second quarter of the nineteenth century, it was by no means alone, as a second representative example, the *Philadelphia Journal of the Medical and Physical Sciences*, demonstrated. When that journal was launched in 1821, its editors paid no special attention to jurisprudential issues, though they did publish in the third volume a ten-page fold-out appendix that listed in chart form the major poisons, their symptoms, their antidotes, and most importantly for present purposes, the "mode of detecting" them. For the mineral poisons, chemical tests were described, though a practitioner would have to know quite a bit about chemistry in the first place to follow the directions. For the animal and vegetable poisons, no means of detection were known. The chart was clearly designed to be detached for handy reference and served both as an indication of the desire to disseminate enough toxicological knowledge to encourage post-mortem examinations, whenever poisoning was a possibility, and as a convenient base line against which to measure the increasing toxicological sophistication of American physicians during the next several decades.[15]

Publication of Beck's *Elements*, however, elicited a dramatic response from the *PJMPS*, further evidence of the impact of that remarkable book. The *PJMPS*'s review of the *Elements* in 1824 read like a manifesto in behalf of medical jurisprudence. Unlike the English tendency to rely on "a free declamatory style" and "arrogant assurance," according to the *PJMPS*, Beck's volume demonstrated the value of practical research in the field and a thorough knowledge of Continental developments, especially French. Out from under England, Americans were free to develop their own medical jurisprudential traditions, independent of the *"misplaced erudition"* and irrelevant material that had long passed for serious work in Britain. The editors of the *PJMPS* commended the *Elements* "to our *American* readers" both because they considered it the best work on the subject and because they now realized that the subject itself was crucially important. They hoped "Dr. Beck's book" would "diffuse a taste for the study of medical jurisprudence" through "the American profession." In an impassioned paragraph, the *PJMPS* reminded readers of many ways in which physicians were the only ones who could "shield the unoffending from injury" and "deliver the wicked up to severe and merited fate." Once realization of the importance of the field spread throughout the United States, proclaimed the *PJMPS*, "our countrymen will hereafter produce works in extension of this desirable knowledge."[16]

The next year, in 1825, the *PJMPS* published R.E. Griffith's "On Medical Jurisprudence," another ringing endorsement of the field. Griffith envisioned medical jurisprudence "serving as a link to unite" physicians and lawyers "in the detection of error, the vindication of accused innocence, and the conviction of guilt." Medical jurisprudence was "a science peculiarly calculated to control the disorders of the social system," and Griffith hoped that publication of Beck's *Elements* would "remove the opprobrium that has too long rested on physicians, when called on by the law of their country to explain and elucidate facts allied to their profession."[17]

The *PJMPS* became the *American Journal of the Medical and Physical Sciences* in 1827 (and eventually the *American Journal of the Medical Sciences*) and rose to a place of national prominence. The obvious commitment of the *AJMPS* to stimulating interest in and spreading the latest knowledge about medical jurisprudence manifested itself in the form of hundreds of articles, reviews, notices, translations, letters to the editor, and essays of various types over the next quarter-century. For several years R.E. Griffith carried the burden of that effort; then in 1841 the *AJMPS* induced none other than T.R. Beck himself, whose *NYMPJ* had ceased publication more than a decade earlier, to become a collaborating editor with particular responsibilities for items relating to legal medicine.[18] From that point through mid-century it was not unusual for a single volume of the *AJMPS* to carry dozens of items related to medical jurisprudence.

The volume for the second half of 1842 was indicative (the *AJMPS* published two volumes to a calendar year during this period): it contained forty-four summary pieces by T.R. Beck, most of them under the heading of "Medical Jurisprudence and Toxicology," and a longer essay by his brother John on the latest research concerning the signs of stillbirth and live birth.[19] The volume for the first half of 1843 contained a feature article by T. R. Beck; twenty-one case summaries of interest in "Medical Jurisprudence and Toxicology," which was a regular and ongoing section of the journal; and a thirteen-page review, written by Charles R. King, of Orfila's 1842 treatise on mineral poisons.[20]

King's review of Orfila's latest research re-emphasized the continuing influence of French models on the leading American champions of medical jurisprudence. After publication of his earlier work on poisons, Orfila had been appointed to the chair in medical jurisprudence in the University of Paris faculty of medicine in 1819 and had published *Leçons de médecine légale* (Medico-legal Lessons) in 1823, the same year Beck published the *Elements* in Albany. In 1830, Orfila wrote a study of post-mortem examinations that was well received in the United States, and he became dean of the faculty of medicine at Paris.[21] During his deanship Orfila did in France exactly what his American admirers were trying at the same time to do in the United States: upgrade both their profession and the role of their profession in the public life of the nation. Under Orfila's leadership pre-medical course requirements at the University of Paris were made far more demanding than they had previously been. Working with his medical faculty, Orfila also managed to introduce the equivalent of licensing examinations. He held the deanship through 1848, when he fell from political favor in the revolutions of that year, but continued to write in his areas of specialization.[22]

In extolling those French developments, which were presented in the United States as major achievements, American medical journals amplified the francophonic tones struck earlier by Stringham and others in their lectures on medical jurisprudence and by Cooper in his *Tracts*. From 1820 to 1850 American journals routinely reviewed French books on all subjects related to legal medicine, often devoting long feature articles to important French work in such key areas as toxicology and insanity. One of the most commonly cited sources of material about medical jurisprudence in American medical journals after 1830 was the *Annales d'hygiène publique et de médecine légale* (Journal of Public Health and Legal Medicine), the strongest voice of French medico-legal activity, which began publication in Paris in 1829.[23]

Many factors sustained American attention to French legal medicine through mid-century. One certainly was the political and cultural residue of the post-Revolutionary era. As young men the physicians who rose to the top of the American medical profession between 1820 and 1850 had disliked, distrusted, and resented the English. They continued to do so.

T.R. Beck, the committed young republican who had tried to enlist in the army to fight the British in 1812, publicly defended distinctively American usages of the English language in an essay published in 1830 and insisted upon hiring only native-born Americans to teach science and mathematics at his Albany Institute.[24] Nor did these American professionals wish to replicate the English professional structure in their new nation. R.E. Griffith in 1824 considered the British medical establishment a decadent group that maintained its position through pretense, exhortation, and the power of the aristocracy rather than through training, merit, or social contribution.[25]

A second factor behind the strong attraction of French medical jurisprudence during this period was related to a more general shift in the focus of American medical attention away from Edinburgh, where it had been during the second half of the eighteenth century, toward Paris, where it remained through the first half of the nineteenth century. This broad shift has been well documented by historians of medicine. Increasing numbers of American medical students traveled to Paris to learn about human tissue from Xavier Bichat, about advanced surgical technique from Guillaume Dupuytren, and about the diagnostic power of René Laennec's new stethoscope.[26] As R.E. Griffith observed in 1824, the English had fallen behind the French "not only in medical jurisprudence," but also in surgery, experimental physiology, and anatomy.[27] Pierre-Charles-Alexandre Louis indoctrinated a generation of American medical leaders with the importance of accurate statistical observation, another French tendency readily endorsed by the American champions of medical jurisprudence.[28] The so-called French Clinical School, with its emphasis on teaching practical applications in actual cases in the hospitals of Paris, as distinguished from theoretical analyses of what diseases were and how they should be understood intellectually, may fairly be said to have revolutionized nineteenth-century medical training.

Champions of medical jurisprudence in the United States were in the forefront of this general shift of attention toward Paris. T.R. Beck carried on French correspondence, regularly translated French articles for American journals, and continued until his death to add the latest French legal and medical books to his personal library.[29] John B. Beck, who also owned an extensive collection of French books, went out of his way in a survey of American medicine published by the New York legislature in 1850 to urge all physicians to learn French, and there is plenty of evidence that many of them did.[30] An especially forceful, though not unusual, testimony to the importance of French material to the American champions of medical jurisprudence during the first half of the nineteenth century appeared in an obituary notice for Amariah Bringham in 1850. Bringham was a friend of T.R. Beck, with whom he sometimes collaborated, superintendent of the New York State Lunatic Asylum at Utica, and founding editor of the *Journal of Insanity*. "In prosecuting his medical studies," recalled his eulogist, Bringham "found that many things which he wanted were locked up in the

French language. [So]. . . he procured dictionaries and without any teacher mastered the French. Nearly one-third of his large library left is in this tongue. . . ."[31] French medical books and articles were regularly cited in American medical texts, in American dissertations on medical jurisprudence, and in American courtrooms through the first three-quarters of the nineteenth century.[32]

American medico-legalists found especially attractive the system in which Orfila and his colleagues worked. The French required all physicians to pass an examination in medical jurisprudence in order to practice medicine. If they later became involved in jurisprudential questions themselves, the profession could rest assured that they had some training in the field. Even if they never became involved in jurisprudential questions themselves, they were at least aware of the chief issues in the field and conditioned to consider the addressing of those issues a central part of their professional identity. The American champions of upgraded medical jurisprudence were hoping to accomplish something approaching the French situation by introducing the serious study of medical jurisprudence into their medical school curricula, even though the Americans were not in a position to require the subject. Indeed, in the absence of functional licensing laws in the United States through the first half of the nineteenth century and beyond, they were not in a position to require anything.

The Americans also admired the fact that the French had established an institutional base for the development and exercise of public health initiatives. In Paris this took the form of the *Conseil de Salubrité de Paris* (Paris Health Council), which had been founded in 1802. Similar councils existed in secondary cities as well. Operating under the prefect of police, these councils, comprised of professionals trained in medical jurisprudence, had extensive powers from 1810 onward, at least in theory, to investigate and act against threats to public health. They had the right, for example, to deny manufacturing permits and force changes upon industries deemed dangerous. In actual practice, for a host of complex reasons analyzed by the historian William Coleman, these French health councils rarely exercised their considerable theoretical powers.[33] But that was difficult to discern from the American side of the Atlantic and ultimately immaterial to the champions of better medical jurisprudence in the United States, who wanted a system like that of the French, whether the French used theirs effectively or not.

One final aspect of the French system received highly favorable notice in American journals: the French rules concerning expert opinions in court. In the determination of cases before the bar, the French permitted judges to call experts on behalf of the court to help settle difficult or disputed questions of a medical nature. Once the expert had ruled (a given wound, for example, did or did not appear to be the cause of death), that ruling had a de facto presumption of truth. Disgruntled parties to the case could attack the ruling, but the burden of proof, because they had a vested interest, was on them. Even though the French system had evolved from fundamentally inquisitorial origins, most American champions of better medical jurisprudence considered it superior in medico-legal matters to the adversarial system they had inherited from the English, in which judges were effectively precluded from summoning neutral experts to settle contested results, either before or after the case had been argued, no matter how arcane the issues might be.[34]

Many of Orfila's most famous cases arose when he was called by perplexed judges to re-examine confusing evidence. The *PJMPS* described such a case in 1825, a murder trial in which the accused was supposed to have poisoned the victim. Though the preliminary testimony indicated guilt, the defense claimed the prosecutor had made more of the medical evidence than was warranted. To settle the matter, the judge called in Orfila, who ended up agreeing with the defense; in his opinion the evidence was not conclusive. Consequently, the judge gave the benefit of the doubt, thus established legally, to the accused. In the view of many American professionals, that was a nearly paradigmatic instance of the way medical jurisprudence could work and should work.[35]

In actual practice, this aspect of the French system did not work as well as its American admirers believed it did. The French system was open to influence-peddling and corruption; sanction was often given to the opinions of physicians who did not merit the confidence of the courts (there were few Orfilas, after all); and the structure was constantly in need of tinkering and reform throughout the century.[36] An insightful French commentator surveying the period from 1810 to 1912 pointed out in 1913 that his country's medico-legal traditions had functioned not as a smoothly operating engine of perfect professional justice, but rather as an evolutionary and imperfect embodiment of what Americans would call the common law tradition *(droit coutumier)*, combining social customs, royal edicts, and ecclesiastical rulings, regardless of what the formal codes might have stipulated.[37] But the American admirers of the French model did not wish to analyze it too closely. For them, the French system could be presented in letters, lectures, books, and professional journals as a reasonable arrangement that might be emulated with appropriate variations in the United States, an alternative more attractive than the English system they inherited.

As medical jurisprudence became more and more visible in American professional life, especially in medical journals, more and more individuals began to see in the field a potential source of research interest and professional advancement. Several factors encouraged them to do so during the first half of the nineteenth century. First was the sheer challenge of a new and exciting field. Before 1800 virtually no local practitioners could test a corpse for signs of poisoning; by 1825 there were plenty of physicians around the United States who could. Second was the professional encouragement they were receiving in medical schools and professional journals to tackle jurisprudential issues. Before 1800 such subjects were seldom raised; after 1825 a flood of literature documented the apparently mounting number of great successes accomplished by physicians in legal situations both in the

United States and abroad. Third was the confidence of having solid professional guidance. Before 1800 there had been essentially nothing available to physicians to help them contribute in legal situations, even if they had the inclination to help; after 1825 they had the *Elements* and an exploding journal literature to follow. Moreover, many of those who attended the nation's growing number of medical schools had been exposed to formal training in the field, and their professors, of course, had urged them to get involved.

Fourth, but by no means least, was the possibility of attaining a professional reputation not easily acquired in any other fashion. Many American physicians dreamed of making a mark in their society. They wanted genuinely to contribute to their fellow citizens and to serve the nation; and they wanted the rewards of contribution and service, both psychological and tangible. Nor was there anything illegitimate or ignoble about those desires; those desires were then and still remain near the center of any professional ethos. When a physician brought his special medical skills and advanced knowledge to bear upon the problems of an ailing neighbor, he had the satisfaction of achieving both those goals (provided the neighbor paid his bill, which was by no means a certainty), at least on a limited scale. Even if a physician performed brilliantly in his private cases, however, any acknowledgment of his contribution was likely to remain quite limited. Most patients did not want their cases to become the subject of public discussion, and the public was poorly equipped to distinguish between a brilliant treatment, on the one hand, and a lucky or routine one, on the other, even if the case was discussed in public. Successful cases, of course, could lead eventually to a large and satisfying practice, which afforded both psychological and financial rewards, but that road was all too often long and bumpy.

Given the circumstances of the first half of the nineteenth century, involvement in medical jurisprudence seemed to offer a rapid route to fame; a dashing and dramatic, yet altogether appropriate and legitimate, avenue of professional advancement. Trials were eminently public events in the first half of the nineteenth century, almost forms of social theater. A triumph in court was not a private matter. The physician who solved a public mystery, rid his community of toxic pollution, identified a dangerous murderer, or saved an innocent local citizen from wrongful conviction became a public hero; and he deserved to be a hero since he had applied to the good of others a set of skills he had worked hard to acquire. Material success seemed bound to follow, directly or indirectly. Involvement in jurisprudential cases thus appeared to be good for the individual, good for the profession, and good for society. Hundreds of physicians in the United States must have wondered to themselves what it might be like to become a regional American Orfila.

A great deal of evidence in the journal literature and in court records indicates that many physicians went beyond wondering about involvement in legal matters. They actively sought opportunities to participate in jurisprudential undertakings, difficult as that might be for modern physicians to imagine, for all of the personal and professional reasons just alluded to.[38]

Some pursued private research on their own because they thought it would have public jurisprudential applications. Others waited for particular situations and specific cases, then tried to tackle the issues they raised. Perhaps the best known story of the way in which medical jurisprudence could establish a person's reputation involved a man who eventually became one of the most eminent surgeons in United States history: Samuel D. Gross.

Gross graduated from Jefferson Medical College in Philadelphia in 1828. Prior to his graduation he had taken a course in medical jurisprudence. The subject clearly intrigued this able and ambitious young medical student, and he thought medical jurisprudence had professional potential. Gross became a great admirer of Beck's *Elements*, and he also kept up with French developments, especially those in pathological anatomy. Gross actually enjoyed dissections and translated for the American market (and for income) some of the French texts he followed on surgery and anatomy. But his career seemed to be going nowhere by 1830. No medical school had offered him the professorship he thought he deserved, and he was unable to establish a financially viable practice in Philadelphia, where he longed to break into the medical elite. Reluctantly, Gross returned to provincial Easton, Pennsylvania, where he had grown up and where he could at least make a living.[39]

Once back in Easton, Gross occupied his spare time with experimentation and dissection, mostly on rabbits and dogs. He was especially interested in the properties of blood, in intestinal wounds, and in the absorption rate of substances by the stomach and the subsequent filtration rate of those substances by the kidneys. Each of those areas of investigation had fairly obvious forensic applications, and each allowed him to hone his surgical skills. The Lehigh Valley was not a healthy place for stray animals during the two and one-half years Gross lived there; his exploration of intestinal wounds alone involved the sacrifice of upwards of seventy dogs. Gross's penchant for experimentation and his strong inclination toward medical jurisprudence combined to make him a logical candidate to participate in local cases that involved medical investigations, and by his own account he "served several times as an expert" in local trials.[40]

Much to Gross's good fortune, a dramatic case arose in Easton in 1833, when a man named Goetter was indicted for strangling to death in the eighth month of her pregnancy a woman whom Goetter had allegedly seduced. The local authorities asked Gross to perform a post-mortem examination of the victim's body, and Gross became the prosecutor's star witness during the flamboyant and nationally publicized trial that ensued. The "great interest" manifested by the general public in this macabre but romantically spectacular case was heightened by the fact that Goetter retained a defense team headed by James Madison Porter, the most prominent and successful attorney in the area and one of the co-founders of Easton's Lafayette College. As Gross put it, Porter was "celebrated for his dexterity as an examiner of witnesses, which, combined with a certain amount of impudence, caused him to be greatly feared."

The Goetter trial reached its climax when Gross and Porter confronted one another for the better part of a day. Gross had made an uncharacteristic slip in not examining anything inside the woman's skull, and Porter tried to exploit the oversight by suggesting that she might well have died of apoplexy, which could be determined only by examination of the brain. She had been, after all, under tremendous stress. But Gross had prepared himself thoroughly on the internal and external signs of strangulation and asphyxia. To supplement the standard texts, he had done additional fresh research of his own on those subjects by strangling and dissecting a dozen rabbits;[41] and he held his ground against Porter and a host of other physicians whom Porter had brought in to testify about apoplexy. The verdict sustained Gross, and the judge sentenced Goetter to death. Again fortunately for Gross, since the case was entirely circumstantial, Goetter confessed to the crime on the eve of his execution, and Gross found himself a professional hero. Indeed, Gross's research on strangulation and his victory in the Goetter trial were quickly incorporated into the next edition of Beck's *Elements*.[42]

The event functioned as a springboard for Gross, who promptly left Easton to accept the first of a series of professorial appointments that would propel him to the top of his profession. Half a century later, Gross still remembered the Goetter case as "the most important event of my professional life at Easton," which made it clearly the turning point in his career.[43] No wonder Gross stressed in his presidential address to the American Medical Association in 1868 not some aspect of the surgery for which he was so renowned, but the need for an effective national system of providing expert medical testimony in American courts.[44] No wonder Gross insisted that medical jurisprudence be included among the subjects recognized in a week-long series of lectures about American medical progress at the centennial celebrations in 1876, when he chaired the committee that put the series together, even though the field had by then fallen upon very different and much harder times.[45]

Finally, medical jurisprudence also affected the American medical profession during the period from 1820 to 1850 by acting as a stimulus to research that in turn produced significant, if sometimes unintended, consequences in other fields as well. Beck himself clearly recognized this important aspect of medical jurisprudence. "[P]atient, laborious, and philosophical investigations" would be needed over the long run, if medicine as a whole hoped to place itself on an "enlightened and learned" foundation. "I am probably blinded by a partiality for a favorite pursuit," he admitted in a lecture at the Albany Institute in 1826, "but I cannot avoid . . . expressing my conviction, that the study of medical jurisprudence will, in some degree, aid in producing" that result. The reason was straightforward: Beck believed that most professionals in the real world responded better to specific problems than to grand theory, and medical jurisprudence would help physicians focus their investigations, precisely because actual lives, properties, and reputations would be at stake. Moreover, any conclusions they deduced would have to stand the test of public challenge. Medical jurisprudence thus represented in early America the "application of analytical reasoning to the science of medicine, in its best form and under the operation of the most powerful incentives."[46]

Many examples of Beck's insight, some trivial and some profound, could be cited. Good examples already alluded to would include the impact on surgery of Gross' experiments with intestinal wounds and the long-term effects on drug therapy of investigations in forensic toxicology. In a similar fashion, efforts undertaken to distinguish human blood from animal blood in court cases during the first half of the century led to a better understanding of the properties of the former.[47] Rape cases advanced the microscopic investigation of seminal fluid by 1850.[48] Overall, however, probably the greatest of what might be labeled the secondary beneficiaries of the medical jurisprudence movement was the emerging field of physiology.

Anatomy, the identification and examination of the human body and its component parts, had in one form or another long been a staple of medical training.[49] But anatomy remained a remarkably superficial field well into the nineteenth century. A medical student in 1825 could probably have identified a human kidney, for example, and probably knew that it functioned as a filtration device in the body, but would not have known how quickly it did its work or whether it filtered some substances better than others. Nor would the student have known in any meaningful sense how the kidney actually worked. The burst of research on poisons and poisoning played a major role in generating answers to those basic physiological questions, and those answers, in turn, permitted twentieth-century science to intervene in kidney disorders in ways that early nineteenth-century physicians could hardly have imagined.[50] The toxicological and physiological findings that resulted from the great burst of poisoning investigations during the first half of the nineteenth century also helped provide a scientific underpinning for the largely chemical-based therapeutic revolutions of the second half of the century.[51]

John B. Beck's lifelong attention to infanticide provided another illustration of the point being made here. He did not set out to advance neonatal physiology; he set out to explore ways in which he might help his profession become more effective in dealing with the jurisprudential questions surrounding an age-old legal problem. Put differently, it was not a specifically health-related question that motivated his research, nor would his research on that subject benefit him in the everyday medical practice that brought him his living. It was his interest in the role of his profession in legal questions that motivated over thirty years of investigations and experiments related to infanticide; but along the way, almost inadvertently, he advanced neonatal physiology. From the writing of his dissertation in 1817 until his death in 1851, his contemporaries considered him the world's expert in the field and provided him with a more or less continuous supply of deceased infants for examination, many of them from New York City's Bellevue Hospital. Though the work was grim, the results were significant.

He was able to discover much about the relationships between birth weight and survival, the causes of suffocation during the birth process, the role of the arteries in the first few moments of life, the rates of oxygenation in newborns, the rapidity of putrefaction in stillborns, and more.[52] The key point here is that medical jurisprudence, not pure science or the hope of future medical breakthroughs, provided the purpose for those undertakings. Moreover, John Beck was certainly not alone, even in the field of infanticide, where such leading medico-legalists as R.E. Griffith also conducted investigations of their own.[53]

In a similar fashion, research undertaken to settle longstanding medico-legal disputes over the length of gestation advanced the physiological understanding of that process.[54] Stringham had confessed to his medical jurisprudential students as late as 1815 that "we know little of the Phenomena of Pregnancy," and that "it is very difficult in Legal Medicine" to "ascertain whether a woman be pregnant or not."[55] But students of medical jurisprudence began to alter that situation from the early 1820s onward. The use of the stethoscope to detect fetal heartbeats in cases of doubtful or feigned pregnancy after 1820, for example, helped to establish the gradual nature of the process of gestation and to undermine the ancient quickening doctrine, which had long considered fetal movement the first legally reliable sign of developing life.[56] Medical jurisprudential concerns were also influential during the 1840s in the systematic evaluation of urine tests as reliable indicators of pregnancy.[57] These and related efforts, though launched by professionals trying to provide answers to specific legal questions, ended up cumulatively helping to provide an underpinning for the formal emergence of the specialty of obstetrics.

The rising interest in medical jurisprudence among American physicians had a major impact during the first half of the nineteenth century on several aspects of American medical history. But the influence of physicians interested in medico-legal issues was not confined to medical history alone. During one of the key formative periods in United States history, physicians interested in medico-legal issues also began to help shape a broad range of American social attitudes. Their efforts would eventually leave an enduring imprint on the nation's social culture and public policies.

CHAPTER FIVE

Medical Jurisprudence and American Society, 1820–1850

The increasing professional interest of physicians in medico-legal matters effected far more than the internal development of the medical profession. Especially during the second quarter of the nineteenth century, the growing involvement of American physicians in medico-legal matters began to produce lasting and important effects on American society itself. Some of the large social changes physicians helped bring about were obvious and dramatic; others were more subtle and more difficult to pin down. Since no one volume, much less a single chapter, could capture all of those changes in detail, three condensed examples will have to suffice: the impact of the new medical jurisprudence movement on the American treatment of insanity; the promising progress of the battle against poisons and poisoning; and a shift in attitudes regarding sexuality and procreation.

Any assessment of the impact of the medical jurisprudence movement during the first half of the nineteenth century must take seriously the subject of insanity because the early champions of upgraded medical jurisprudence saw in that subject, long a problem for physicians and jurists, a field of great potential advancement and professional contribution. In 1810 Benjamin Rush had selected the general subject of insanity to illustrate the future promise of medical jurisprudence in the new republic. T.R.Beck had entered the field a few years later with his doctoral dissertation on insanity. Countless other young professionals shared the enthusiasm of those pioneers and followed similar paths through mid-century. Francis Wharton, co-author of the general treatise that finally supplanted Beck's *Elements* after 1855 was but a single excellent example. He, too, had first entered the field through his fascination with and writings about the legal aspects of insanity.[1]

Virtually every lecturer in every course on medical jurisprudence in the country addressed the subject of insanity. Virtually every publication on medical jurisprudence that claimed any intention of being comprehensive also dealt at length with that subject. Hundreds of articles in medical journals discussed various aspects of insanity, the vast majority of which had explicit legal implications. Most of this large literature drew directly or indirectly upon theories first propounded by French writers, especially Philippe Pinel and François Fodéré, but tried to apply those theories to the circumstances of the new United States.

Throughout the early writings of American medico-legal experts on insanity ran a pair of recurring themes: mental disease underlay and explained a much greater proportion of aberrant behavior than most people realized; and ordinary citizens should be made far more aware than they were that insanity of various sorts and degrees was frighteningly widespread. At one level, those themes were clearly self-serving. If the problems were more subtle and more nuanced than most people thought, the medical profession, which had traditionally been called upon to deal with them, could anticipate more latitude, more training, and more social influence. And if the public could be convinced that the problems were more widespread and disquieting than most people perceived, the public would be more likely to implement policy changes of the sort the medical jurisprudents favored. But their position was not simply one of professional aggrandizement or cynical manipulation. Beck and his contemporaries really believed that professionals could help the republic deal with this problem.[2]

Toward that end, the champions of improved medical jurisprudence stressed two principal areas of medico-legal interaction within the general subject of insanity. The first was the social treatment of insanity. Most early American physicians and medical jurisprudents probably considered insanity part of the medical police branch of their field rather than the criminal law branch. Through the late 1830s, Beck and his contemporaries focused comparatively little attention upon specific questions of criminal responsibility. They were primarily concerned instead about insanity as a public health question, and they were optimistic about their ability to address the question in general terms.

Their program was straightforward and attractive. Insane persons should be removed from county almshouses or the back rooms of families who did not know what to do with them to places of refuge, to asylums. There trained professionals could apply the humane therapies that so captured the sympathies and admiration of T.R. Beck as a young medical student. The early advocates of humane treatment in asylum settings anticipated high rates of what they consistently and optimistically called "cures." Because individuals could not build and maintain asylums on their own, the state should support the effort. The advocates of state-supported asylums probably believed themselves, and they certainly allowed the public to believe, that their advancing and ever more scientific understanding of mental diseases would in this fashion ultimately reduce the burden of insanity upon society as a whole, notwithstanding the outlay of public funds in the short run, by reducing the number of mentally debilitated citizens in the long run.

Beck's own writings, especially during the 1820s, resonated with those assumptions, and so did the lobbying efforts of others like him in state capitals throughout the country.[3] Deftly combining a sensitive and caring attitude toward individuals with a faith in scientific rationalism and the role of the state, the early asylum movement came close to epitomizing the sunny Enlightenment hopes of the early republic. No wonder so many of the champions of active medical jurisprudence found the field so attractive during that period and no wonder so many of them, including Beck himself, actually took a turn at asylum-keeping at some point in their careers. And notwithstanding the spectacular breadth of Beck's work, which included pathbreaking efforts in forensic toxicology and international fame as a medico-legalist, he was best remembered by state politicians after he died for his efforts in behalf of the insane.

The closest the state of New York ever came to memorializing T.R. Beck, in fact, involved a legislative proposal in 1865, ten years after his death, to build another new state insane asylum and to name it in his honor. When Beck's friend Sylvester D. Willard, another Albany physician and another strong proponent of humane, state-supported treatment for the insane, collapsed and died suddenly in front of an Assembly committee "while making one more passionate appeal for the [Beck] asylum," a stunned state legislature altered the bill at the last minute and named the institution instead for Willard.[4] Beck, though his long-range impact on many of the social policies of his state may have been unmatched in New York history, was in the end never publicly recognized.

Much debate has raged over the virtues of asylums. Many people, including most of those who first endorsed asylums in the nineteenth century and most of those who still vote tax money to maintain them in the twentieth century, have considered asylums, for all their imperfections, fundamentally beneficent institutions wherein the state assumes the burden of caring for people who can neither cope for themselves nor be coped with by others under ordinary circumstances. Asylums provided an institutional setting in which the insane could receive therapy from experts who knew more about the treatments for and problems of insanity than friends and relatives did, and the public as a whole could help share the financial burdens involved.

In the last few decades, however, a substantial number of critics have come to see asylums as insidious vehicles for overt social control, institutions whose chief purpose all along, implicitly or explicitly, was the removal and incarceration of citizens whom emerging industrial societies did not wish to accommodate. Around this latter premise analysts like Michel Foucault have constructed broad-gauged and influential social critiques.[5] Others, including the historian David Rothman, have taken a more subtle position. In their view the early asylum-builders, at least in the United States, probably began with a sincere desire to aid those citizens who could not function effectively in society. The reformers may well have allowed themselves a hopeful, if naive or even self-serving, faith in the possibility of rehabilitations. But because so many of the cases they encountered proved so intractable, the institutions they created evolved easily and quite quickly into human holding tanks, better perhaps than the county jails and miserable almshouses in which mentally troubled citizens of the eighteenth century had endured a horrible existence, but hardly models of effective social action.[6]

This is not the place to settle the difficult historical argument over the fundamental character of asylums, but it is the place to add another perspective to it. Among other things, the asylum movement may be seen as an important early example of state medicine. Had asylums functioned as Beck's generation envisioned them, they would certainly have been powerful examples of medical jurisprudence at its best, since they combined state support and a number of complex legal issues (including commitments, the respective responsibilities of all parties involved, and the terms of release) with medical expertise, both psychiatric and conventional. It is certainly no historical accident that asylums arose in the United States during the great push by influential physicians for more effective medical jurisprudence, and it is no accident that Benjamin Rush and T.R. Beck, among many others, saw in the treatment of the insane a nearly paradigmatic example of why their republic needed active professionals engaged in a strengthened tradition of legal medicine.

The early champions of medical jurisprudence also placed heavy stress on a second dimension of the insanity issue as well: the question of mental competence in the disposition of material wealth. This generally, but not always, took the form of trying to determine whether a person had been of "sound mind" when he or she signed a contract or a will. For people trying to stabilize a democratic republic based in large part upon the assumption that each individual was rationally able to act in his or her own best economic interests, the question of competence was no trivial matter. Since most twentieth-century analysts have become understandably fascinated with the almost philosophical problems of human responsibility, modern scholarly discussions of medico-legal insanity have seldom dwelt upon this eminently practical question. But in the first half of the nineteenth century the vast majority of the insanity-related cases that physicians actually encountered under normal circumstances involved property disputes of one sort or another; in most of them the person whose sanity was being adjudicated had no personal stake in the outcome whatsoever because he or she was dead. Most of these cases were challenges to wills, and much could hinge upon whether a given testator was retroactively determined to have been competent or incompetent to dispose of property.

The elder Duncan's original lectures at Edinburgh had treated insanity primarily as an issue in civil law rather than criminal law, as a practical matter that usually involved money rather than a theoretical matter of when and whether to hold someone responsible for a criminal action.[7] "There are few Particulars which are more frequently the Subjects of Investigation before Courts possessing a Civil Jurisdiction," Duncan told his students in 1798, "than Insanity, and they are very often of the greatest Importance."[8]

Stringham, Rush, Beck, Griffith, Dunglison, and most of the other early champions of medical jurisprudence in the United States all shared that frame of reference. As late as 1855, even though the criminal responsibility of the insane had been a subject of hot debate for more than a decade by then, Wharton and Stillé devoted only about twenty-five pages of the first edition of their influential new *Medical Jurisprudence* to that aspect of medico-legal insanity; they devoted over two hundred pages to cases that involved questions of medico-legal insanity in the context of contracts and wills.[9] Through the medico-legal question of insanity, physicians saw a way to involve themselves more and more significantly in matters of property.

Rush had proclaimed their position straightforwardly in his 1810 exhortation "On the Study of Medical Jurisprudence." In this public lecture, the one Rush had urged Jefferson to read as soon as it was published and the one Rush considered an illustration of why the new nation needed better medical jurisprudence than it had, Rush envisioned physicians playing a large role in the process of inheritance. A physician, he pointed out, should always "assist a dying patient in disposing of his property in a correct manner." The doctor should tell the family to tell the patient to draft a will (the doctor would not want to tell the patient himself because the patient would know the doctor had no more hope). "We owe this duty to [the patient's] family and to society," he argued.[10] The reason for this duty quickly became clear.

In Rush's view physicians could help ensure for families and for society the orderly and predictable transfer of economic assets. On this subject the Revolutionary politician and radical physician was profoundly conservative. For him the insanity laws should be used to guard against whimsy, caprice, idiosyncrasy, and the last-minute fits of poor judgment sometimes associated with critical illness or old age. "Should a man [in what would now be called a state of depression] bequeath the whole, or the greatest part, of his estate, to a church, or any other public institution, or to a stranger," said Rush by way of illustration, "to the injury of a family of children who had never offended him, and whose necessities, or rank in life, as well as their blood, intitled [sic] them to be his heirs, he should be considered as morally deranged; and his will should be set aside as promptly as if he had disposed of his estate in a paroxysm of intellectual derangement. The laws, and the voice of nature, in such a case, should silence a volume of reports in favour of a contrary practice."[11] That was an extremely strong position: a will deemed inappropriate by the courts should be set aside "as if" the testator were insane.

Needless to say, this position forced Rush to take an unusually inclusive view of what constituted the signs of mental incompetence. The easier it was to prove insanity, after all, the easier it would be for physicians to play the role of community arbiters and help set aside on grounds of mental incompetence wills they or those who retained them did not consider appropriate; and the greater would be the legal power and social role of physicians. Almost anything would do as an indicator of insanity. New hatreds, taciturnity, loquacity, prodigality, economy, liberality to public institutions, cunning, and even "the evolution of talents of wit and rhyming," according to Rush, could legitimately be used retroactively in court as signs of mental disorder. And if those did not prevail, Rush laid down the ultimate doctrine: "There are instances in which madmen talk rationally, but write incoherently." In other words, the document itself could be used as evidence of insanity, and hence set aside by the court, even if there were no other signs of derangement present.[12]

In 1812, the year before he died, Rush further adumbrated his broad view of insanity in a major study of *The Diseases of the Mind*.[13] In that book he continued to expand the public consciousness of insanity as a pervasive and easily induced disease. It could result from normal bodily processes, especially those associated with reproduction in women; from revolutions in government, which had obvious implications in a recently established republic; and from changes in social habits. More traditional causes, of course, such as masturbation, continued to obtain as well. Rush also suggested that the United States, because it was a Protestant nation, was at risk for widespread outbreaks of insanity because its citizens no longer had faith in the old Roman Catholic ability to "relieve their minds from the pressure of guilt, by means of confession and absolution."[14] Physicians would have to guard society against the potential disruptions of mental disease.

Though his opinions were characteristically bold, Rush was by no means alone. Griffith and Beck both paid close and specific attention to the role of physicians in willing property. Griffith pointed out that even Sir William Blackstone, who had wanted to minimize the involvement of physicians in legal processes in England and the colonies in the eighteenth century, had conceded doctors a role in the area of wills. The English commentator thought all physicians should at least know the proper forms and procedures in order to help patients and their families in emergencies.[15] T.R. Beck devoted a section of the *Elements* to "the state of mind necessary to constitute a valid will," and his emphasis, like that of Rush, was upon the wide variety of afflictions that might incapacitate a testator. Beck also explained for his readers and students the legal regulations governing nuncupative, or verbal, wills. In these dispositions of property, physicians might play an enormous role, for the courts were often forced, in a literal sense, to take the doctor's word for it. Nuncupative wills were not uncommon in cases of emergency and among the illiterate.[16] Dunglison told his students at Virginia in the 1820s that "old age—debility of mind induced by old age—may render a person unfit to manage his own affairs," and he devoted a lecture to the subject of challenging wills.[17]

On the first day of his class in medical jurisprudence at Berkshire in 1824, Stephen W. Williams addressed the issue directly:

> We are often called upon to decide upon that state of mind whereby a man is capable or incapable of making a will. In proving a will the question is always asked by the judge, whether the deceased was of

> sound and disposing mind and memory. This question is many times
> difficult to solve. . . . upon some subjects a man may be of perfectly
> sound mind, while upon others he may be a complete lunatic. . . . If
> under this delusion he dispose of his property, his will cannot be valid.
> . . . No department in your profession requires more patient and ac-
> curate investigation. If in all other departments of medical jurispru-
> dence great care is necessary in forming and giving in our opinion, how
> much more necessary is it in these cases. . . .[18]

Williams's students could not have missed the importance of this aspect
of the insanity question. Nor could they have failed to see that their own
advantage lay in promulgating a broad interpretation of mental disorders,
which they would then be able to interpret. At Yale, medical students were
getting the same message from Nathan Smith. In his course on medical
jurisprudence, he berated his own state of Connecticut for being too supportive of wills as written; in Smith's view, doctors should be able to dis-
qualify bad ones more easily than Connecticut's courts had been permitting
them to.[19]

The champions of more aggressive and influential medical jurisprudence made remarkable headway on this second insanity-related campaign,
especially during the second quarter of the nineteenth century, just as they
did on their first front, the asylums. The evidence, however, was less tangible than the creation of state-supported asylums and less systematic, from
a historian's point of view, than it might ideally have been. It consisted
primarily of a heightened awareness of the role of physicians in the disposition of other people's property, an awareness clearly evident in medical
journals, and an increasing number of well-publicized cases that involved
the application of flexible concepts of mental incapacity to the adjudication
of wills.[20]

Among those cases was the drawn-out battle over the estate of John
Randolph of Roanoke. A year before he died in 1833, Randolph had executed a will that nullified his previous testament of 1821. At stake was a
great deal of property for rival beneficiaries and the freedom of some 400
slaves: by the will of 1821 the latter were to be freed and resettled; by the
will of 1832 they were to be sold. The case dragged through the Virginia
courts for twelve years before courageous physicians and lawyers finally
succeeded in setting aside the 1832 document. The Virginia Court of Appeals ruling in 1845 recognized the slaveholder's sanity at the time he granted
emancipation and his insanity at the time emancipation was revoked. Randolph's trustees subsequently arranged to resettle the slaves in Ohio.[21]

One of the most tangled of the will cases, one which resulted in an
essentially political decision that many medico-legalists disliked, made its
way through the courts of New York during the late 1830s and early 1840s.
The case attracted a great deal of attention because a great deal of money
was involved. At stake was the estate of Alice Lispenard, who died in 1836
at the age of fifty-five. Though she possessed extremely limited mental abilities and had been considered an imbecile in her father's will, Lispenard

had not only inherited substantial principal in trust from him but had also fallen legal heir, as next of kin, to estates amassed by other relatives as well. Before she died, Lispenard had put her mark to a will that left her entire holdings to her brother, Alexander L. Stewart. On the one hand, Stewart had certainly been in a position to influence Lispenard, who was not only diminished mentally but allowed by her brother to indulge her alcoholism; on the other hand, Lispenard's desire to bestow her entire fortune upon Stewart may have been the legitimate consequence of Stewart's providing care for Lispenard most of her adult life. The lawsuit arose when other potential beneficiaries challenged Lispenard's competence to dispose of her property at all. If she were ruled of unsound mind, the will would be set aside, and they would split some of the estate.

In 1838 the challenging parties, resting their contentions upon the testimony of physicians, succeeded in having the Lispenard will set aside at the local level, as had been done with many less famous wills under similar circumstances. Stewart thereupon appealed to the Circuit Court, where he lost; then to the Chancellor's Court, where he lost again. Stewart, who had powerful political friends, finally appealed in 1841 to the Court for the Correction of Errors, his last resort. Under the state constitution, this body consisted of the New York State Senate sitting as a court, guided by the justices of the state Supreme Court. None other than the attorney general of New York, Willis Hall, represented Stewart before the Court of Errors, and two of the most influential senators then serving, G.C. Verplanck and J.B. Scott, managed Stewart's case. Verplanck defended the pro-Stewart will in part by arguing that the disposal of property was "not a mere institution of positive law, but a natural right." Unless the testator were entirely devoid of all mental ability, and not merely suffering from some degree of diminished capacity, he or she should be allowed to exercise that natural right.[22]

The Court of Errors voted 12 to 6 to reinstate Lispenard's will, and Stewart emerged victorious. Though T.R. Beck knew and admired Verplanck personally, he was dismayed that "no judge of the Supreme Court gave an opinion on the case, and that the decision of it constantly remained with the *lay members* [his emphasis], as they are called," or in other words, with the elected senators.[23] Beck had come to view the determination of mental competence in inheritance cases as a professional preserve, not a lay matter. He disliked both the intervention of the politicos and Verplanck's implicit denial of professional authority.

Beck need not have worried; the Lispenard case proved to be one of the last major cases of its sort. The state's highest political bodies, after all, were not likely to involve themselves regularly with such matters, and even in the Lispenard case every court beneath the state senate had sustained the power of the physicians. Especially after 1840, physicians asserted growing authority over the disposition of estates. Lawyers delighted in doctrines that allowed them to rewrite the testaments of the dead in behalf of living (and paying) clients, and they needed physicians to justify the process with *ex post facto* diagnoses of incompetence.[24] Fees offered to doctors in large will cases were alleged to be much higher than those offered in other sorts of medico-legal proceedings.[25] By the 1860s, John J. Elwell, then the nation's leading authority on medical evidence in court, was able to state flatly that "no class of witnesses dispose by their testimony of larger amounts of money than [medical witnesses]. The greatest fortunes ever collected together by financial ability, have been distributed by medical men upon the witness stand, in contests over the validity of wills. . . . The law books are full of illustrations of this fact."[26]

The celebrated Parish will case, which was under appeal when that line was written, ultimately confirmed what was happening. The case involved the estate of Henry Parish, a New York City businessman whose assets in real estate and corporate securities easily exceeded a million dollars when he died in 1856. Parish had originally directed the disposition of his property in a detailed document drafted and attested by his attorneys in 1842. A total of three codicils were added in 1853 and 1854, however, which redirected the disposition of about $400,000. Although the codicils were also drafted and attested by Parish's attorneys, they were challenged at probate by the superseded benefactors.[27]

The challengers claimed that Parish was not of sound mind when the codicils were executed. He had suffered a stroke in 1849, which left him extensively paralyzed, unable to speak or to write (though he apparently could gesture agreement or disagreement, conduct his affairs through his wife, and make a mark in lieu of a signature), and, in their view, almost certainly impaired mentally. According to the challengers, Parish's wife had taken advantage of her husband's diminished capacity to persuade him to alter his will, at the expense of his own brothers and for the benefit of hers. A titanic legal struggle ensued, involving several of New York's top lawyers, a number of charitable foundations (which stood to gain or lose handsome bequests), two of the city's most economically influential families, and a great deal of testimony from physicians on the question of mental soundness.

The New York City Surrogate heard testimony about the codicils for two years before accepting the first of them and rejecting the other two. That decision was sustained by the New York Supreme Court and appealed to the New York Court of Appeals, then the state's highest bench. After hearing the case argued and reargued, the appellate judges, in a sharply divided decision, also sustained the Surrogate's ruling.[28] Since Parish had been unable to express himself in a manner that might have permitted an objective assessment of whether he had lost any of his mental acuity, the majority was implicitly giving great weight to the theoretical arguments of those physicians who claimed expertise in such matters. Editorial comments, legal texts, and judicial opinions all around the country made explicit the conclusion thus confirmed in the Parish case: using their new theories about insanity, American physicians had established a major role for themselves in the adjudication of wills.

Indeed, the power of physicians to overturn wills through retroactive rulings of testamentary incompetence eventually became so great that several states later in the nineteenth century moved to restrict what they regarded as an "epidemic of contests of wills." Ordinary citizens feared undue infringement of the long-standing rights of perfectly sound citizens to dispose of their property as they wished. Michigan legislators would eventually take the lead in this effort by passing a law in 1883 that allowed testators to approach a circuit judge or a judge of probate and have their will formally certified in advance of their death. The act authorized the judge to hold a hearing for all interested parties and attest to the validity of the will in a special decree. That decree, in turn, would "have the same effect as if made by said court after the death of the testator . . . and such will having been so established shall not be set aside or impeached on the ground of insanity or want of testamentary capacity."[29]

Developments related to toxicology offer a second major illustration of the impact of the early medical jurisprudence movement on American law and society. Though various rulers through the centuries had taken various measures to try to deter the incidence of poisoning, the state in reality remained relatively powerless to do much about it through the middle of the eighteenth century.[30] Even into the first decade of the nineteenth century there were few reliable tests for poisons of any sort and little research going forward to find better tests or to understand the actions of various poisons on the human body. Lecturing in 1815, Stringham had considered poisoning a "very dangerous method of committing murder as it is easily concealed—and consequently frequent."[31] Accidental poisoning was also common, since even apothecaries made many mistakes with lethal substances; indeed, that was one of the reasons the editors of the *New York Journal of the Medical and Physical Sciences* had called for regulation of the sale of arsenic as early as 1822.[32] Citizens feared death from poisoning and considered the incidence of murder by poison to be quite high in the United States through the first half of the nineteenth century. Even after the Civil War, one of the nation's best-known authorities on medical jurisprudence still surmised that poisoning was America's "most common form of homicide."[33]

Post-mortem examinations were sufficiently imprecise and ordinary physicians so poorly informed about forensic toxicology prior to 1820 that formal investigations often produced as much confusion and debate as scientific clarification, even when people's lives were at stake and even when the highest public authorities got involved. A case in point took place in 1817 in Montgomery County, New York, hardly a backwater area. Circumstantial evidence suggested that a man named Abraham Kesler might have poisoned his recently deceased wife with arsenic. Local physicians disinterred the woman's remains two months after she had been buried and performed a superficial series of observations and chemical tests. At the ensuing trial, they testified that the woman had indeed been murdered with arsenic. The jury found Kesler guilty and the judge sentenced him to death.[34]

When Kesler's attorneys appealed to the governor, the state's chief executive ordered his own independent reassessment of the medical evidence. The governor's experts in New York City concluded forcefully that postmortem observations of the woman's stomach were meaningless, given the extensive putrefaction that had taken place during two months of burial, and that the local physicians had not conducted the proper chemical tests for arsenic. The governor thereupon stayed the execution and sent the case to the state legislature, urging the legislature to exercise the constitutional power it then had in New York to pardon Kesler. The Courts of Justice committee of the legislature, in turn, proceeded to take yet another round of medical opinion on the case and the daily newspapers in Albany tossed in their opinions as well. The legislature's doctors eventually decided that they had no quarrel on the whole with the original local procedures, and the legislature passed an act overriding the governor's stay. Kesler was executed in 1818.

The situation began to change during the 1820s, however, as the champions of better medical jurisprudence began to disseminate toxicological information in their lectures, articles, and books. In his classes on medical jurisprudence at the College of Physicians and Surgeons of New York, for example, John B. Beck went through the Kesler case specifically to illustrate the importance of careful procedures, the advantage of conducting several different types of forensic tests at the very beginning of an investigation, and the human tragedies that could result from cursory efforts.[35] Conditions did not shift suddenly. Several poisons, headed by mercury compounds and arsenic, continued to be used medicinally, for example, and according to the *New York Medical and Physical Journal* in 1824, "illiterate prescribers . . . not unfrequently and most suddenly" killed people with their "audacious" therapies.[36] At the end of the decade, the short-lived *Maryland Medical Recorder* could still complain with much justification that most doctors did not know the standard antidotes to common poisons.[37] But progress was being made, both in research and in public perception.

By 1832 John K. Mitchell, who was then teaching medical chemistry at the Philadelphia Medical Institute, could list with confidence several reliable tests for arsenic. Though each might be challenged by itself separately, the coincidence of positive results from all of them "would amount to a miracle."[38] In combination with supporting evidence from a well-conducted post-mortem examination, which paid careful attention to the characteristic "morbid appearance" of tissues affected by arsenic, American physicians had the potential of rendering arsenic murder virtually impossible to get away with as a purely scientific question by 1830.[39] Just as importantly, effective forensic investigations would make erroneous convictions less likely.[40]

The general public became aware of the progress being made in forensic toxicology through a number of well-publicized criminal cases that seemed to illustrate nicely the way a strong system of medical jurisprudence could and should work. One of them occurred in a small village just outside Philadelphia in 1828. There a man fell ill and died, despite treatment by Samuel Jackson, a former president of the Philadelphia Board of Health and a leading medical educator. Though Jackson considered the death a result of the dead man's heavy drinking, village rumor blamed the man's wife. The wife was thought to have been too friendly with a neighboring man, and she was alleged to have purchased arsenic before her husband fell ill. The villagers pushed the local coroner for an inquest. "It seldom happens that reason is listened to amidst popular clamour," Jackson noted after the fact; "hence the coroner [proceeded] with his inquest."

The coroner empaneled four local practitioners, who conducted crude liquid tests for arsenic, and unanimously concurred that the man had been poisoned. On the basis of that finding, the coroner turned the case over to the grand jury. Jackson himself then re-entered the case, for among other things, Jackson was a national expert on medical pharmacology.[41] The Philadelphia professor challenged the validity of the old-fashioned tests conducted by the local panel and upbraided them for failure to send the viscera to Philadelphia for more conclusive investigation under better conditions by people who knew what they were doing. Jackson, not by accident, was among the nation's most fervent advocates of French medical methods, and he pointed out that local results on the Continent were routinely double-checked at central laboratories. Clearly, in his view, professionals should be doing the same thing in the United States. The grand jury voted 23 to 1 not to indict the woman, and the case was dropped. Jackson saw this incident as a good example of the way medical jurisprudence ought to work in the republic. Science had triumphed over gossip; an innocent life had been saved. Lest the lesson be lost, he published the story in the *American Journal of the Medical Sciences*, being careful to list by name the four practitioners whose lack of medical jurisprudential skills might in an earlier era or in a less sophisticated region have sent the wife to the gallows.[42]

Eight years later another Pennsylvania case illustrated neatly the continuing progress that seemed to be under way in the general field of forensic toxicology. John Earls, an illiterate laborer and fish-trapper from the remote hamlet of Muncy Creek in Lycoming County, a still-rugged area of north-central Pennsylvania, was indicted for killing his alcoholic wife Catharine shortly after the latter had delivered a child. Earls maintained impoundments for the fish he trapped and used arsenic in large quantities to try to poison the minks and otters that raided his ponds. He was accused of using some of that arsenic in hot chocolate and tea to kill his wife as she recovered from childbirth. He had probably hoped people would take the death as a case of childbed fever, but they did not. The marriage was known to be unhappy, and Earls's plans to head west with his mistress quickly came to light. Accordingly, he was taken into Williamsport, the county seat, to stand trial for first degree murder.[43]

The county coroner asked three physicians to conduct a post-mortem examination of Catharine Earls's remains. They took their assignment seriously; collaborated with the local apothecary, who provided the chemicals they needed; ran the three best tests available to them; and kept good notes from which to testify. Each of their tests proved positive for arsenic in large concentrations. Even so, they sent part of the contents of Mrs. Earls's stomach to the laboratory of the Medical Institute at Philadelphia. Physicians there spent the better part of four days testing for poisons by five different methods, all of which pointed to the presence of arsenic.

The trial lasted two weeks. The prosecutor's physicians performed professionally and effectively. When challenged on the authorities they had followed, they cited Beck, Orfila, and Christison. Even John Earls's lawyer commended the job they did, and the best he could do in rebuttal was to assert "the time has not yet arrived when the presence of [arsenic] may be certainly affirmed in a *post mortem* examination of the human stomach."[44] Maybe she died of cholera, he suggested lamely, though that disease had not been present in her community for years.

The presiding judge was fully persuaded by the expert witnesses: "The court have no doubt whatever upon [the poisoning] part of the case," he instructed the jury, "and, as it belongs to the department of medical jurisprudence, we have deemed it our duty to express the clear conviction which this evidence has produced in our minds."[45] To the physicians themselves he offered personal congratulations. "The duty of giving evidence in Courts of Justice is one of the most irksome and responsible duties which belong to the medical profession," he acknowledged, for the physicians had spent considerable time and trouble on the post-mortem, attended the trial at least intermittently for two weeks, and realized full well that a man's life almost certainly hung upon their testimony. But in this case they had brought medical science admirably to the service of justice and they were "entitled to the commendation of the community."[46]

John Earls was convicted, subsequently confessed, and was hanged in May 1836. The story of his trial was put into book form and circulated nationally, another triumph for forensic toxicology. Well-trained professionals had acted splendidly, even in a remote area; lest anyone harbor doubts, they had subjected their results to the independent assessment of the Philadelphia laboratories; Earls's confession confirmed that justice had been done. Even the one note of challenge in the case, that no single test for arsenic could be conclusive, was removed the same year Earls was hanged by the development in England of a further refinement of one of the tests the Lycoming physicians had employed. From 1836 onward the so-called Marsh test would be considered conclusive by itself, even if the other tests conducted in the Earls case were not done.[47] In short, forensic toxicology appeared to be an area in which the new interest in medical jurisprudence was paying genuine dividends for the medical profession, for the legal system, and for American society. Forensic toxicology seemed to epitomize medical jurisprudence at its best.

American medical journals probably published more articles on poisons and their detection during the second quarter of the century than on any other aspect of medical jurisprudence, and medical school courses in medical jurisprudence probably spent more time on toxicology than on any

Fig. 36.

Fig. 35.

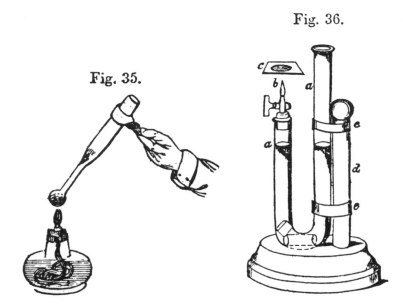

Two pieces of apparatus for determining the presence of arsenic. The U-shaped tube in Figure 36 was used in Marsh's Test. From the American edition of Christison's *Dispensatory*, edited by R. Eglesfeld Griffith (Philadelphia, 1848).

other subject.[48] Long learned articles like T.R. Beck's thirty-three-page review essay in the October 1841 issue of the *AJMS* were not at all unusual. In that piece he led his readers through recent advances in France and England that permitted the forensic detection of much more minute quantities of metallic poison than had previously been the case.[49] Hundreds of toxicological articles by scores of different authors could easily be cited.

The champions of medical jurisprudence were so fixed on the discovery and dissemination of information about forensic toxicology that T.R. Beck even used a tragic incident in his own household to test the new findings he was in the process of summarizing for the profession in 1841. A maid he employed became pregnant by a local married man, and Beck dismissed her. The maid thereupon committed suicide by taking arsenic, and Beck treated the grim business, in part at least, as an unusual opportunity to double-check against the latest work in the field exactly how long the arsenic had taken to act, precisely what the post-mortem symptoms of arsenic poisoning were in an almost controlled situation, and how known doses of arsenic dispersed in the body.[50] T.R. Beck was a legendarily sensitive and humane man, but he published the results of his autopsy in this case without apparent embarrassment. Reliable first-hand facts in the field of forensic toxicology took precedence over any personal awkwardness.

Toxicological interests also lay behind pioneer efforts to expose the adulteration of foods and drugs. Lewis C. Beck, the younger brother of T.R. and John Beck, published a volume in 1846 entitled *Adulterations of*

Various Substances Used in Medicine and the Arts, with the means of detecting them.[51] The only other study of its sort had been published in England in 1820, but that volume failed to address some of the problems that most affected consumers in the United States, especially the adulteration of milk.[52] Lewis Beck, who was then teaching chemistry and pharmacology at Albany Medical College and at Rutgers (in different terms), concentrated on the ways that physicians could determine whether the medicines they bought were up to standards, but his detailed discussion of milk and how to test for its adulteration helped touch off what became the first large-scale socio-political battle in American history over pure foods and drugs: the so-called swill-milk wars in New York City that lasted from the late 1840s through the late 1860s.[53] Surprisingly little serious literature was destined to appear in the United States on the subject of pure foods and drugs prior to the twentieth century; it is no accident that the one towering exception, Lewis Beck's 1846 volume, emerged in a decade of intense toxicological activity among the champions of medical jurisprudence.

Ongoing attention to poisons and poisoning proved in the long run to be among the most sustained results of the early surge of interest and involvement in medical jurisprudence. By the late 1850s Americans were beginning to make significant breakthroughs of their own in forensic toxicology, after years of following and refining European research. In 1856 the so-called Palmer murder trial in England raised an international stir when expert witnesses were unable to detect strychnine once it was masked by morphine. Two able young Americans who were interested in forensic toxicology, T.G. Wormley, then living in Ohio, and John J. Reese, a resident of Philadelphia, independently turned their attention to the problem. Wormley published the results of his research in 1859, and Reese, spurred on by a poison case of the same sort in Perry County, Pennsylvania, published his in 1861.[54] A toxicological problem that had baffled the great Alfred S. Taylor and his colleagues in England was thus at least partially solved by the Americans.[55] After the Civil War, when most other aspects of medical jurisprudence as it was embraced during the first half of the nineteenth century were going into eclipse, Americans still maintained a lively interest in forensic toxicology; and it was significant that most of the leading individuals who would remain active practitioners in the shrinking field of medical jurisprudence as the century wore on, including both Wormley and Reese specifically, were experts in that specialty.

Along with insanity and toxicology, issues related to sexuality and procreation constituted a third large area in which the champions of upgraded medical jurisprudence made a significant long-term difference in American life and law. Sexuality and procreation had been subjects of special interest in medical jurisprudence since classical times, and when Americans tried to revive medical jurisprudence and re-adapt it to their circumstances in the second quarter of the nineteenth century, they continued to feature those subjects in their writings and their lectures. Their approach appeared to be straightforward: enlightened science should triumph over both ancient legal precedents and entrenched folk perceptions. The way they dealt publicly with the question of rape, an issue previously alluded to in the context of medical jurisprudence inside the medical schools, illustrated their approach.

Under old English common law, rape had been extremely difficult to prove and was punished technically as a damaging of goods.[56] Both emission on the part of the attacker and resistance on the part of the woman generally had to be proved. As direct heirs of both the Scottish and the French Enlightenments, however, American physicians tended to present the crime of rape as an uncivilized act of aggression in and of itself.[57] Most of them argued strongly, for example, that penetration alone should be enough to convict; demonstration of emission should not be necessary. That opinion appeared over and over in jurisprudential writing and lecturing during the first half of the century. Nathan Smith was typical, explaining to his Yale Medical School students in 1827 that Connecticut still required proof of penetration and emission, but "penetration ought to be sufficient."[58] Stephen Williams was roundly censured by fellow physicians when he defended the old emission standard in the 1830s.[59]

American medico-legalists also attacked the English standard of demonstrable resistance by the victim in rape cases. Both the *Elements* and the Wharton/Stillé *Treatise* agreed strongly by mid-century, in the words of the *Elements*, that "fear or terror may operate on a helpless female—she may resist for a long time, and then faint from fatigue, or the dread of instant murder may lead to the abandonment of active resistance."[60] In other words, a woman could be free of violent signs on the rest of her body and still be the victim of a rape. Juries might continue in practice to look somewhat suspiciously upon women who could not demonstrate some form of resistance, but at least the formal English requirement that their bodies bear the evidence of their resistance was being steadily undermined.

American professionals remained sensitive to the dangers of false accusations of rape. In New York City in 1800 a man named Levi Weeks had been accused of a rape he did not commit. Convinced that Weeks was guilty nonetheless, a mob threatened to tear down the home of the attorney who won Weeks's acquittal on criminal charges, and in the ensuing atmosphere of popular intimidation, Weeks lost a companion suit for civil damages on essentially the same charges. That civil defeat sent Weeks to prison and cost him "a very enormous sum," before his obvious innocence could be reestablished by the discovery and release of additional evidence. Weeks's much-publicized case was cited repeatedly in medical jurisprudence textbooks through the rest of the century as an example of what could happen in these emotionally explosive matters.[61]

But on the whole, the medico-legalists of the first half of the century attacked the old English burdens of proof with the intention of allowing the crime to be more effectively prosecuted.[62] By mid-century they had clearly affected public policy. Some states, including Indiana and Tennessee, had followed Illinois by stipulating explicitly in their statutes that penetration alone would constitute the crime; other states, including Pennsylvania and

South Carolina, moved in the same direction through court decisions; while still others decided to follow T.R. Beck's 1823 suggestion to bring indictments for assault in rape cases, thereby finessing the old English standards of proof.[63]

Concerns about rape, a crime "by no means unfrequent in different parts of our country," according to Samuel Gross, also stimulated additional research on related subjects. For purposes of increasing conviction rates in those states that still required proof of emission, and for purposes of acquitting men falsely accused of rape by women who used various materials to simulate seminal stains on their undergarments, Gross introduced chemical methods of identifying dried semen in the *Western Medical Gazette* in 1834. Gross had come across the techniques in a newly revised edition of Orfila's *Lessons.*[64]

Champions of improved medical jurisprudence battled more than old English precedents, however, when they formulated and presented their views on the subject of rape, for they were forced to confront the tenacious folk perceptions that underlay those precedents. A good example was the widespread and legally accepted popular belief that conception could not take place without "a certain degree of enjoyment" on the part of the woman, and the conditions for female pleasure would be unlikely to exist unless the woman had acquiesced.[65] Physicians could finally demonstrate convincingly by the second quarter of the nineteenth century that pregnancy was not a matter of volition. Women had conceived while under the effects of narcotics and anesthetics; they could also have a pregnancy forced upon them by a rapist. All of the leading authorities in the field of medical jurisprudence were in agreement on this point by mid-century.[66] Yet the old notion did not die easily, as cases during the Civil War demonstrated, and large portions of the public continued to suspect that there was some relationship between female orgasm and conception.[67] By maintaining a constant and nearly unanimous drum-fire of testimony in rape cases to the effect that pregnancy could follow a rape, American physicians were self-consciously crusading in behalf of science and rationalism against what they considered barbaric anachronisms inappropriate to an enlightened republic.[68] Only in the late nineteenth century, however, were they able to all but eliminate that long-standing British excuse for acquittal.

Much to the dismay of the nation's leading medical jurisprudents, too many other myths, fears, and unscientific misconceptions hung on among the common people of the United States in the sensitive and psychologically freighted areas of sexuality. Robley Dunglison, for example, reminded his students in the 1820s that "a common opinion amongst the lower classes" held that intercourse with an uncontaminated female could cure gonorrhea. Rape, especially upon young women, because they were the least likely to be diseased, might be rationalized as a form of self-therapy, given that assumption.[69] Dunglison urged the nation's physicians, now that they were getting involved in the legal process, to disabuse the citizens of such irrational notions.

An excellent illustration of their ongoing efforts occurred in 1836, sixty years after the beginning of the Revolution. Thomas W. Blatchford, a prominent and aggressive New York physician, was asked by defendant's counsel in a slander suit to prepare formal written medical testimony "with reference to the understanding of an ordinary jury" on the question of whether a woman could become pregnant by a dog and bring forth pups or any other issue as the consequence of "such unnatural intercourse."[70] Like so many other members of his generation of physicians, Blatchford had found medical jurisprudence intriguing. Twenty years earlier he had chosen a medical jurisprudential subject for his dissertation, and he now agreed to prepare the testimony requested of him.[71] Abjuring "technical phraseology," he wrote a short paper explaining the impossibility of hybridization across species as distant from one another as humans and dogs. Because it was not germane to the charge of slander, however, the lawyer for the other side conceded the medical point without a fight, and Blatchford never had a chance to present his material in open court.

Neither Blatchford nor "several gentlemen of both the medical and legal professions," however, wanted the matter dropped. The latter "expressed a desire" to see Blatchford's effort at popular instruction "receive . . . a more extensive circulation" because they were convinced that "popular sentiment [was] notoriously adverse to the position" Blatchford had taken, and they wanted to counter that popular sentiment. Blatchford obtained the lawyer's permission to publish the piece separately, and the Rensselaer County Medical Society agreed to underwrite its dissemination. In the 1840s the Medical Society of the State of New York still considered the essay sufficiently worthy of public attention to have it reprinted at the state's own expense.[72]

The ongoing battle against folk beliefs was real, and more intense than many students of American history might suspect. Because they left few records of their beliefs about such matters, it is easy to overlook the fact that substantial portions of the general public harbored suspicions and fears more appropriate to a medieval peasantry than to citizens of a post-Enlightenment republic. Deliberately pitting themselves against the persistence of those folk traditions, the champions of medical jurisprudence crusaded self-consciously as the agents of applied science.

Taken together the illustrations in this chapter suggest at least tentatively a final overarching observation. During the second quarter of the nineteenth century, a key formative period in the social history of the United States, physicians were already playing an important role in the formation of what is commonly assumed to be the modern American world-view; and it was their self-conscious commitment to medical jurisprudence, even more than their role as healers, that motivated and sustained their early activities. Under the banners of logic and science they battled what they considered to be outdated attitudes, medieval precedents, folk perceptions, and irrational policies. Conflicts were most likely to surface publicly in cases at common law, which were fought out in local courtrooms all around the nation. As more and more physicians grew more and more committed to the discovery and establishment of professionally defensible resolutions to those conflicts, they became, consciously or unconsciously, among the most significant and influential shock troops in a great campaign that ultimately solidified and confirmed an American version of rationalism, rooted in logic and science. The campaign was vast, largely uncoordinated, full of ambiguities, imperfectly understood even by the participants on the front lines, and still dimly perceived a century and a half later. But it was one of the most crucially important and essentially invisible crusades ever launched in the United States.

CHAPTER SIX

Medical Jurisprudence
and the State,
1820–1850

Approximately at mid-century, professional interest in medical jurisprudence, especially among physicians, began an abrupt and surprisingly precipitous decline. Young professionals, many of whom had been intrigued by the possibilities of a career in medical jurisprudence before mid-century, either abandoned the field or stopped entering it. Medical journals, which had heralded the triumphs of medical jurisprudence during the second quarter of the nineteenth century, grew defensive during the 1850s and started to complain about the field rather than celebrate its potentials and achievements. Following four decades of proliferation and expansion in American medical schools, courses in medical jurisprudence started to contract and disappear after 1850; by the beginning of the twentieth century they were either gone altogether from most medical curricula or pushed so far to the periphery of professional training as to be little more than pathetic remnants of what once had been a central, progressive, and exciting aspect of medical and legal life in the United States. Needless to say, the reversal had profound long-term effects not only upon the history of the professions but also upon the history of the country.

The reasons for this far-reaching turn of events were complex and interrelated, but for the sake of analytical clarity they may be separated somewhat artificially and dealt with sequentially. The first factor, the subject of this chapter, was the failure to create a firm economic base for medical jurisprudence at the state level. People like T.R. Beck were able to exercise considerable personal influence over state social policy, as will become apparent, but were unable to bring into being an American version of the Continental system of state-supported legal medicine. Subsequent chapters will explore the other large factors that came together near mid-century to reverse the progress of what had been a surging and successful field for almost half a century: the mounting problems encountered by medico-legal experts in court; a socio-political backlash against the new view of insanity;

76

the impact of the nation's first malpractice crisis; and a general loss of confidence even in the key field of toxicology.

The early champions of medical jurisprudence assumed that governmental authorities would welcome and support what they were trying to accomplish. Their hope and optimism sprang from two basic sources, one theoretical and the other personal. At the theoretical level, virtually all of the young professionals who entered the field during the first quarter of the nineteenth century believed that their efforts were perfectly consistent with the goals of the republic. Hence it followed that the state should sustain them; theirs was a public service.[1]

On a personal level, the early champions of medical jurisprudence constituted something of a professional elite. Many of them either came from or married into powerful, well-established, and influential families; others quickly developed strong political and social ties on the basis of their professional credentials. Educated physicians interacted routinely with educated attorneys in a host of settings, both casual and formal. Doctors and lawyers, in turn, regularly moved in and out of governmental and quasi-governmental positions.[2] The United States remained a rough-and-tumble, overwhelmingly agrarian, emerging nation through the first quarter of the nineteenth century, and professionals capable of operating effectively at the interface of law and medicine were in a position to command attention, much as in developing nations today. And it is worth remembering that social policy in the new republic was made overwhelmingly at the state level, rather than the national level. At the state level, where prominent professionals often knew one another personally, men who would probably have occupied secondary provincial positions in Europe could often exercise tremendous primary power in the United States. Indeed, the personal position of the early champions of medical jurisprudence, rather than the theoretical ties between their new professional field and the role of the republican state, produced the first and most lasting links between medical jurisprudence and American government. Those links were epitomized in the process known as code revision.

The situation in New York illustrated these early developments in a paradigmatic and significant fashion: paradigmatic because what happened in New York was repeated over and over again with local variations in most of the other states, and significant because policies and principles adopted in powerful New York were invariably taken seriously and often copied directly by other states through the rest of the nineteenth century. Like each of the other states after the American Revolution, New York wrestled at length with the problem of adapting English common law to the ideologies and actual conditions of a democratic republic. Some of the problems involved grand theory and great amounts of economic power. To what extent, for example, should property rights that evolved from centuries of feudal privilege be modified to meet the needs of an aggressively entrepreneurial and fiercely individualistic society? Other problems were far more

practical. Exactly which of the old English and old colonial regulations were
still in effect and which were not? Even lawyers found it impossible to
obtain a complete and accurate compendium of the statutes and rules that
were supposed to obtain in a given jurisdiction.[3]

Early efforts to define New York's criminal and procedural policies had
been made in 1786 and 1788, but those efforts caused as much confusion
as clarification during the next two decades.[4] The situation remained so
tangled through 1821 that delegates to the New York state constitutional
convention that year felt compelled to try once again to clarify the status of
the state's laws in the document they were drafting. As a result, the new
constitution formally "abrogated" all parts of the colonial common and statute law that were "repugnant" to the republican principles it was trying to
establish.[5] But no one quite knew what that meant in actual practice, so
even the ratification of the new constitution failed to resolve the problems.
In 1824, pressed by the public in general and by the legal profession in
particular, state lawmakers decided that they could no longer limp along
with such an ill-defined understanding of what policies were actually in
effect in New York. Continued confusion threatened the orderly development of the state and ultimately the rule of law itself.

The legislature of 1824 created a three-man committee to prepare a
compilation of the state's laws and gave the committee authority to "alter
the phraseology" of statutes, especially old ones, that seemed to conflict
with the fundamental principles of the new constitution. In 1825, T. R.
Beck's close friend DeWitt Clinton became governor and urged the legislature to go even further. Because "our jurisprudence requires revisal, arrangement, and correction," Governor Clinton argued in his annual message to the General Assembly, genuine codification and changes of real
substance ought to be considered. The committee should be allowed to
draft a "code founded on the salutary principles of the common law, adopted
to the interests of commerce and the useful arts, the state of society and the
nature of our government, and embracing those improvements which are
enjoined by enlightened experience." Among the reasons Clinton advanced
for favoring compilation and revision was the need to "elevate a liberal and
honorable profession," by which he presumably meant lawyers, whose responses to the prevailing uncertainties seemed more and more technical and
confusing in the eyes of ordinary citizens. In 1826 the legislature agreed
with the governor and granted the committee "powers to redesign, refor-
mulate, and redevelop the whole body of New York statute law." This was
a mandate, in the words of one legal historian, "totally without precedent
in Anglo-American legal history."[6]

According to their own report, the committee members believed themselves in a position to pick and choose from old English, old colonial, and
modern republican statutes; to arrange and rearrange laws into headings
and categories; to eliminate contradictions; even, and most important, to
recommend the inclusion of new material. New policies would have to be
consistent with the state's recently ratified constitution, consistent with the

governor's sense of "enlightened experience," and ultimately consistent with what the legislature was willing to enact, since the legislature reserved to itself the right to alter or reject the committee's final product. Nonetheless, the process offered an unusual opportunity for thoroughgoing structural reform of the state's fundamental legal policies. Ideas would not have to be embodied in separate bills and fought piecemeal through the tedious legislative process. They could be included in a coherent package, where they might be deemed essential to the whole, where the burden would be on removing them rather than including them, and where they might be presented as minor, logically acceptable propositions. Although the codification process was defended in populistic phrases, the revisers and those people in a position to influence them, including the governor himself, who believed that the emerging professions should play an influential role in deciding what the state's citizens should be allowed to do and not do, could hardly have designed a better vehicle for themselves than the process of code revision on this model.

In 1824 the legislature had asked Erastus Root, Benjamin Butler, and James Kent to serve on the committee of revision. The first two, both of whom were politically prominent attorneys, accepted the invitation. Chancellor Kent, the jurist who had written Beck to thank him for the *Elements*, the man regarded as the state's leading legal scholar, and the person the legislature probably counted upon to direct the committee's efforts, declined. John Duer, one of the state's best private lawyers, took Kent's place, then sided with Butler in support of Governor Clinton's successful efforts in 1825 and 1826 to widen the committee's charge. Root, who had favored compilation and order but seemed uncomfortable with the possibility of thoroughgoing revision, accepted a pension arrangement and stepped aside. His place was taken by United States Supreme Court reporter Henry Wheaton, who served for about a year. When Wheaton resigned from the committee for personal reasons, John C. Spencer, an able young attorney from New York City, joined Duer and Butler. During 1826 and 1827, those three produced the draft version of a new state code.[7]

Though last to join the committee, thirty-nine-year-old John Canfield Spencer quickly became its driving force and did most of the actual work. Indeed, Spencer might reasonably have been listed as the author-editor of what became the *New York Revised Statutes of 1829*, with a note that he was aided in minor ways by the other two members of the committee. The legislature itself later acknowledged as much publicly.[8]

Spencer's background and career in law paralleled T. R. Beck's background and career in medicine to a remarkable degree. Just three years older than Beck, John Spencer had also been born into a prominent family in the Albany area. John's father, Ambrose Spencer, had gone first to Yale before graduating with honors from Harvard. When John was born, Ambrose Spencer was practicing law in Hudson, New York, where he also served as a local judge. Ambrose entered regional politics during the 1790s, and by the beginning of the nineteenth century had become one of the most powerful political chieftains in the state. Though he espoused the Federalist party during George Washington's presidency, Ambrose went over to the Democratic Republicans in 1798. Like the Beck family, the Spencers were thereafter very close to the Clintons; Ambrose's second and third wives were both sisters of Governor Clinton.[9]

John Spencer graduated from Union College in 1806, one class ahead of T. R. Beck, whom he almost certainly must have known as a fellow undergraduate, fellow townsman, and fellow young friend of DeWitt Clinton. Like Beck, who seized the opportunity that would launch him to the top of his profession by accepting a job at the Western District Medical College, John Spencer also moved to the booming western part of the state to build his early career. There, aided by the political connections of his influential father, John became district attorney for Western New York by 1815, and was elected to Congress as a Clintonian the following year, though he was only twenty-eight years old. An unsuccessful bid for the United States Senate removed him temporarily from national affairs (he would return in later life to Washington, first as Secretary of War and then as Secretary of the Treasury under President John Tyler), but he remained active at the state level. Spencer served three years in the assembly (1820–22) and four in the state senate (1825–28). His friend and step-uncle, Governor Clinton, plucked him from the latter body to take charge of the revision committee. Spencer would later return to the floor of the state senate to direct discussion, carpenter amendments, and ensure passage of his committee's efforts.

Spencer was an extremely hard-working man, with a near legendary grasp of detail. Like Beck, he also had a knack for synthesis and organization; the same ability to draw together, to codify, and subtly to modify that Beck had so magisterially demonstrated in the *Elements* five years before Spencer began his own quite similar great work in the law. John's father, moreover, who had sat for two decades on the New York Supreme Court, was also well known for his efforts to construct what might be called an American common law on the basis of state court rulings; he often overrode English precedents in favor of what seemed to him to be commonsensical decisions appropriate to the circumstances of the new republic. John was prepared to carry on in that tradition, and he was in a splendid position to do so.[10]

As he worked his way through New York's basic legal policies, Spencer turned to T.R. Beck for advice and counsel on medically related subjects. None of Spencer's fellow revisers was expert in matters medical; Beck was, and had an international reputation to prove it. Beck was also one of Albany's leading citizens by the middle of the 1820s, a man with almost unlimited social entree and enormous personal prestige.[11] Beck's correspondence during the 1820s included confidential letters of trust on professional and political matters from local and national powerbrokers.[12] Even as the code revisions were pending in Albany, for example, Edward Livingston, a nationally prominent advocate of legal codification who would soon become secretary of state under President Andrew Jackson, wrote to Beck about the growing importance of the "mutual connection" between "law and physic."[13] Finally, Beck was elected president of the New York State Medical Society in 1827, even as Spencer was drafting the revised code.

Though most of their business was almost certainly conducted face-to-face, at least one piece of direct evidence of their close collaboration survived among the Beck Papers now housed at the New York Public Library: a brief letter written in a singular, almost illegible script, which was probably saved for its distinctive signature, because the Beck brothers collected autographs. Addressed to T. Romeyn Beck, it read in full as follows:

Albany, Sept. 11, 1828

I have prepared various Sections against medical malpractice according to your Suggestions, particularly the improper use of instruments, capital operations in Surgery, selling poisons &c. which when examined by Mr. Butler I will have edited and sent to you. In the mean while I want you to prepare the public and particularly the Legislature, by communications in the different newspapers, by extracts from approved writers on such subjects, and by such other means as occur to you, for a favorable examination and discussion upon our provisions. I have neither the time nor ability to do it.

Yours very respectfully,
J. C. Spencer

Leaving aside for a moment the intriguing and unusually early use of the word malpractice, a subject that will be addressed later, the letter makes clear the fact that Beck was given a reasonably free hand to try to insinuate into the proposed code any medically related provisions he wanted. Spencer was obviously deferring to Beck's prior suggestions on subjects about which Spencer personally knew little or nothing, provided Beck took responsibility for persuading the members of the legislature to enact them. As it happens, in this instance, the legislature did eventually balk at some of the restrictions Beck tried to impose on the practice of major surgery, which he quite rightly considered extremely dangerous in the early nineteenth century, and some of those restrictions were removed.[14] But scores of other Beck-inspired provisions scattered in various sections throughout the revised code survived intact to become parts of New York's basic body of social legislation and were widely copied in other states. These included sections that defined rape as penetration (whether ejaculation took place or not), made the administration of poisons a statute offense, proscribed the "poisoning" of food and water, and made abortion after quickening a crime in New York.[15] Most important in the long run, however, was not which specific provisions survived in New York in 1829 and which failed, but rather the nature of the process itself, which Spencer's note to Beck revealed like the tip of an iceberg.

Working together on the New York Revised Code of 1829, Beck and Spencer epitomized one of the most profoundly influential forces operating to shape American society during the formative decades of the nineteenth century: the developing professions, especially medicine and law. As the separate states remolded the British polices they had inherited into a Socio-legal culture of their own, professionals were interested simultaneously in contributing their expertise to the development of an idealistic republican social order and in defining social arrangements, especially crimes and punishments, that would ensure them continued influence in the future. They saw these two goals as logically interrelated, good not only for themselves but also for the United States.

Sometimes the two perspectives of law and medicine were embodied in a single person, like Thomas Cooper in South Carolina, who was discussed earlier, or William Kilty in Maryland, a former physician who had executed for his state at the end of the eighteenth century some of the earliest and most effective revisions made anywhere in the United States on one of the early medical jurisprudents' favorite group of subjects: the rules relating to testaments, executors, and guardianships.[16] From the 1820s, however, the pattern of policy-making that largely determined at the state level what the underlying legal foundations for subsequent institutional development and personal behavior would actually be in the United States usually resembled the paradigm so neatly illustrated in New York by the collaboration between Spencer and Beck: a committee of legal professionals rendered the official revisions, while taking advice from influential medical professionals upon whom they relied heavily.

In some states the process did not involve full-scale code revision, but took the form of drafting omnibus bills about crimes and punishments or compiling territorial policies in preparation for statehood. Local and regional circumstances varied substantially and certainly affected policies. But the basic patterns of professional influence and policy-making were similar across the several states, which helps explain both the mosaic nature of nineteenth-century American social policy and the large degree of consistency among the mosaic's separate tiles. Moreover, patterns of policy-making established under those circumstances often persisted to the end of the century and beyond.

Codification has generally been depicted as a vaguely Jacksonian, vaguely utopian public reform movement that reached its high-water mark between 1820 and 1850, but ultimately failed in its efforts to bring coherence, system, and simplicity to American law. That characterization is not unreasonable, if codification is considered primarily in the context of its grand Benthamite origins.[17] Less closely studied has been the apparently more prosaic, but ultimately more successful and crucially important process of code revision, particularly during the second quarter of the nineteenth century, when the emerging field of medical jurisprudence also reached its high-water mark. The process of code revision became a professionals' policy vehicle par excellence during that key formative period, and the revised codes of the several states themselves, which suddenly become anything but dull in this context, may be read as quintessential statements of what doctors and lawyers wanted American social policy to be. Surprisingly little work has been done on the role of the professions in shaping American social policy, much less on why the professions chose the policies they did. When more work is done, the revised codes will play a strong documentary role.[18]

As the collaboration in New York also illustrated, the influence of the early champions of medical jurisprudence was essentially personal, as distinguished from institutional or structural or corporate. People like Beck in New York, and scores of others similarly situated in other states, could influence policy because they could claim unusual levels of expertise in areas where few Americans could claim any knowledge at all, and because they often knew personally their legal counterparts at the state level in what remained, at least through the Civil War and at least at the top, a highly personalistic society. That, however, was quite different from the formal support and institutional underpinning for medical jurisprudence they hoped eventually to gain from the state, along lines that might combine republican principles with modified Continental structures.

The early champions of medical jurisprudence had established a modest and at least temporary base in the nation's developing medical schools, where students enrolled in medical jurisprudence courses in sufficient numbers to spread the field throughout the country and increase the number of professorships devoted in whole or in part to medical jurisprudence. They found support as well in a somewhat vague, but high-minded sense of the roles appropriate to practicing professionals in a republic, and, presumably, in contemplating the rewards commensurate with those roles. But they hoped ultimately for structural changes that would sustain further development of their field and give them a secure economic foundation. To effect those structural changes they had from the beginning of the century looked to the state.

In 1823 Beck had summarized the arguments for state support in his introduction to the *Elements*, where he stressed both the long heritage of governmental support for medical jurisprudence on the European continent and the negative consequences of the lack of governmental support in the English tradition.[19] Those themes went back to Stringham and Rush and appeared in the writings and lectures of virtually every one of the early champions of medical jurisprudence. In a passage typical of dozens of similar statements penned by the others, Griffith characterized medical jurisprudence in 1825 as a field "peculiarly calculated to control the disorders of the social system, to rescue innocence from infamy and death, and to lead to the detection and punishment of crime," all of which should be governmental functions in the new democratic republic. Griffith looked forward to the time when medical jurisprudence would be "publicly recognized, and its assistance legally required."[20]

Because the field seemed to be advancing so rapidly among the nation's leading physicians, Griffith and others were buoyantly, if somewhat naively, confident that swelling popular support and appropriate legal changes were close at hand. In 1826 the *NYMPJ*, which the Beck brothers and their friends dominated, called first for special medico-legal schools on the French model, then for official designation of "a set of men . . . particularly educated as examiners in medical cases—and, of course, as witnesses." The latter could "enlighten the bench" in court cases.[21] John B. Beck likewise urged his students in New York City during the late 1820s to call upon the state for "patronage and superintendence."[22]

In his widely circulated 1828 presidential address to the New York Medical Society, Beck made explicit what he and many of his contemporaries ultimately wanted: an American version of the French system they so admired. State-supported medical jurisprudence, Beck maintained, had "led to the diminution of crimes" and aided "the distribution of equal justice" in Europe. Though he acknowledged German and Austrian precedents, Beck stressed the attractiveness of the French structure, which he traced back to Henri IV. Like the French, Americans should designate "medical men in a county, a district, or a part of the state, who shall be specially charged" as medico-legal officers for their areas. Those individuals would perform both forensic and public health duties for their areas; prepare and publish formal reports, in the fashion of the *Conseil de salubrité de Paris;* and "also appear in a judicial capacity" in court, thus assuring society a high and consistent level of medical expertise and relieving ordinary practitioners from the burdens of doing so. Such a system, in Beck's view, would "lead to the more accurate study of the science [of medical jurisprudence]. . . . afford numerous and favorable opportunities of improving it. . . . [and] in a great degree, prevent that disputation of facts, which produces so many unpleasant collisions in courts of justice." Assuming these medico-legal professionals were paid by the state, such a system would also, of course, undergird the entire field of medical jurisprudence in the United States with a network of secure posts, because "the incumbent, if assigned to a sufficiently large district," would be a full-time public health officer.[23] Though they would never achieve it, the champions of medical jurisprudence would continue to press for such a system over the next half-century.

Beck must have been optimistic in 1828 about the long-term prospects of state support for medical jurisprudence. Only a year before, the New York legislature had conferred real power upon the state medical society, which Beck now presided over as president, by allowing the society to certify physicians and by declaring the unauthorized practice of medicine a misdemeanor. That law was considered a great victory for the state's so-called regular physicians, those associated with the better medical schools and those committed to scientific research as the best method of advancing medical care in America.[24] Beck and his fellow medical society members viewed the 1827 law as an improvement even over New York's so-called Anti-Quack Act of 1819, and they no doubt felt that the legislative tide was running in their direction.[25]

But the rapid deployment of a small army of state-supported medico-legal and public health experts would be such a major and massive undertaking, especially in a society still so consistently and almost reflexively suspicious of governmental encroachments, that Beck decided in 1828 that "the time ha[d] not yet arrived for such an arrangement" in its entirety.[26] The system would have to be developed in stages. Consequently, as a first stage, Beck turned his attention to the short-term objective of forcing medico-legal expertise upon the most likely set of officers the state already had in place: coroners.

New York, like the other American states, had inherited the office of coroner from the British colonial system. The office had been introduced formally throughout England late in the twelfth century as part of the legal reforms associated with the reign of Henry II. The Latin title of this officer, *custodes placitorum coronae*, revealed nicely what the king had in mind: an agent on the local scene who would look out for the crown's interests, especially in criminal matters. Because the king could confiscate animals and objects that caused accidental deaths, and because the king could lay claim to various sorts of theoretically forfeited goods in cases of accident and wreck, his agent was instructed to hold inquests on the bodies of persons who died "suddenly, accidentally, or by foul play," in addition to his other duties.[27] To assist him, the coroner had fairly strong powers of attachment (subpoena), and he was expected to use them to summon juries to examine and record evidence while the evidence was still fresh. The coroner could not render verdicts himself, but his so-called rolls, the records he made of his evidence, were given heavy weight in subsequent proceedings, especially in the king's own courts.[28]

The investigatory nature of the coroner's job often prompted him to act as an unofficial medical examiner, and thereby on occasion to perform duties administratively akin to those assigned state physicians on the Continent.[29] Some analysts believe this may be why the British government never felt the need to establish formal medical officers in the manner of the other chief European powers, despite urgings to do so.[30] But coroners were most unlikely to be physicians and the quality of what went on under coroners' auspices was legendarily suspect.[31]

The coroner had always been a political officer, not a medical officer, and his chief duty was substantiation of the king's interests, as distinguished from the determination of truth, the preservation of public health, or the assurance of justice. The coroner could order and supervise various sorts of medical examinations, including post-mortem examinations, but he was not required to undertake them and did not actually perform them himself. Instead, he used his powers of subpoena to force local physicians to perform autopsies, run chemical tests, or whatever else he, the coroner, thought appropriate, again as distinguished from what the impressed physicians might have considered important. In England this awkward situation had produced centuries of tension between coroners and local physicians.[32]

When the American states broke from the British empire, they retained the office of coroner, though the very name was odd in the new republic. In Beck's New York, for example, the constitution of 1777 gave the newly created Council of Appointment, which consisted of the governor and four state senators, the right to name coroners all around the state.[33] While those officers might in theory have looked out at the local level for the legitimate interests of the new state government, just as their predecessors were supposed to have looked out at the local level for the interests of the crown, coroners in fact became little more than local political agents of whatever party controlled the Council in Albany. The office of coroner thus became a highly partisan patronage post, and citizens often joked that the average American coroner had never seen a dead body. By 1820, the state of New York had 630 coroners, at least on paper, all appointed by the ruling party in Albany for annual terms.[34]

When New York revised its constitution in 1821, the Council of Appointment was eliminated, but the office of coroner was not. Each county would henceforth elect its own coroners, up to four of them per county, if the legislature permitted the county that many. The coroner now served a three-year term and could not succeed himself.[35] The fact that he could not succeed himself suggested that the framers of the constitution of 1821 continued to view the coroner not as an elected expert for whom a long tenure would be desirable, but as a politician for whom rotation in office would be salutary. And the framers proved correct, for the essentially political character of the office persisted. Even in New York City, a center of medical education and medical activity, no one with medical training of any sort served as coroner until 1841.[36] In Boston, notwithstanding the considerable influence of medical leaders there, no physician was appointed coroner until 1853.[37] Nor were political coroners unique to New York or Massachusetts.[38]

This, then, was the situation that Beck confronted in 1828. Coroners themselves were certainly not medical officers, and it seemed unlikely that they would very quickly be transformed into medical officers. But they held constitutionally mandated offices, they were charged with overseeing a number of medically related functions, and they were organized in a fashion strikingly similar to the network of public medical officers that Griffith, Beck, and others hoped someday to persuade each of the states to implement. What was needed as a first step was leverage both to force coroners to avail themselves of the medical jurisprudential expertise that already existed and to force physicians to render that expertise when called upon. The former would push the office of coroner closer to that of a regional medical officer with legal duties; the latter would enhance the importance of medical jurisprudence within the medical profession. And by no accident, the pending New York code revisions, in two directives clearly marked "new" by the revisers, made it explicitly "the duty of the coroner to cause some surgeon or physician to be subpoenaed" whenever the coroner conducted an inquest involving death or severe wounds, and made any witnesses called, including physicians, subject to punishment if they did not answer their summons.[39] Those sections carried without comment in the legislature and became part of New York's basic law after 1829.[40]

Even as this first step toward state support for medical jurisprudence was taken, however, the political climate in New York and elsewhere around the nation began to shift dramatically. An era of reasonably friendly relations and close ties among doctors, lawyers, and the state came to an abrupt end about 1830, as ordinary lay people began to fear what they perceived to be growing concentrations of power in what was supposed to be an egalitarian republic. Historians have long recognized this peak of anti-monopolistic suspicion, alternately celebrating it as an appropriate expression of populistic democracy (and more recently as an era of emerging class-consciousness) or condemning it as a reactionary burst of anti-modern, counter-productive anti-intellectualism. The idea of a great socio-political watershed in the 1830s is also consistent with the theory that the American polity shifted in some profound fashion during that period from one primarily driven by concepts of classical republicanism to one increasingly informed by what might be called democratic liberalism and entrepreneurial capitalism, the world of the modern marketplace. Indeed, if the presidential election of 1828 is taken as the first, or most symbolic, manifestation of the new American paradigm, as many distinguished historians have done, the timing for the history of medical jurisprudence in Beck's New York is almost too strikingly coincidental to be believed. This is not the place to resolve the huge analytical problems that surround this epochal transition, but regardless of how they are characterized, the political sentiments of the new polity helped fuel a virulent anti-professionalism that quite quickly and unexpectedly put the best-educated, best-organized and most scientifically oriented physicians, including virtually all of the serious advocates of medical jurisprudence, on the defensive.

Health care in the United States from the founding of the republic through the 1830s had been and continued to be an amorphous, overlapping, often ad hoc, and extremely uneven business. Americans could choose among many sorts of healers and frequently employed several of them either simultaneously or sequentially. Many citizens simply cared for themselves and their friends, either instinctually or from home medical manuals; neighbors provided long-term nursing and health advice; midwives presided at births and deaths; herbalists continued medieval traditions; itinerant folk prescribers wandered from village to village dispensing what they claimed to be Native American and African lore.[41] Somewhat more systematic healers of several sorts, including Hydropaths (the "water-cure" doctors), Botanics, Thomsonians, and Eclectics also practiced widely among the general population. Homoeopaths, who had their own sectarian colleges, tended to have well-established practices among well-to-do Americans. All of the foregoing, known collectively as "irregulars," coexisted uneasily with the formally educated and scientifically oriented "regulars," who dominated most medical schools, controlled most formal medical societies, and considered themselves at the top of the profession.[42] Even among the latter, however, a wide range of theory and therapy still prevailed.

Irregular healers of all sorts took full advantage of the anti-monopoly sentiment of the period to protect their position in the emerging market. And the general public, for perfectly good reasons, supported the irregulars' desire to remain fully viable medical alternatives, since in actual practice the regulars could not demonstrate more effective results than the irregulars. Indeed, the reverse may sometimes have been the case, depending upon the ailment. The herbal tea administered by a Botanic, for example, may not have done the patient much good by modern standards, but it probably did not do much harm either. The powerful purgatives favored by the regulars, in contrast, did not do the patient much good either, but could have by modern standards some frighteningly undesirable side effects. Though the regulars' commitment to scientific medicine would eventually benefit both themselves and their society, those benefits were far from obvious in the great professional turmoil of the 1830s.

By the early 1840s, between 30,000 and 40,000 people in New York alone were said to have signed petitions opposing any form of exclusive control over the practice of medicine in the state; between 15,000 and 17,000 people were said to have done the same in neighboring Connecticut.[43] While they disagreed with one another fiercely, the irregulars and their allies all concurred that no single organization, especially the New York Medical Society, which the irregulars collectively hated and resented, should have an exclusive, government-sanctioned say over the practice of medicine in the state. These were the same years President Andrew Jackson was waging political and ideological war on the "monster" Bank of the United States, and the parallels were striking: many of the state and local bankers who backed the president hated each other, but none of them wanted a government-sanctioned national bank controlling their business.

In the face of such confusing claims and counter-claims, and operating in the anti-monopoly atmosphere of the period, the New York legislature gutted the Medical Society regulations of 1827 in 1830, temporarily reinstated them later in the mid-1830s, then destroyed them once and for all at the end of the decade.[44] As a result, New York, which seemed in 1828 to be well on the road toward consolidation of its medical regulations under the leadership of the regulars-dominated State Medical Society, instead emerged from the decade of the 1830s with what contemporaries aptly labeled a free trade in medicine. Anyone who wished to could still try to make a living as a healer. Nor was New York alone. In fact, most other states never even enacted the sort of regulations that New York revoked during the 1830s. In 1841 Massachusetts reaffirmed the legal right of "any person" to collect charges for performing medical services "good or bad."[45] In 1842 legislators in Michigan passed an act formally granting Thomsonians the same rights as regular doctors, and Alabama legislators did substantially the same thing in 1843.[46] In Pennsylvania, where lawyers gained the right to sue their clients for unpaid fees, regular doctors lost it.[47] The New

York legislature reaffirmed its earlier position in 1844, explicitly authorizing anyone to "prescribe for or administer medicine or specifics, to or for the sick."[48] In 1845 Mississippi courts declared the state's local medical boards unconstitutional and made explicit the fact that all citizens could "practice physic or prescribe medicine in any way that may suit their convenience."[49] That same year the South Carolina legislature repealed an old exclusion law, thereby opening the medical profession to anyone who wished to practice.[50]

In the United States as a whole by mid-century, medicine had become an overtly unregulated, unlicensed, overcrowded, doctrinally incoherent, and fiercely competitive profession.[51] A navy physician who had experienced medical practice in many parts of the country summarized the situation as he saw it in 1849:

> It is well known, that all efforts to limit the exercise of the profession of medicine to those who have the abilities and acquirements essential to its proper understanding, have utterly failed; and ignorant and impudent pretenders, under a great variety of humbugging titles, come before the public with equal rights, and a better chance for popular favor, than the regular practitioner. The public, unfortunately, seems to consider all efforts to limit the practice of medicine to those of scientific attainments, as the attempt of a sect to monopolize rights, and to infringe upon the largest liberty. Under this latitudinarian license, we have Indian doctors, urine doctors, root doctors, water doctors, steam doctors, and homoeopaths, preying upon the community; and each has his representative [in judicial processes].[52]

Rush and Beck had dreamed of a society guided by the cooperative interaction of scientific physicians, broad-minded attorneys, and the people's representatives working through the state. Four decades into the nineteenth century that dream began to look increasingly unrealistic, even un-American. In the new America it would not only be every profession for itself, but every professional.

Needless to say, the regular champions of medical jurisprudence made no more progress toward their goal of state support during that tumultuous era, even though the field was attracting the serious attention of many of the profession's most able talents and was making unprecedented progress on a number of research fronts. In New York state the law governing coroners' inquests remained unchanged from 1828 through 1847; the only change in the revised code of 1848 allowed coroners to conduct inquiries with smaller juries than Beck and Spencer had thought appropriate.[53] While coroners were still supposed to summon physicians in most cases, the state had no way to force them to do so and no desire to get into the awkward position of constantly second-guessing the judgment of its own officers whenever coroners decided full-scale inquiries were unnecessary. As Beck himself was forced to admit in the 1838 revision of the *Elements*, ten years after he and Spencer had altered the state code to try to require medical investigations,

"It cannot be denied, that a full and satisfactory medico-legal examination is avoided as often as public sentiment will permit; and even when judicially ordered, its proper objects are often thwarted, or not fully accomplished."[54]

Even more disastrous from the point of view of those who had looked to the state to underwrite medical jurisprudence was the issue of compensation for the public medico-legal examinations that were conducted. In 1828, Beck had called for "adequate compensation" for physicians pressed into service in behalf of the government, and he expected payment to be forthcoming.[55] But the New York code had not formally stipulated any special professional pay when it mandated coroners to subpoena the services of physicians, presumably to avoid the appearance of offering a financial incentive on the government's side when prosecuting its own citizens. In the absence of formal provision, however, most coroners, especially during the anti-professional 1830s, were refusing to pay physicians more than the slender travel expenses allowed any other subpoenaed witness, even though the physicians were called upon to perform duties rather than relate what they knew or what they were a direct party to or what they had seen. By 1835, Beck himself was clearly worried.

> . . . no compensation is allowed to the surgeon for the dissection, nor to the chemist for his analysis, while he incurs at the same time the responsibility of deciding on the guilt or innocence of the accused. Certainly, no plan could be suggested more effectually to deter all and every medical man from engaging in these thankless investigations.[56]

And he now had little hope of legislative remedy, given the dramatically altered political atmosphere. With good reason, he was increasingly afraid that suggestions "will pass unheeded by those to whom [they are] principally addressed. I refer to our lawgivers, with whom alone it remains to give a new and proper impulse to the science of medical jurisprudence, and to make that infinitely more available to the ends of justice and the prevention of crime than it has ever yet been in this country."[57] That perception proved accurate. The New York legislature of 1840 sustained the principle of paying modest travel expenses and a small daily allowance to witnesses subpoenaed for various court proceedings, but made no provision to pay physicians more than ordinary witnesses and forbade fees altogether to government witnesses in criminal cases, presumably to continue to avoid the appearance of conflicts of interest.[58] By 1842 Beck was reduced to wondering whether the state might hold physicians liable if they decided to protest by withholding their services until they were adequately compensated.[59]

The problem for many prominent New York physicians went well beyond occasional annoyance. James Webster of Geneva Medical College complained bitterly about "the constant liability of physicians to be called upon as witnesses in court . . . at their own personal expense, with the loss of time and business." He told his students about the time in 1846 when he was summoned from Rochester to Cayuga County, "compelled to go under the auspices of the Sheriff," even though Webster was "in feeble health" at the time, and testify in two cases he knew nothing about. He calculated his "forced sacrifice" at "nearly one hundred dollars, a sum which I was not able to afford." Zealous Cayuga authorities had also summoned physicians from New York City, Albany, Utica, Auburn, and Geneva for those same cases. During 1849 Webster "was compelled to break in upon my course at great inconvenience, and leave in company with the Sheriff of Wyoming county, as medical witness in the trial of Shadbolt for murder."[60] Webster hoped the legislature would do something about the situation, but despite active lobbying from T.R. Beck and others, the legislature did not. In a published series of lectures on medical jurisprudence in the *New York Medical Press* in 1859, Judge H. John Anthon reminded the state's physicians that "your attendance is compelled by subpoena, and here no fees are allowed for your attendance, save the compensation of fifty cents per day fixed for other witnesses."[61]

In Pennsylvania, notwithstanding the power of the medical profession in Philadelphia, the situation was not much better. The prominent physician Washington L. Atlee had to sue Lancaster County in 1844 to try to establish the principle that he should be paid a fair professional fee for conducting medical examinations at the behest of the county authorities.[62] George Watt, another physician, had to do the same thing in Pittsburgh a few years later. Watt's case against Allegheny County went to the Supreme Court of Western Pennsylvania, where Chief Justice Gibson allowed Watt's fee of fifteen dollars to conduct a post-mortem examination he had been ordered to do for free by the county coroner.[63]

But even in Pennsylvania, much less in the rest of the nation, that sort of ad hoc proceeding was small practical solace for ordinary practitioners, who had neither the time nor the resources to make symbolic court challenges every time the local coroner wanted to lean on them for an official opinion with little or no compensation. Only widespread changes in state law would help the vast majority of physicians, as members of the New York State Medical Society argued before the state legislature in Albany in 1850.[64] But neither New York nor the vast majority of the other states altered their systems. In the eyes of many prominent professionals, American state governments collectively had created by mid-century a system that could impress medico-legal skills but did not reward or support them. Not only were the advances in medical jurisprudence not being underwritten, there had evolved a disincentive to participate on the government's side in medico-legal proceedings.

Protests quite literally from Boston to New Orleans went largely unheeded by state and local governments at mid-century.[65] The Illinois State Medical Society even put into its constitution and code of ethics in 1850 its strong belief "that the public should award [physicians] a proper honorarium" whenever "legally constituted authorities" called upon the latter "to enlighten" them about "the science of medical jurisprudence"; but nothing happened.[66] In 1851, four years before he died, a deeply disappointed Beck joined the chorus: "It is quite time that the medical profession in this country should rouse itself to a demand of its just rights" in these situations.[67] But the only states that responded by 1860 were Virginia, where, significantly, code revisers inserted a "reasonable compensation" clause into the section requiring coroners to call upon physicians to "render services incident to [their] profession"; and Georgia, where the legislature actually stated specific sums for specific duties ($20 for a dissection prior to interment. $50 and expenses for chemical analyses, and so forth).[68]

Elsewhere the problem continued to fester. Most physicians on the eve of the Civil War almost certainly shared the frustrations outlined in an angry letter to the *New York Medical Press* in 1860. "We call for legislation upon this matter. Make it legal for the judge alone to call for 'experts'; and if, in his judgment, they are necessary, let him be empowered to pay them from ten to a hundred dollars per day."[69] In the correspondent's home district, expert fees were restricted to one dollar per day. Government compensation of medico-legal expertise would remain a serious problem through the rest of the century, and would eventually provoke a series of ugly crises after the Civil War. In the meantime, the last thing many struggling physicians wanted was a reputation as a good medico-legal examiner. Local coroners would constantly be impressing their skills, while the real source of their livelihoods, their everyday practices, suffered first from the time, travel, and attention lost to the investigation and to the coroner's inquest; then from the time, travel, and attention lost to any ensuing court proceedings; not to mention what might subsequently happen to their reputations in the course of those proceedings.

By mid-century, in short, the champions of stronger medical jurisprudence had to face the fact that state support would not soon be forthcoming. In economic terms, the client they had sought and thought they deserved, the state, was not prepared to pay for their services. Notwithstanding the considerable influence they managed to exert personally on nineteenth-century social policies, largely through the code revision process, the champions of medical jurisprudence were unable to win from their governments, particularly in the anti-professional climate of the 1830s and 1840s, the state-supported economic base they had hoped to obtain. Indeed, they not only failed to create a modified French system of medico-legal officers, they even failed to adjust the existing coroner system to their own advantage. They did not suddenly despair of winning state support in the future, and they would fight on into the 1880s with a host of proposals and suggestions. But fundamental socio-legal patterns, as it turned out, were beginning to harden.

Alternative sources of support were at least in theory still available to the champions of active medical jurisprudence. They could earn fees in private civil actions, for example, and also in separately compensated efforts to help defendants. But in those situations they served individual clients, as distinguished from the public good, and they faced, as will become apparent in the next chapter, a separate set of debilitating professional problems. They also still retained at mid-century the network of professorships that had been established in American medical schools. Yet these too would be eroded after mid-century, once the demand for their subject matter began to plummet among the students, who understandably enough favored those subjects that promised income and professional advancement, such as therapeutics and surgery, over those subjects with little economic promise and plenty of professional problems, like medical jurisprudence.

Under such circumstances, medical jurisprudence no longer looked like the promising field it had once appeared to be. An entire generation of physicians had to face the fact by mid-century that their efforts to secure the support of the general public for medical jurisprudence had failed. Though they had spread medical jurisprudence through the medical curriculum, pushed their researches into exciting new scientific areas, and influenced American social policy on a personal basis, they ultimately failed during the second quarter of the nineteenth century to establish a firm base for their enterprise. They thus learned by mid-century a bitter but enduring lesson in the history of American professions: inherently useful new services or theoretically good new ideas have not by themselves determined the directions of professional development, regardless of what the professions themselves would sometimes like to believe. The creation of inherently useful new services and theoretically good new ideas have no doubt been necessary to professional development, but they have not been sufficient by themselves. In the end, American professions have made major advances only into those areas where someone has been willing to pay for their inherently useful new services or theoretically good ideas.

CHAPTER SEVEN

Medical Testimony in Court
to 1860

The people who pushed medical jurisprudence to the forefront of American professional life during the early decades of the nineteenth century initially paid almost no attention to questions of legal procedure. They hoped that medical professionals could generate and disseminate reliable knowledge, appropriate skills, and credible tests upon which to base medically related policies and judgments; but they did not foresee difficulties persuading their fellow citizens to use the knowledge, skills, and tests as they became available. Pioneers like Rush, Cooper, Caldwell, Stringham, and T.R. Beck had all recognized the challenges presented by research and education; yet none at first even considered the possibility that applying the results of research and education might also prove challenging. None of the surviving student notebooks from the first two decades of the nineteenth century contained instruction about how the information being conveyed to the students was supposed to be presented in actual courts of law. In 1823, when T.R. Beck galvanized the field by publishing the first edition of his *Elements*, it did not occur to him to include anywhere in his two thick volumes any discussion whatsoever of the subject of medical evidence. The early champions of better medical jurisprudence seem to have assumed that the application of what they had to offer, provided it was scientifically sound and appropriate to circumstances in the new republic, would be a straightforward matter. That proved to be one of the most naive assumptions, or monumental oversights, in American professional history.

R.E. Griffith was among the first to sense that the application of professional knowledge in courtroom situations, even upgraded and widely disseminated knowledge, might prove more difficult than most of his colleagues seemed to assume. There was a traditional "disinclination in the medical profession to appear in a court of justice as witnesses in a case," he reminded his colleagues in 1825, and that traditional uneasiness would have to be surmounted. Griffith believed that physicians were hesitant partly because the responsibilities placed upon them in court were so weighty (the

94

lives and property of friends and neighbors often hung upon their opinions), and partly because many of them lacked the "necessary knowledge"
of "many facts . . . whose practical applications are solely confined to the
purposes of jurisprudence, and are therefore entirely overlooked in the usual
routine of medical study." Griffith was confident that both those sources of
hesitancy could be overcome in the United States once medical school courses,
journal literature, and books like the *Elements* spread a sound knowledge of
medical jurisprudence through the profession. But so far, he warned, too
many physicians remained "unacquainted with the forms of judicial inquiry, unversed in the history of criminal courts," and hence unable to
advance the cause of medical jurisprudence as effectively as they might.[1]

By 1828 T.R. Beck had also come to the realization that the question
of actually delivering medical evidence in court was far too important to
continue to ignore. That was the year his colleagues elected him president
of the Medical Society of the State of New York. Beck was, of course,
deeply involved at that time in battles to secure medical regulation, revise
the criminal code, and gain state support for medical jurisprudence; and as
expected, he alluded to each of those subjects in his presidential remarks.
But Beck surprised his audience by choosing "amidst the multiplicity of
subjects that present themselves for selection, and which might with propriety be noticed at this time," the subject of "medical evidence in courts
of justice" as his chief topic.[2] Under the circumstances, that decision was a
dramatic indication of how significant he now considered the subject to be.

Though the subject Beck confronted in 1828 had been emerging in fits
and starts for half a century, remarkably little attention had been paid to
the status of experts of any kind, let alone medical experts, in American
courtrooms. Most American jurists of the early national period clung,
sometimes loosely, to a British judicial practice that recognized and admitted two different types of testimony and two different types of witnesses.
One type involved the direct reporting of what an individual had actually
seen or directly experienced; the other type involved the reporting of accepted principles, established rules, or standard assumptions in fields not
generally understood in detail by ordinary judges and jurors.[3] The concept
of the expert witness arose in conjunction with the latter.

Through the first two decades of the nineteenth century, the most
common use of expert witnesses probably occurred in commercial cases. If,
for example, a ship captain was defending himself in a damage suit for not
sailing on an appointed day, because he considered the tides too low to
allow his vessel to get out of the harbor safely, he would probably present
both eye-witnesses to the height of that day's tides and an "expert" who
would know how much draught was considered necessary for a vessel of
the type and load involved in the case. The latter was needed because judges
and jurors could not reasonably be expected to know the intricacies of ne-
gotiating various types of vessels through shifting navigational channels and
would, therefore, have to be informed about the settled rules and procedures of maritime operations by someone who knew them in detail: an ex-

perienced harbormaster, for example, with no apparent personal interest in
the outcome of the case. Guilt or innocence, or in this case liability, was
still up to the court to determine and might hinge on other considerations
or extenuating circumstances (Was bad weather predicted? Had the captain
been instructed to risk it anyway in a close call? Should those who hired
him have known he had a reputation for caution?), but at least the court
would have the basic "facts" available: the water was so many feet deep
that day and those who were expert in the field did or did not consider that
much water safe to sail upon under the circumstances.

Unfortunately, however, adjudicated situations were seldom as
straightforward as that hypothetical case might suggest; if they were, they
would probably not have come to court. All too often, the purported experts disagreed. In the example given, the party bringing the suit might call
in harbormasters from nearby areas to testify that the captain's expert did
not really know what he was talking about because he had never sailed a
newly designed vessel of the sort involved in the case, or to testify that the
rules and procedures in the harbor at issue were archaic or erroneous. That
sort of testimony would not only confuse the issue in the eyes of the jurors,
but suddenly give the original harbormaster a vested interest in the proceeding, for he might be removed as harbormaster if he really was outdated
or in error, and his harbor might lose future commercial business if the
other side were believed. So back he would come to rebut, and the battle
would be on. Moreover, there might be particular judges or jurors who had
some maritime experience themselves, or had a friend or relative who did,
and consequently felt sufficiently qualified in that field to draw conclusions
independent of either side's purported experts. And all this would be over
a question that might be considered relatively objective and capable of precise measurement.

Consider the logical extension of this sort of situation into a field like
American medicine in the early nineteenth century. The practitioners
themselves disagreed widely and wildly over genuinely fundamental principles. Conditions that one healer might treat with herbs and alcohol, because he considered their cause to be dietary, might be attacked surgically
by a second healer, because he considered their cause to be structural, and
treated chemically by a third, because he considered their cause to lie in a
humoral imbalance. Each of the three would be thoroughly and passionately convinced that he alone was the real expert; the others were misguided
or malicious or both. The potential for confusion in the minds of judges
and juries can easily be imagined in medically related proceedings, and most
of the sorts of situations that can be imagined found their way into court
in real cases. Moreover, virtually every judge and juror had some personal
experience with poor health, injuries, birth, death, weak-mindedness, and
the like, or had some friend or relative who did, and might therefore rather
draw his own conclusions in any given case, regardless of what the purported experts had to say. Indeed, it was that world of contradiction and

confusion that the champions of better medical jurisprudence hoped to correct.

The first piece of advice Beck offered physicians who went into court as expert witnesses had to do with the use of professional language. When in doubt, he urged, try to state the facts plainly and directly. Some medical and scientific terms were essential for accuracy and precision, of course. "But there is a medium in all this," counseled the world's leading expert in the field. At the very least, he hoped, most parts of the body might "be named by their common appellations, and the appearances observed designated by words in ordinary use."[4]

A substantial literature now exists on the extent to which arcane language is or is not necessarily and inherently a hallmark of professionalization in any given field, and there is a long-standing debate over the extent to which professionals consciously or unconsciously perpetuate and exploit specialized terms as a way of mystifying what they actually do.[5] Beck and his colleagues in medical jurisprudence were already fully engaged in those tough issues in the 1820s, and they feared the tendency of vulnerable and insecure practitioners to try to impress the public with a show of verbal pyrotechnics. That all-too-obvious tendency, which was well documented in countless trials, was bad enough, certainly, and Beck wanted overtly to caution his colleagues against the tendency. When physicians behaved like that in court, the whole profession looked silly, and serious medical jurisprudence got lost in defensive obfuscation and pedantic showmanship. But Beck believed that the problem was ultimately solvable, at least in theory: as physicians grew more knowledgeable and more sure of their place in the new republic, they would presumably understand better what they were talking about in any given case and have less reason to try to dazzle either their potential rivals or their potential patients.

Whether the knowledge base of the profession will ever reach that optimistic but theoretically possible level remains to the present day an open question. Even if it did, however, the profession would still face a related and more serious problem that was not obviously solvable, even in theory. Ironically, the difficulty resulted from the very nature of the movement Beck and his colleagues had launched: the more progress they made during the 1830s and 1840s in sophisticated scientific areas, the more difficult became the choice between technical terms (which would be hard to explain to ordinary and often incredulous jurymen) and common language (which would not, in a literal sense, do justice to the fine points of understanding that researchers were beginning to reach in fields like forensic toxicology). Griffith cited an excellent specific example of the problem in an area of research where the champions of medical jurisprudence were making real progress. "There is probably no science so little understood, and of which even the technical names are so little known at the bar," he observed in 1832, "as Physiology; hence in a great measure arise those perplexing scenes which not unfrequently occur on the examination of medical witnesses."[6]

Though Beck barely alluded to this aspect of the language problem in 1828, many of the professionals he inspired would be calling openly by mid-century for the empaneling of special medical juries capable of understanding ever more complex professional testimony.

Beck's second piece of advice followed from his first: once the plain facts had been stated clearly, stand by them. "Physicians are not sufficiently firm in expressing their sentiment," Beck feared, and are too apt to yield to the "decisive tone" of a judge or a cross-examining attorney.[7] Though he had again put his finger on a serious problem for physicians testifying as expert witnesses, he again could not have foreseen the circumstances that rendered the problem even more troublesome than his early admonitions might suggest. Physicians, after all, were testifying in an adversarial setting, where rebuttal and contradiction were considered normal, even essential. What lawyers viewed as a positive good, physicians took as unprofessional bullying. Stories of ill-treatment in court at the hands of skillful or unscrupulous lawyers were still quite rare in medical journals when Beck first addressed the question of expert testimony, but they would increase dramatically by the 1840s.

The third piece of advice Beck gave his colleagues was to take careful notes when conducting any sort of forensic investigation and refer to the notes in court. If the judge allowed it, in fact, try to submit findings in the form of written reports. Medical witnesses, Beck observed, too often got carried away in the competitive atmosphere of the courtroom and overstated their findings. "Pressed by perplexing questions, and probably irritated in his feelings," a doctor "is apt to make declarations more strongly corroborative of opinions that he had formerly advanced, and as his examination advances, he may incur the charge of being *biassed [sic]*, more than facts will warrant."[8] Written reports, prepared in advance of the legal battle, could serve as forms of insurance and reassurance. Virtually every writer on medical jurisprudence throughout the rest of the nineteenth century followed Beck by repeating this advice, usually in strong terms of exhortation. Both their tone and their frequent complaints, however, suggested that the advice was seldom heeded.

Fourth, Beck urged American physicians to take better advantage of one of the significant ways in which court practice in the United States had diverged from traditional British procedure. In the old English system, expert witnesses were generally on their own in the witness box; they were quite literally deemed to be expert on whatever question was at hand, and were therefore not allowed to introduce other people's opinions or the work of alternative authorities. Even if a medical witness was not fully versed in every detail of the question under examination, he was not allowed recourse to reference books. Consequently, he could easily end up looking shabby and unsure, since the attorneys grilling him certainly could and did refer to standard texts. This aspect of the British system had tripped even the great surgeon John Hunter in 1780, when "he found himself a good deal embarrassed" in the widely publicized Donellan poisoning trial.[9]

By contrast, expert witnesses in the new United States, perhaps in part because the level of professional knowledge was so thin and so poorly diffused, were routinely permitted to refer to specific passages from specific texts. Most of the time in most jurisdictions they were even permitted to read aloud on the witness stand from whatever volumes they wished to cite, though these procedural rules of evidence would slowly change later in the century.[10] Putting aside Beck's personal interest in this doctrine (his own book, after all, was quickly becoming the almost universal reference in American courts on all questions of medical jurisprudence), he was correct that physicians could avoid many foolish mistakes if they would only be less reluctant to arm themselves with standard authorities. Unfortunately, too many American doctors would continue through mid-century to be heroic solo practitioners on the witness stand, just as they wanted to be in their practices.

The fifth piece of advice Beck offered was to take seriously the concept of the whole truth. Expert witnesses, like all other witnesses, were necessarily called by one side or the other, and consequently they were open to the charge of being a partisan. In order to avoid those imputations every physician should introduce all the facts he had, even those not favorable to the side who summoned him. Beck believed that the whole truth would ultimately be more persuasive than one-sided presentations, and hence good for the side that called the physician. But even if that were not so in every specific case, the profession as whole would be elevated to the level of neutral truth-seekers by consistently giving all the facts. That was a noble ideal, to be sure, in 1828, but by mid-century it would begin to founder on the shoals of openly purchased and highly selective testimony.

Finally, Beck pleaded, "medical witnesses" must learn to treat "each other with respect."[11] Ugly public showdowns, after all, embarrassed both the profession generally and the cause of medical jurisprudence specifically. To discredit contradictory evidence in the minds of judges and juries medical witnesses not infrequently attacked the personal and professional standing of physicians on the other side. Yet Beck was again hopeful that this problem could be solved, or at least muted, in the coming decades. After all, the most powerful and influential state in the young nation seemed to be moving in 1828 toward professional consolidation and regulation under the leadership of Beck's own New York State Medical Society.

As outlined earlier, however, the ensuing decades brought dissension and deregulation rather than consolidation and control over who would be allowed to try to earn a living as a healer. American courts, moreover, had never had clear methods of determining exactly who was or was not an expert for the purposes of offering expert testimony. Each judge and each court made that determination on whatever grounds seemed appropriate to the specific case before them. Prospective expert witnesses typically offered their credentials, which could vary from university degrees and years of intense experience, on the one hand, to the growing and selling of herbs that seemed to make the neighbors feel better, on the other, and the court was free to accept or reject their claims to special knowledge on whatever grounds the court wished to apply. Since there were no functional licensing laws to regulate the practice of medicine, no formal educational requirements, and plenty of deep-seated disagreements over what constituted effective health care, American courts during the second quarter of the nineteenth century tended more and more often to err on the side of inclusion in medically related cases. Anyone with a plausible argument for expert status would likely be heard, though the judge and jury, of course, were free to weigh the opinions of some experts more heavily than those of others. Untrained practitioners whom serious medical jurisprudents held in contempt were thus afforded an open and equal chance to persuade juries to cling to folk perceptions and superficial appearances over often arcane and difficult-to-explain scientific conclusions.

The result was devastating to the champions of better medical jurisprudence in the United States: the very concept of the expert witness, which in theory should have been enormously attractive and advantageous to them, was in practice undercutting their efforts by perpetuating the notion that all healers and all forms of medical knowledge had equal standing before the bar. "Doubtless there is too little discrimination exercised in receiving all who are called *doctors*, as witnesses," observed a much chastened Beck in 1835, already striking by then a more pessimistic note than any he had sounded in his original discussion of medical witnesses seven years earlier.[12] His altogether justified pessimism rested on a development, the importance of which can hardly be overstated: by 1835 the arena in which medical jurisprudence had its greatest public visibility was fast becoming an arena that made the medical profession look unprofessional.

An otherwise sympathetic article in the *American Jurist* put the situation plainly in 1841: "It is a matter of common remark, that medical men, even when possessing considerable reputation, make but a sorry figure on the witness-stand, and the fact is regarded, on account of its frequency, as reflecting some discredit on the profession itself." Physicians were "breaking down" in court. To make matters worse, the American system of medical jurisprudence, "especially in the country," too often seemed to allow "feelings of personal animosity" to "usurp the place of a conscientious regard for truth, and the witness-stand becomes the scene of professional collisions in which ignorance generally triumphs." But all the author could do was to call once again upon state legislatures in the United States to create "a distinct class of medical men examined and licensed by proper authorities" who would serve as independent and exclusive medico-legal experts in American courts, the plan already so "practically made use of in France."[13]

By mid-century the bickering and squabbling of medical witnesses in American courtrooms would become legendary, a common cliché. Virtually every writer on medical jurisprudence for the next seventy-five years would comment on the problem and urge physicians to stop fighting in court, both for the good of justice and for the good of the profession. Medical societies even entertained resolutions that would mandate expulsion of any member who controverted another member in court. Yet nothing seemed to work. Courtroom confrontations, which had been a relatively minor irritant to the profession through the end of the eighteenth century, became a major problem by the middle of the nineteenth century. Indeed, physicians not only continued to confront each other as hostile third-party experts, but soon turned to direct actions upon one another as well, a frightening phenomenon addressed in the following chapter.

From the point of view of those who wished to raise the standards of the medical profession generally and of medical jurisprudence specifically, the often *ad hominem* and sometimes vicious bickering of physicians on the witness stand posed a special set of problems. One was the ruination of individual careers. If that resulted most of the time in purging the weaker members of the profession, it might have been tolerable. But there was no evidence that was happening. In fact, the contrary seemed increasingly to be the case. Strong members of the profession were often the ones most likely to try to do their duty and confront error where they saw it, and they often ended up instead as victims of the process. Though Samuel Gross launched a great career in the witness stand, many others sank there. Beck had foreseen the danger even in 1828, and he gave it special emphasis: "The fact cannot be too distinctly stated, that a *man may be a judicious, correct, and excellent practitioner of medicine, and yet not competent as a witness*" in areas he seldom dealt with or knew little about.[14]

As the situation deteriorated, physicians grew more and more resentful of the role of lawyers, judges, and juries; especially lawyers. In 1825 Griffith had cast lawyers as almost heroic partners with physicians in the court process: their "acuteness and ready comprehension . . . the versatility of their genius . . . and their rapid discernment" kept physician-witnesses on their toes and ensured the highest caliber of testimony.[15] Stories of outrageous treatment at the hands of lawyers were rare in medical journals during the 1820s and uncommon into the 1830s, but began to appear with increasing regularity by the 1840s.

Symptomatic of the mounting sense of frustration and disgust was the report of a case tried in Binghamton, New York, in 1843. There a man named Benjamin Turpening died suddenly and without apparent cause. The public authorities persuaded a committee of the city's leading and most scientifically knowledgeable physicians to conduct a post-mortem examination of Turpening's body, and the doctors found large amounts of arsenic in the viscera. The group had absolutely no doubt that the arsenic had killed him, and they were quite certain that the arsenic had been administered in two successive doses. A number of suspicious circumstances pointed to Turpening's wife Elizabeth, who had earlier accused her husband of carousing with "negro wenches." Elizabeth was indicted for murder.

At the trial the defense attorneys berated and belittled the physicians involved. Mrs. Turpening's lawyers alleged that no real proof of arsenic had been presented (though it had been), that the toxicological tests employed were inconclusive and inaccurate (they were not), and that physicians generally were a class of men not to be trusted. The defense team "unhesitatingly set the whole medical faculty of witnesses down," reported the primary victim of this verbal assault, "as stupidly ignorant, and of course wholly unfit to enter upon such investigations." Doctors were accused of recklessly dispensing poisons themselves and of filling the city's graveyards in order to rob them for bodies. Worst of all, the physicians could do nothing about the "solemn mockery," willful misrepresentation, individual vilification, and character assassination that went on in court, since the court looked after its own. "The slightest impeachment of the integrity of the judge or jury would be considered a contempt of court," so the medical witnesses for the state would face incarceration themselves if they protested.[16]

The only thing that distinguished this particular case from hundreds of others reported to medical journals and medical societies was the fact that the chief physician involved in this case was the effective young professionalizer Nathan S. Davis, who emerged outraged and disillusioned from his attempt to implement the dreams, the exhortations, and the medico-legal skills of those who had taught him in medical school. The Turpening case had cost the field of medical jurisprudence a potentially valuable recruit: just six years later Davis would be among the most active and influential founders of the American Medical Association and, twenty years after that, its president. But the larger point was more important than the loss of a specific individual: when physicians went into court, they were getting battered. Forced to play by a set of rules they could not change, they were being made to look ridiculous, even when they were on strong ground, even when they appeared at the specific behest of responsible local officials, and even when their efforts were undertaken in the public interest.

By mid-century, evidence mounted that physicians were consciously avoiding jurisprudential situations. An editorial in the *New Orleans Medical and Surgical Journal* in 1852 noted that doctors were fleeing scenes of trouble and refusing to treat people injured in street skirmishes, lest they end up in court.[17] Even when physicians got involved, the system seemed more and more frequently to thwart and disillusion them. From Memphis came an all-too-typical report. There the coroner asked the professor of anatomy in the local medical school to disinter and re-examine the body of a man allegedly shot to death by an Irishman. The Irishman had already been convicted of murder and sentenced to hang, but the coroner harbored doubts. The professor of anatomy, A. K. Taylor, reluctant to see the city execute a man who might not be guilty, enlisted the aid of his predecessor at Memphis Medical College, and the two anatomy professors conducted the postmortem as requested. They both agreed that the gunshot wound had been superficial and that the man died of unrelated peritonitis. Yet the court refused to take their evidence seriously and would not reconsider the verdict. The lawyers involved in the case behaved, in the eyes of these two medical professors, heinously. Taylor, obviously bitter about the way expert testimony was being received in local American courtrooms, was forced into the awkward position of applauding the fact that the Irishman escaped from jail before the authorities could hang him.[18]

One of the most pointed statements about the way court procedures and the behavior of lawyers seemed to be undermining medical jurisprudence by mid-century came from David Humphreys Storer, the prominent Boston physician selected to give the Massachusetts Medical Society's prestigious annual address in 1851. Storer had already established a strong reputation, especially in obstetrics, and would later become dean of Harvard Medical School and founder of the American Gynecological Society.[19] He took the occasion of the 1851 annual address, however, to present a retrospective overview of the field of medical jurisprudence, a field he knew well.[20] He had taught the subject for many years, and he had written on medical jurisprudential topics. He was also at this stage of his life helping his son, Horatio Robinson Storer, try to carry on his own efforts in the uncharted, increasingly dangerous professional zones between medicine and law.[21]

David Humphreys Storer had been involved in a large number of actual court cases himself, some of which had been nasty and professionally damaging encounters. Perhaps the worst of them had occurred a decade prior to Storer's mid-century retrospective in the poisoning trial of Hannah Kinney, indicted for murdering her husband. That case had rocked the Boston medical elite, for they ended up disagreeing with one another on the witness stand, feuding openly with the Boston legal establishment, and creating a situation in which a doctor who was not a member of the Massachusetts Medical Society looked good in the eyes of the public. Storer had been attacked personally in the columns of *Chandler's Law Reporter*, a legal monthly; he had been scored by Harvard faculty members in their class lectures; he had been rebuked by the influential *Boston Medical and Surgical Journal*, which compared his efforts most unflatteringly to those of Orfila; and he had been driven to defend himself in the *Atlas*, a Boston daily newspaper.[22] At one stage in the journalistic debate Storer had summarized in two sentences his sardonic view of the process of giving expert testimony: "It is the duty of a witness on the stand to state the truth. It is the business of legal counsel to distort and suppress the truth, except so far as it suits their own purpose."[23] The whole sorry affair must have seemed like a precursor of the sorts of problems that were becoming increasingly common around the country by mid-century and the subject of widespread concern among American physicians interested in medical jurisprudence.

Storer began his 1851 address by lamenting what seemed to him to be a national trend away from formal course work in medical jurisprudence, even in the better medical colleges. Storer considered the trend a professional disaster, both because unprepared young physicians could find themselves testifying before courts and legislatures whether they wanted to or not and because medical jurisprudence was the branch of medicine that permitted potentially the most important interactions between "the profession" and "the community." But physicians were withdrawing from the field, both intellectually and in daily practice. Echoing the editorial from Louisiana, Storer noted that in Massachusetts, too, "it is not an uncommon thing for [doctors] to refuse to attend a post-mortem examination, however much they may have been interested in the case, if there is the slightest probability that a judicial investigation will follow."[24]

Why were physicians turning their backs upon medical jurisprudence? Why did the hopeful and progressive field that attracted him as a young physician now find itself in retreat and disarray? In Storer's view the chief reason was clear: medical witnesses were being treated shamefully in American courts. Reputations were being ruined, characters smeared, and professional confidences breached under duress. Medical testimony was "reviewed, ridiculed, doubted," and perverted. Attorneys behaved unconscionably. "I have known a distinguished member of the bar, while addressing a jury, indirectly to impeach the veracity of a Fellow of this Society," remembered Storer. His friends in the audience almost certainly realized that he was probably referring to his own trauma ten years before. "That hour has long since passed; but the wound then inflicted will never heal."[25]

Samuel Parkman, a surgeon at Massachusetts General Hospital, echoed Storer's concerns a year later in a lecture he gave to the Boston Society for Medical Observation. The *American Journal of the Medical Sciences*, in turn, considered the lecture sufficiently important to share with a national audience. Physicians had come to dread the process of giving testimony in court, Parkman believed in 1852, because they now supposed they were

> about to be subjected to an ordeal from which they can hardly expect to escape unscathed. The medical man alleges that, on the stand, he is liable to be browbeaten by ingenious and unprincipled counsel—to have his opinions misrepresented by the demanding of a degree of accuracy which is impossible—or be entrapped into statements seemingly contradictory by artfully devised questionings; that, in fact, he is in various ways subjected to treatment which he has a right to consider unfair and illiberal. The lawyer is regarded by the medical practitioner as a species of grand inquisitor, who, although he may not have at his command the means of physical torture, by which evidence of old was extracted from an unwilling or incapable witness, has still the power to stretch the unlucky physician upon a kind of intellectual rack. . . .
>
> Such, it cannot be denied, is the general feeling with which a medical man approaches a court of justice; his only desire and hope is to escape from it without a blunder, or the appearance of one; and he considers any subterfuge lawful by which he is freed from such an annoyance. In a word, a doctor is apt to look upon a lawyer as his natural enemy, against whom his only defence is that of the hare against the hound, viz., flight.[26]

Moreover, in Parkman's opinion, lawyers tended to concentrate their fire on physicians precisely because the latter came into court as professional experts. Ordinary witnesses might be doubted by the jury or dismissed in a skillful summary. But expert witnesses, because their testimony was often so crucial to the other side's case and because they had the imprimatur of "expert," had to be thoroughly and relentlessly demolished in cross-examination.[27] As a Cincinnati attorney acknowledged in 1859, "The lawyer fears the doctor, not knowing how far an otherwise plain case may be damaged by medical ambiguity and technicality. The doctor fears the lawyer, lest a cross-examination may distort his meaning and place him in an absurd position." The results, according to this lawyer, all too often damaged them both. "No scene can be more amusing to the spectator, and more grievous to the professions, than that of an ignorant attorney eliciting evidence from a pompous doctor."[28]

The dangers of testimony seemed especially terrifying to young physicians just entering the field. James Wynne began his introductory lecture to the incoming class at New York Medical College in 1859 by warning them that

> . . . it is quite possible that your character as medical men may be fixed, in the community in which you may take up your residence, by the extent of information you may possess in the first medico-legal case to which you are called, and in the absence of regularly established officers for this purpose, this may occur immediately upon your entrance into your professional career.[29]

Medical opinion had swung by the 1850s almost 180 degrees since the optimistic era when Rush and Beck envisioned ever more knowledgeable and public-spirited physicians eagerly playing ever more influential and positive roles in the nation's system of justice. Instead of enhancing the status of the expert, actual practice seemed to belittle and diminish it; instead of driving inferior healers from the field, court rules afforded them de facto equality; instead of working with the legal profession in pursuit of truth, physicians found themselves openly attacked in a public forum. By mid-century they were clearly shocked and repulsed by a prospect and a partnership that once intrigued and excited them. To repeat Parkman's pithy summary: "a doctor [was now] apt to look upon a lawyer as his natural enemy."[30]

As concern increased in the medical profession about the sinking prospects of the expert witness in American courts, medical societies and medical schools sought the advice and counsel of lawyers. The latter, in turn, obliged with a series of lectures, papers, and articles that tried to explain to physicians why they were having so much trouble in court. Indeed, articles of explanation, instruction, and exhortation from lawyers became staples in American medical journals after mid-century, and the genre has persisted through the twentieth century. Much of the commentary was superficial and repetitious; some of it was downright patronizing. But the chief points the attorneys made were worth taking seriously, for they confirmed the fact that the entire concept of the expert medical witness underwent profound scrutiny in the United States in the middle decades of the nineteenth century.

Among the most influential and insightful lawyers to address the mid-century crisis of the medical witness was Allen G. Thurman. Thurman rose to the top of the Ohio bar as a relatively young man, served in the U.S. House of Representatives during the 1840s, and had only recently stepped down as chief justice of the Ohio Supreme Court when he was asked in 1857 to speak at the spring commencement ceremonies of Starling Medical College.[31] Located in the state capital, Starling Medical College had been endowed by a lawyer-entrepreneur at its founding ten years earlier and was basking in the glory of a newly completed building as Thurman spoke.[32] Thurman chose medical jurisprudence as the subject of his address; he told the graduates that he thought speakers should stick to something they knew well, and medical jurisprudence was the area in which his own knowledge and experience overlapped the concerns of the new doctors.

Thurman quoted Beck's expansive definition of medical jurisprudence, then paraphrased it as "the administration of law enlightened by medical knowledge."[33] As might be expected of the former state chief justice, however, Thurman believed that the real impact of medical jurisprudence on American life, and the key to the future of the field, depended upon the ability of physicians to deliver sound and persuasive medical evidence in courts. A surprisingly large number of cases in American courts turned upon medical testimony, in Thurman's view, and American juries, though almost "wholly ignorant" of medical matters and "not qualified by any previous education to judge" medical opinions, generally paid close attention to the professional testimony they heard.

For all its imperfections, Thurman considered the legal situation in the United States at mid-century a long stride forward from the "dens of barbarism, miscalled Courts of Justice" in old England and the colonies before the Revolution. Justice was then, more often than not, the "mere instrument" of the "arbitrary will" of a tyrant or one of his minions. Since those tribunals were not primarily interested in truth or justice in the first place, especially for individuals without power or influence, there had been little reason for accurate medical evidence in any given case. No wonder, in Thurman's view, "that it was not until a comparatively recent date that the science [of medical jurisprudence] received any great development and became a distinct branch of medical and legal study" in the United Kingdom. Fortunately for Americans, the old British fetters binding true justice had been more thoroughly smashed in the United States than elsewhere in the English-speaking world, and hence it followed as no accident that medical jurisprudence had produced in America "wonderful growth" and "glorious result" during the first half of the nineteenth century.[34]

But what about the crisis? What good was progress in medical jurisprudence if those trained in the field could not prevail in court? Why not let medical experts, or some subset of them, sit as special juries in cases where their knowledge might be brought to bear? Why should judges perpetuate what Thurman aptly characterized as "the most perfect free trade in medicine," when they knew full well that some of the "experts" testifying, for example, in a poisoning case had studied toxicological and forensic chemistry and others had not? These were, Thurman recognized, profound questions. They went to the heart of the American legal structure and to the basic relationship between it and the medical profession.

In reply, Thurman first made a number of practical observations. Juries of experts would be difficult to assemble in many jurisdictions, even if they were theoretically desirable. There were too few reliably trained medico-legalists. Second, if physicians could decide all medically related cases, then merchants should decide all mercantile cases, farmers all agricultural cases, and so on. Third, what Thurman labeled "esprit du corps" (we might today label it professional consciousness), envy, and rivalry within the medical profession would almost inevitably cloud results and make the public distrustful. Ultimately, however, Thurman objected to expert juries because the concept of experts operating above the ordinary rules of law conflicted with the open, adversarial principles upon which the American legal structure was ultimately based and upon which Thurman's own legal profession had solidified its increasingly powerful place in American life.[35]

In the American system, only grand juries operated in a manner even remotely close to a star chamber, and the former chief justice of Ohio implied in no uncertain terms that he thought grand juries presented altogether too many "false indictments" as it was. Juries of experts, operating almost exclusively on *ex parte* testimony, would make things worse. Evidence must be rendered in open session for all the community to judge, whether they were fully capable of understanding the esoteric points or not. They would at least be assured that the procedure was fair and the whole case presented. Finally, this influential judge did not believe that juries took medical evidence as blithely or as foolishly as many physicians thought they did. "I have never, in a long experience," Thurman declared near the end of his talk to the new graduates, "known a verdict rendered by a jury upon a scientific question, against the clear, decided and unshaken testimony of a respectable body of scientific witnesses." Even should that occur, he informed the young doctors, judges had the right to set verdicts aside.[36]

That last observation, of course, was part of the problem from the physicians' point of view. The legal profession fully intended to retain control over the processes of justice. Lawyers had no intention of surrendering power, real or symbolic, to rival professional collectives. When doctors entered American courtrooms, they did so under rules established, interpreted, and administered by lawyers. Thurman's summation must have come as no surprise to the graduates and as little consolation to their professors:

> I am satisfied that the present mode of trial is substantially correct, and
> that the idea of a trial by experts is altogether impracticable, and were
> it not so would in general be found inexpedient. That there is room for
> improvement of the present mode, I am quite ready to admit, but that
> it will, or ought to be, radically changed, I do not believe.[37]

Thurman tried to conclude on a hopeful note. Each physician would continue to be a "welcome witness" in court. The medical expert would be "sought with eagerness, listened to with respect, considered with care, and when he and his brethren unite in judgment, they, in effect, decide the cause." [38] Unfortunately, fewer and fewer physicians still believed those sentiments by 1857.

The optimism of the 1820s had disappeared and the medical profession after mid-century began to adjust to the situation that actually existed, as distinguished from the one their predecessors had hoped would develop. More and more physicians refused to go into courts as experts in civil litigations unless they were well paid, usually in advance, by one side or the other. If they were going to do partisan battle, whether they wanted to or not, they might as well exact mercenary fees, the higher the better. This was a far cry from the notions of disinterested medical expertise at the service of the state and available to all citizens, the notions that so fascinated medico-legalists at the beginning of the century. But it was a perfectly logical accommodation on the part of regular practitioners to the situation that actually existed in American professional life by mid-century.

CHAPTER EIGHT

The Emergence of Medical Malpractice

Issues surrounding medical malpractice have come to dominate discussions of medical jurisprudence in the United States in modern times. Indeed, for a surprisingly large number of contemporary Americans, especially physicians, malpractice and legal medicine have become all but synonymous. A medico-legal world in which malpractice was not a prominent problem now seems to them both fancifully idealistic and almost inconceivable. It may come as a shock to many contemporary doctors and lawyers, therefore, to learn that medical malpractice litigation was not a serious medico-legal concern in the United States before 1840, even among the leading scholars of medical jurisprudence. But with striking speed thereafter, medical malpractice broke dramatically into American popular and professional consciousness to become a major issue for the nation's medico-legalists. Indeed, combined with the problems they were already encountering as witnesses in other types of cases, medical malpractice actions would begin after 1850 to alter the basic way physicians approached the whole subject of medical jurisprudence.

The basic concept of professional malpractice had existed in Anglo-American legal theory prior to the American Revolution, for William Blackstone referred specifically to malpractice in the famous *Commentaries on the Laws of England* he published during the 1760s. Moreover, Blackstone had linked the concept explicitly to the medical profession by including, under *mala praxis*, "Injuries . . . by the neglect or unskilful management of [a person's] physician, surgeon, or apothecary . . . because it breaks the trust which the party had placed in his physician, and tends to the patient's destruction."[1] The *Commentaries* were widely read in the colonies and remained influential through the early national period. But as a practical matter, actions for medical malpractice were seldom initiated in American professional situations through the first third of the nineteenth century. And even at a theoretical level, the concept of medical malpractice had been so arcane and unimportant in the United States that American writers on medical jurisprudence, those most likely to be interested in the subject as an aspect of legal medicine, did not bother to address it through the first four decades of the nineteenth century. Beck's *Elements* never mentioned malpractice from its first publication in 1823 though its mid-century editions, though the latter began to approach 2000 pages in length and were considered encyclopedic in the breadth of their coverage. Neither did standard legal treatises on evidence and proof.[2]

As late as 1834 R.E. Griffith, one of the best-informed medico-legal writers and editors in the country, noted the total absence of any American study of "medical responsibility," by which he meant the standards of competence appropriate to various types of cases and various geographical regions. In fact, like many other physicians of the early period, he complained that the legal doctrines governing malpractice were too murky and unenforceable; complete charlatans could probably plead ignorance and escape the consequences of whatever harm they might do to fellow citizens.[3] In 1855, the first edition of Wharton and Stillé's *Medical Jurisprudence*, which supplanted Beck's *Elements* as the dominant treatise in the field during the third quarter of the nineteenth century, still contained no reference to medical malpractice, though by then it probably should have.

This is not to say that medical malpractice cases were completely unknown in the United States before 1840. In 1827, for example, the Beck brothers' *New-York Medical and Physical Journal* reported a case of obvious and special interest to those who urged closer cooperation between the medical profession and the government. The events that led to the case had taken place in 1824. That spring the City of New York hired physicians to canvass Manhattan by districts and vaccinate at public expense anyone who had not already been protected against a cresting epidemic of smallpox. One of the physicians hired, a young practitioner named Gerard Banker, vaccinated some 870 citizens in his district, many of whom were children. One of those children, a two-year-old, subsequently died a hideous and horrible death from the disease, and the child's father sued Banker for inflicting smallpox upon the child through a bad inoculation.[4]

Though Banker was acquitted when other city physicians testified that the child was probably coming down with the disease at the time Banker performed the vaccination, the case might have had a chilling effect upon future cooperation between the medical profession and public authorities had the decision gone the other way; that was no doubt the reason the *NYMPJ* publicized the case. Moreover, Banker's defense attorney had also tried to make as plain as possible to other physicians the potential danger of this sort of accusation. "The case is of vast importance to the defendant," he argued, because the young doctor had "chosen a profession, to the study of which, he has already devoted many years of his life, and a verdict in this case against him, is his professional death."[5] But that last aspect of malpractice law had hardly begun to dawn upon the vast majority of American physicians.

Other scattered cases occurred during the 1820s. Two obscure practitioners in Maine, for example, were sued in a case involving the treatment of a hip injury incurred in 1821. That case dragged on nearly five years, gained national attention, and eventually pitted John Warren, a leader of the Boston medical establishment, against Nathan Smith, a New England rival who helped establish both the Dartmouth Medical School and the Yale Medical School, at least in part to offset the dominance of the Harvard-based Boston group. Yet reports of the case revealed clearly that one of the chief reasons for its notoriety lay in its novelty. Indeed, attorneys in the case were not sure exactly how to phrase the court action they were trying to take.[6] Later in the decade Nathan Smith told his medical jurisprudence class at Yale about that case and about a small handful of other malpractice actions that he was aware of in Connecticut during the 1820s. But Smith, who had been personally involved in the most famous medical malpractice case in the nation's history to that time and who was in a position to know such things, remarked to his Yale students that he "Never knew but one case sued for Malpractice in medicine [as distinguished from surgery]," and he seemed to suggest that more aggressive legal activity on the malpractice front might prove salutary for the medical profession in the long run, since under the doctrines in force in Connecticut in 1827, "the most egregious Quacks must escape punishment."[7]

Notwithstanding the foregoing examples, then, malpractice cases involving physicians were sufficiently few in number through the first fifty years of the republic to be reasonably characterized as isolated, though sometimes troubling, curiosities.[8] Certainly medical journals, even though they had a *prima facie* interest in malpractice developments and even though they evinced a strong and growing interest in most other types of medico-legal topics after 1820, rarely mentioned malpractice cases prior to 1840 and did not betray any special misgivings about the isolated ones they happened to come across. The precise number of medical malpractice actions at any given point in the century cannot be determined. Even if armies of patient researchers were available to survey all legal actions in all jurisdictions at all levels, many, if not most, of the records were never saved in the first place or have subsequently been lost or destroyed. Consequently, despite obvious drawbacks, legal historians have used state appellate cases as a sort of statistical surrogate in situations of this sort. By that measure, only 2 percent of the medical malpractice cases to reach American state appellate courts between 1790 and 1900 were reported in the period before 1835.[9] Kenneth De Ville, who has made the most recent and most thorough assessment of those cases, also noted that 1790 to 1840 was the only period in American history in which the rate of population growth easily exceeded the rate of increase in medical malpractice cases.[10]

After 1840 the frequency of malpractice actions shot suddenly upward, and well-established physicians, not charlatans, found themselves the targets of an almost revolutionary and certainly unprecedented surge in malpractice accusations. As a result, what had appeared for half a century to be a potentially beneficent curiosity was transformed in the perception of well-educated regular American physicians in less than a decade into an anti-professional specter of high visibility and ominously destructive power. That change in the role of medical malpractice in American professional life, in turn, quickly proved to be yet another of the mid-century developments that widened the gap between law and medicine and pushed the field of medical jurisprudence farther toward the margins of American professional development.

Though historians have only begun to explore this striking and intriguing transition, some of the broad outlines of what happened are relatively clear. The same socio-political and ideological ethos that blocked state support for medical jurisprudence during the 1830s had begun by the 1840s to transform physicians from community helpers into contract agents. Doctors no longer looked like designated healers or well-meaning neighbors who served their local communities as best they could in an interactive and organic social system that involved mutual trust and obligations. Instead, doctors looked more and more like individual entrepreneurs in an intensely competitive marketplace. Under those altered circumstances, increasing numbers of patients decided that the physician-agents they retained could have and should have done a better job than they did. Rather than pay their doctors for doing as well as they could under the conditions at hand, an increasing number of patients instead sued their doctors for failing to prevent or for apparently inflicting permanent disabilities and deformities; for failing to deliver on an implied contract of full recovery or restoration.

Shifting public attitudes may also have been fueled by perfectionist health and fitness movements that swept the nation during the 1840s, for those movements almost certainly raised people's expectations of what was considered normal in matters of health and made people more sensitive to physical well-being. Some historians argue that the era also experienced a corresponding decline in the number of people still prepared to dismiss bodily suffering in a religiously fatalistic fashion. A surge of aggressive and flamboyant medical advertising during the late 1830s and early 1840s proffered the general public a host of false promises, further adding to general expectations. The steady nationalization of the new medical marketplace probably also played a role in the advent of widespread malpractice litigation, for standards of care once considered not only adequate but uniquely appropriate to a particular local region began to seem inferior and erroneous in comparison with results claimed or obtained elsewhere. Changes in the technical rules of legal pleading during this same period, moreover, had the effect of further easing the process of bringing malpractice actions in the first place.[11]

In any event, the new "contagion" of lawsuits, as physicians characterized the phenomenon in a typically medical metaphor, seemed to become virulent almost overnight. At first centered in western New York State, a sharp surge in the frequency of malpractice cases was evident throughout New England and the upper Mid-West by mid-century. Even though exact numbers for the period remain impossible to calculate, and even though the rates of malpractice actions were probably lower than they have come to be in the twentieth century, the evidence is overwhelming that "the profession and the country crossed over the most critical threshold in the 1840s and 1850s."[12] Malpractice cases carried to state appellate courts roared ahead 950 percent between 1830 and 1860, while the nation's population increased 144 percent, and almost all of the increase in malpractice appeals took place after 1840.[13] Medical journals, after decades of barely noticing malpractice on the medical horizon, reacted defensively with strong and frequent articles and editorials.

The public's increasingly frequent recourse to medical malpractice suits in the 1840s may be seen in retrospect as a perfectly reasonable response to the marketplace professionalism which was then emerging in the United States. Anti-monopolistic sentiment during the 1830s, after all, had precluded the creation of professional structures that might have permitted some degree of self-regulation by the medical profession: structures such as licensing qualifications to ensure minimal competence or government-appointed physicians to provide a public standard. Halting experiments designed to encourage internal settlements within local medical societies proved quickly and utterly ineffectual in the face of intense personal rivalries inside the societies and accusations from healers outside the societies.[14] Consequently, individual practitioners, one at a time, would have to be held to standards deemed acceptable by those who retained their services. Quality control would come not from self-policing by medical providers, since that was too dangerous for other reasons and historically ineffective in any event, but from the people who paid the bill. Indeed, if the concept of medical malpractice had not already existed in Anglo-American legal theory, Americans might have been forced to invent it; in seizing upon an arcane doctrine and changing the rules of pleading to ease its employment, Americans essentially did just that.

At least in theory, the nation's strongest physicians might have welcomed the sudden and dramatic increase in the number of malpractice suits as a useful method of driving charlatans and amateur hacks from the field. The general public and the legal profession might have been enlisted as allies in an effort to improve medical care. The early champions of medical jurisprudence, after all, had cautiously endorsed the positive potential of malpractice litigation and envisioned lawyers not as hostile attackers but as partners in a process of professional purification. Over and over during the 1840s and 1850s, however, the nation's best-educated and most professionally minded physicians observed with a sort of defensive incredulity and disbelieving horror that many, if not most, of the burgeoning numbers of malpractice suits were being lodged not against charlatans and amateur hacks, but against others like themselves: successful regular doctors. What early commentators like Griffith and Smith once considered a potentially useful mechanism had somehow quickly and alarmingly come to be a means of persecuting the best physicians then practicing.

Several factors help explain why the best-educated and most successful physicians, rather than the nation's army of amateurs and alternative healers, became disproportionately frequent targets for malpractice suits in the 1840s. First, they became ironic victims of their own medical advancement. The vast majority of the lawsuits that constituted the first great wave of malpractice litigation at mid-century involved orthopedic cases in which a limb had healed to a shortened, deformed, or frozen position following compound fracture. Patients found themselves with an unambiguous, easily demonstrated, and obviously measurable problem and sued the doctor who set the bone fragments and dressed the wound. What made this situation ironic was the fact that twenty years earlier most compound fractures would have been amputated. The patient would have no limb at all, but no malpractice case either, since the doctor would have been following safe and standard procedures. Improved techniques and more careful training produced an advance; but because the consequences of the advance were often imperfect, those who tried to save limbs in difficult cases often found themselves being sued.

Second, the better the physician, the more likely he would be to take a difficult compound fracture case and the more likely he would be to try to save the limb, even if it survived in less than perfect shape. The techniques involved in saving compound fractures in the 1830s, while still avoiding the dangers of internal infection that previously made amputation necessary to save the life of the patient, required sophisticated knowledge of wound dressing and bone setting that amateurs or inexperienced healers would never pretend to possess.

Third, amateurs and alternative healers delivered what patients came to them for, be it hot baths or herbal teas, and could not be sued for undesirable results (in theory they could have been sued for concocting their own teas erroneously, but in practice they claimed no standard recipes and made a virtue of treating each case individually). Regular physicians, on the other hand, could have the very body of educational texts and advanced manuals they were steadily producing used in court against them as standards or norms from which they could be accused of deviating. William Rothstein and others have pointed out the sometimes deceptive truism that *malpractice* is virtually impossible to demonstrate in the absence of *practice*; no one can be convicted of doing established procedures poorly, if no procedures have been established.[15] Writing from Erie, Pennsylvania, in 1849, William Wood, a U.S. Navy doctor, understood the frustrations of that principle all too well. "It is better to be without a diploma," in the current climate, he concluded ruefully, because then a "practitioner can say, 'I make no pretensions, I offer no certificate of ability, and only gave my neighbour in his sufferings such aid as I could.' "[16]

Finally, patients had little or no incentive to sue marginal healers with few assets, but substantial incentive to sue the most prosperous physicians, from whom they might actually collect. That incentive, superimposed upon the anti-elite, anti-monopoly, and anti-professional ethos of the 1830s and 1840s, gave the nation's first medical malpractice crisis a distinctly class-oriented aspect. Physicians near the top of their profession certainly saw class as a factor in the crisis. Many of them thought that the vast majority of malpractice suits were initiated by poor patients either trying to escape paying for a job they considered less than perfect or trying to turn a misfortune into cash at the expense of a wealthy professional. Medical societies reconsidered their obligations to treat the poor; impecunious patients were made to post bonds against subsequent legal actions before receiving medical treatment; and medical spokesmen railed against the use of a long-dormant legal doctrine for the purpose of shaking down the nation's better physicians, since a doctor often found it easier to forgive the bill or settle a claim out of court than to fight the accusation and risk his reputation and his whole practice.[17]

In a most revealing comment, Walter Channing at Harvard was appalled at reports of "a certain county, of a certain State, [where] the jury in all suits for malpractice give their verdict for the plaintiff; and that same county, it is said, tries more of such cases than all the others of the *Commonwealth* put together."[18] Under the circumstances, Channing's pointed emphasis of the word commonwealth was almost certainly intended to be mocking. The concept of society which that hopeful word once evoked for republican state-makers in an earlier era, Channing was suggesting, no longer seemed to exist in the United States by the middle of the nineteenth century.

Channing had become convinced that the only antidote to the malpractice contagion would be the creation of special medical juries to try malpractice accusations. Other professions already enjoyed that perfectly reasonable and logical privilege in the Anglo-American legal tradition, he argued. "In both army and navy, officers are tried by their peers—by themselves," and clergy, when challenged on questions "relating to their profession," were judged by other clergy. But the citizens who ended up on ordinary American juries were in no sense peers of the physicians whose efforts they were now being asked to assess. Common juries tended not to evaluate physicians, but to attack them.[19]

The malpractice crisis of mid-century also widened the gap between physicians and lawyers. That gap had already been opened by previous professional confrontations over expert medical testimony, but became a chasm in the context of malpractice. Many prominent physicians believed that the general public, and especially the poor, would not be attacking the doctors who helped them, often for little or no fee, unless they were incited by self-seeking and professionally irresponsible attorneys. By mid-century the *Boston Medical and Surgical Journal* was referring to geographical areas where actions for malpractice proliferated as "law-infected districts."[20] And there is some evidence that lawyers did encourage one another to keep expanding what appeared to be a new growth market for their services. In 1849, for example, the *American Law Journal* noted with disgust that the death of a patient during neck surgery had been ruled accidental. The *Journal* suggested that the same standards of liability should apply in medical cases that applied in any other dangerous trade. The editor likened physicians to boiler mechanics: the former should be as liable as the latter if clumsiness or lack of knowledge led to an explosion.[21] The *Journal* likewise considered deaths and complications that followed the administration of anesthetics, which were just beginning to come into widespread use among American physicians, a potentially fertile new field for lawyers to cultivate more aggressively.[22]

Physicians particularly deplored the contingent fee system, which lawyers began to employ frequently in the middle decades of the century in malpractice cases. Under that system plaintiffs risked nothing in bringing charges, then split with their attorneys some portion of any judgment they were able to win in or out of court. Physicians denounced those arrangements and tried repeatedly to have them declared illegal or unethical. But they gained little headway in the face of egalitarian arguments that every citizen had the right to bargain for legal representation on the best terms available, whether cash was in hand or in prospect. By the 1880s the American Medical Association regarded "a large proportion" of malpractice actions as having "no other foundation than a desire to extort money from the defendant sufficient to secure a good fee for the prosecuting counsel."[23] Medical journals likewise castigated what they considered to be illegal fishing expeditions long after the fact, since litigants during the 1840s were beginning to receive large settlements for alleged suffering that occurred years after the operation at issue had been performed.[24] Physicians were appalled in the early 1850s when lawyers also began to sue physicians for what they did *not* do, thereby cashing in on an implied responsibility to treat the public that popular newspapers of the 1850s also asserted.[25]

The expression of anti-lawyer sentiments, which had not been a strong theme in doctors' discourse before 1840, became both common and blatant after mid-century whenever physicians discussed malpractice. To cite a single prominent example, Eugene Sanger, a physician whose 1878 survey of medical malpractice in Maine was one of the most systematic of the early sources of information about the growing phenomenon, believed that malpractice attorneys "follow us as the shark does the emigrant ship."[26] Many of his fellow physicians before him and after were less metaphorical and less subtle. It would be easy to fill several hundred pages full of vituperative, anti-legal rhetoric from medical journals after mid-century, but there is little reason to do so here. In the twentieth century, Americans have become accustomed to strained relations and strong opinions whenever physicians discuss lawyers in the context of malpractice. Suffice it to say that the origins of those now axiomatic sentiments lie in the period between 1840 and 1860.

The malpractice crisis also began to reshape the teaching of medical jurisprudence in medical schools. To oversimplify, medical students no longer wanted their professors of medical jurisprudence to tell them how to become more effectively involved in the nation's legal system; they wanted to know how to avoid involvement altogether or at least how to escape with minimal disruption if they became involved. A near perfect illustration of that long-term shift within medical schools occurred at the Geneva Medical College exactly at mid-century.

The place, the professor, and the date all seemed symbolic. Geneva Medical College, then a prominent institution with a faculty considered among the most able in the nation, was located squarely in the middle of western New York, the area in which the malpractice crisis seemed to originate.[27] By the middle of the 1840s, in fact, western New York had already gained a legendary reputation, in the oft-quoted characterization of the *BMSJ*, as "dangerous ground for a surgeon."[28] An especially nasty malpractice case in nearby Cortland in 1841 had dragged on for years and disrupted the region's local medical societies.[29] Frank Hamilton, the well-educated and prominent physician from Buffalo who would eventually publish data demonstrating statistically predictable variations in compound fracture cases in order to undercut what he considered to be the unrealistic claims of those whose healing had been less than perfect, estimated that nine out of every ten physicians in western New York had been charged with malpractice by mid-century.[30] The students at Geneva, many of whom no doubt hoped to practice themselves in the otherwise prosperous and economically attractive districts of western New York, could not have been unaware of the malpractice crisis.

The professor who taught medical jurisprudence at Geneva through most of the 1840s was James Webster, a prototype of the able young professionals who had been drawn to the field in the 1820s and 1830s. Webster had earned his M.D. degree from the College of Physicians of Philadelphia (University of Pennsylvania) in 1824, one year after Beck first published the *Elements.* In the afterglow of Rush, Caldwell and Cooper, and under the direct influence of Griffith, Webster wrote his dissertation on medical jurisprudence. His thesis summarized the field as it then appeared to an enthusiastic student. Webster thought medical jurisprudence in 1824 had "assumed a more imposing aspect" than it ever possessed before and was becoming recognized as an "indispensable" element of future professional training in the United States.[31]

For twenty-five years, through 1849, Webster maintained his commitment to medical jurisprudence as Beck and Griffith had conceived of it. He taught the subject in Philadelphia through 1835 and in New York City from 1835 through 1842, where he delivered a course of lectures on medical jurisprudence to the Bar of New York. In 1842 Webster went to Geneva as professor of anatomy and medical jurisprudence, and when asked to deliver the ceremonial introductory lecture shortly thereafter, he had, in his own words, taken "the occasion to endeavor to impress upon the minds of a former class, my sense of the deep importance of a clear and accurate knowledge of the principles of Medical Jurisprudence to the practising physician and surgeon."[32]

In the spring of 1850 Webster was again asked to deliver the ceremonial lecture that opened each term. And as he had in the past, Webster

again took up the subject of medical jurisprudence. But this time his tone
shifted dramatically. Until he came to Geneva, Webster stated, he had never
encountered a malpractice case, though he had frequently been an expert
witness in medical cases of almost every other sort. In recent years, however, the subject of malpractice had come to overshadow all other aspects
of legal medicine. As a result, the optimism and excitement that Webster
himself had enjoyed as a student when he contemplated the possibilities of
combining medicine and law in the public interest had come to be replaced
in the minds of his Geneva students twenty-five years later by fear and
misgiving. Consequently, responsible teachers of medical jurisprudence in
western New York in 1850 could no longer afford noble dreams, Webster
suggested to his students; the time had come to face up to the fact that
medical jurisprudence courses had to address "the darker side of your professional prospects."

Once a champion of active involvement, Webster now felt obliged to
suggest "a remedy" for aspiring physicians to avoid "the attacks of the un-
principled, . . . escape persecution, and protect yourselves from the assaults of the unworthy upon your professional reputations, as well as your
peace and comfort, to say nothing of your property, if you should be so
fortunate to accumulate any."[33] His advice was to refuse fracture cases among
the poor. If the graduates proved unable to "sacrifice . . . the best feelings
of your nature," and took such cases anyway, counseled Webster, at least
make certain that "judicious witnesses" wrote down everything you did and
kept independent ongoing records of the case.[34] What a far cry from the
idealistic hopes, humane sentiments, and cooperative assumptions that in-
fused the *Elements* a quarter of a century earlier and drew Webster himself
to the field.

What happened at Geneva exactly at mid-century was repeated in less
dramatic ways throughout the United States in the decades that followed.
Legal medicine became so intertwined with the question of medical malpractice that students and professors alike began to emphasize not the positive interactions envisioned in previous decades, but practical tactics to
minimize the involvement of physicians in legal processes. Practitioners grew
less tolerant of idealistic exhortation about the ways in which law and medicine ought to cooperate and more demanding of tactical advice about staying out of legal trouble.

Two books that appeared in 1860 neatly epitomized the transition. The
first was the eleventh edition of the Becks' *Elements*. Prepared by friends
and colleagues of the late Beck brothers, the eleventh edition contained a
good deal of new material added by a number of experts in their particular
areas of interest.[35] Edward Hartshorne, a distinguished scholar of medical
jurisprudence himself and the American editor of several English texts on
the subject, reviewed the new eleventh edition for the *AJMS*. He knew "no
single work on a subject relating to medical science . . . so full of varied
and absorbing interest to every class of readers," as the *Elements*. Moreover,
the book remained "the most comprehensive and complete upon its subject

in the English language." But Hartshorne stressed twice in his relatively short discussion the telling fact that the *Elements* had become essentially "a work of reference." Hartshorne expressed the hope that future teams of editors and revisers would keep the *Elements* up-to-date and in print as a reference tool, primarily because the material it contained should be kept "within the reach of medical jurists."[36]

Hartshorne's observation that the eleventh edition of the Becks' book was useful principally to "medical jurists" was in a subtle way quite damning; by implication the book was no longer central to the concerns of most ordinary practitioners. In fact, there would be only one more edition, the twelfth, published in 1863, and it was essentially a reprint of the 1860 edition with a couple of small additions. From a virtual manifesto in 1823, the *Elements* by 1860 seemed ponderous, old-fashioned, and somewhat marginal. In its place appeared a book with an altogether different tone: John J. Elwell's *A Medico-Legal Treatise on Malpractice, Medical Evidence, and Insanity, Comprising the Elements of Medical Jurisprudence.*

Citing the surge of malpractice actions in the previous fifteen years and stressing the fact that the malpractice crisis seemed to be spreading, not receding, Elwell wanted "to strip the subject [of medical jurisprudence generally] of all . . . profitless details" and "speculative themes" in order "to furnish the medical man that necessary information respecting his legal responsibility as a practitioner and witness which he has been hitherto unable to obtain, except by the general study of law."[37] If a previous generation of doctors had needed and responded to Beck's idealistic and erudite suggestions about interesting ways to get involved with the law, the nation's physicians now needed something much more pressing: knowledge to "protect themselves from unjust prosecutions while in the legitimate pursuit of their calling."[38] Some medical societies had been calling openly for such a study during the 1850s;[39] and, using excerpts from recent malpractice cases, that was exactly what Elwell tried to give his readers. His *Malpractice*, the first serious study of its sort in the United States, thus became the first book in what would eventually be a long tradition of defensive medical jurisprudence.

Numerous review essays and an outpouring of testimonials demonstrated that Elwell had touched a nerve as sensitive in his era as the one Beck had touched in his. Walter Channing, who had long taught medical jurisprudence at Harvard in the tradition of Rush and Beck, now wrote Elwell to congratulate him on "this important addition to our professional literature" and prepared a pamphlet to alert other physicians to the excellence and significance of Elwell's volume.[40] John Ordronaux, who would shortly rise to the top ranks of New York's medico-legal experts, hailed Elwell's *Malpractice* as an outstanding work that met the most "pressing deficiency in any department of medico-legal literature."[41] The aging Robley Dunglison recommended the book to his class at Jefferson Medical College.[42] Dozens of others, including lawyers and judges, joined the chorus. The *BMSJ*, the *Cleveland Medical Gazette*, the Cincinnati *Lancet and Observer*, the Cincinnati *Medical and Surgical News*, the *Chicago Medical Journal*, the *New York Journal of Medicine*, the *American Medical Gazette*, the *American Journal of Pharmacy*, the *Boston Law Reporter*, and a surprisingly large number of regular daily newspapers, including the *New York Herald* and the *New York Times* praised the important professional job Elwell had performed.[43]

And even as the grand old *Elements* began to fade from view, the standing of Elwell's *Malpractice* soared. A second edition was issued in 1866, a revised third in 1871, and a revised fourth in 1881. Discussions of Elwell's *Malpractice* confirmed the existence of the growing gulf between law and medicine, a gulf that the early champions of medical jurisprudence had either not foreseen or tried to bridge. The *New York Medical Press*, for example, thought Elwell's book signaled an important new departure in the literature on law and medicine because it faced straightforwardly the reality that now presented itself. Law and medicine had evolved into mutually incompatible professions. Consequently, "It is . . . *necessary* that [a doctor] knows what he should say and do in a contingency which may happen, and unexpectedly, any time," especially in "civil suits for malpractice." Unfortunately, "none of the medical jurisprudences [i.e. previous works on the subject] have been at all sufficiently practical" in such matters and the medical profession, as a result, was suffering. Old idealistic efforts to bridge what Elwell saw as the "chasm" between law and medicine had become too dangerous to continue; Elwell wanted to help doctors avoid falling in. The *Press* considered Elwell's material valuable for lawyers, but absolutely "paramount to our medical brethren."[44]

Even those few experts in medical jurisprudence who disliked Elwell's approach to the subject acknowledged the fact that he and his book signaled something of a new era for the field. Stephen Smith, a medical activist, public health crusader, and politically minded professional who embraced broad views of professional interaction and became influential in New York City health policy and New York State medical reform after the Civil War, was among Elwell's few unenthusiastic reviewers. Smith may simply have been disappointed that Elwell got there first, however, for Smith had been at work on a similar volume himself.[45] Nonetheless, Smith ended his long analytical discussion of *Malpractice* with a begrudging recognition that Elwell had "done much to establish the principles which are to lead to the development of malpractice in medicine as an important branch of medical jurisprudence."[46] Smith could hardly have known how prescient that was.

Elwell's work was quickly joined in the medico-legal marketplace by nationally important and well-received studies that accepted most of his priorities and tried to improve upon his understanding of malpractice. The best of them was Ordronaux's own book, *The Jurisprudence of Medicine in Its Relation to the Law of Contracts, Torts and Evidence*, which appeared in 1869. Like Elwell, Ordronaux held formal degrees both in law and in medicine, having graduated from Harvard Law School in 1852 and studied medicine later in the decade with the specific purpose of taking up medical jurisprudence as a specialty. He was appointed to a chair in the subject at Columbia

Law School in 1861 and continued to teach there until the end of the century. Also like Elwell, Ordronaux projected a distinctly cautious and defensive attitude toward his own specialty.[47] Milo McClelland's popular *Civil Malpractice*, which appeared in 1873, further emphasized the fact that the dangers of litigation had become the central concern of medical jurisprudence.[48]

By the end of the nineteenth century medico-legal experts were lionized in the medical profession not for helping physicians interact with the law in socially progressive ways, but for keeping physicians out of legal entanglements and defending them against charges of malpractice. The well-known *National Cyclopaedia of American Biography* specifically recognized in its index only four individuals prominent during the late nineteenth and early twentieth century for their efforts in the field of medical jurisprudence. One was Ordronaux (1830–1908). Another was James T. Lewis (1865–1935), who engineered a merger of New York's two rival medical societies in the early 1920s and "defended many of the most prominent medical men in the state and argued cases before many courts. The successful defense of over 1000 medical malpractice actions earned him general recognition as a man with a unique combination of medical and legal talent."[49] The small number of people whose chief fame resulted from medical jurisprudence was striking enough in itself, but even more significant was the fact that half the tiny group, Ordronaux as a theorist and Lewis as a practitioner, owed much of their fame as medico-legal experts to their involvement in the question of malpractice.

The great wave of malpractice suits that broke upon the shores of American legal medicine near mid-century never really ebbed. If anything, the swell increased, since malpractice actions continued to rise both in absolute numbers and in rates relative to population. Initial panic abated somewhat as physicians moved to counter the specific accusations associated with orthopedic surgery, largely through statistical analyses of reasonable success rates. Physicians also began to experiment with various self-protective mechanisms, including medical society legal defense funds, medical society pledges of mutual defense, and the first malpractice insurance schemes.[50] In that context, the rise of malpractice litigation at mid-century certainly helped accelerate cooperation and consolidation among American physicians.[51] But the surge of malpractice actions at mid-century dealt the field of medical jurisprudence a heavy blow to be sure, a blow that still staggers American professionals.

CHAPTER NINE

Toxicology on Trial: The Hendrickson Case

In 1841 T.R. Beck began a major article in the nationally prominent *American Journal of the Medical Sciences* by observing that two areas of activity had in recent years emerged as "the primary objects in legal medicine." The two were "the detection of the principal mineral poisons in minute quantities" and "the nature of insanity as excusing from the responsibility of criminal acts." The occasion of his observation was a long review essay that surveyed the nine most recent publications of significance on the first of those two subjects, poisons and their detection. He wove through the essay "a condensed historical view of the discoveries and improvements that have been made" in forensic toxicology, and he was clearly proud and excited about what he regarded as solid advances. A professional field he had helped cultivate for the previous twenty years seemed to be yielding ever richer harvests.[1]

During the next twenty years, however, both the subject of forensic toxicology and the subject of medico-legal insanity would encounter grave difficulties in the United States. Instead of continuing as sources of advancement for the general field of medical jurisprudence, and instead of encouraging further professional involvement in medico-legal issues, those two "primary objects in legal medicine" would themselves begin to raise crippling problems. In the field of forensic toxicology the problems surfaced most dramatically in a famous court case that broke shortly after midcentury, symbolically enough, in the aging Beck's own city. Before it was over, this case would rivet the attention of professionals interested in medical jurisprudence as few trials in American history had done to that point, and it would expose to the public in stark terms many of their worst nightmares.

First public notice of the case could hardly have been less sensational. Tucked in the "local items" column of the *Albany Evening Journal* for March 10, 1853, along with the arrest of a twelve-year-old boy for stealing chickens, the spring flow of ice on the Hudson, and other events of comparable magnitude, was an announcement that a man named John Hendrickson, Jr., from the nearby village of Bethlehem, was being held on suspicion of having murdered his wife four days earlier. The circumstances surrounding his wife's demise were sufficiently muddled that the Albany County sheriff had decided to let the man attend his wife's funeral before serving the warrant for his arrest. But further investigation was under way. The *Journal* attributed the prisoner's predicament in large part to "the suspicions of the neighbors"; the man's marriage had apparently been rocky, and some of the citizens of the outlying hamlets wanted an inquiry when his wife expired suddenly and without obvious cause.[2]

Hendrickson was twenty years old; his wife Maria had been nineteen. The couple had been married for two years, but in a relationship that was far from idyllic. Maria's father, Lawrence Van Dusen, had served as Albany County Clerk and was widely assumed to be a wealthy man; Maria's mother was a respected and religious matron. Young Hendrickson, by contrast, had acquired a well-deserved reputation for flirting and fighting. Though the Van Dusens opposed their daughter's desire to marry Hendrickson, they did not prevent the wedding in January 1851.[3]

Since Hendrickson had no job, the couple lived with the Van Dusens in the town of Clarksville. Maria became pregnant almost immediately. While his wife was approaching term, Hendrickson committed "a gross assault" on another young woman who lived in the Van Dusens' village, and Hendrickson bolted half in flight and half in banishment to Corning, New York, in the western part of the state. Hendrickson returned to his wife shortly after the birth of their baby and promptly communicated to her a venereal disease he had picked up in Corning. To make matters worse, the infant was found dead in bed with John and Maria under circumstances that were inexplicable. Though this may have been a tragedy rather than a crime (SIDS was neither recognized nor understood, and infant death from many causes was an all-too-common phenomenon in nineteenth-century America), it did not make Hendrickson look good. Maria's father had had enough. He ordered Hendrickson out of his house and redrafted his will in such a way that his son-in-law would never benefit from his substantial estate. Hendrickson returned to live at his own father's house, and the couple remained separated but in touch with one another through 1852.

During January 1853 John and Maria reconciled. In February Maria left her parental home, where her husband was neither comfortable nor welcome, and moved into the Hendrickson household in Bethlehem, a village four miles away. Owing in large part to her venereal disease, Maria was unwell and uncomfortable. Hendrickson, not one to be deterred, repaired to the arms of others, including a bar strumpet in Schenectady to whom he pledged marriage complete with an exchange of rings and tintypes, in return for a night in her bed. By the end of February, Maria was apparently planning to leave Hendrickson for good and intended to move back in with her recently widowed mother at the end of the first week of

March. Before she could do that, however, she was found dead in the bed that she shared with her husband.

Witnesses would eventually establish the sequence of events on the night Maria died, as well as what followed during the next several days. John and Maria retired to an upstairs room by themselves on the night of Sunday, March 6. Maria may or may not have been feeling poorly; that was later disputed. At about 2:00 a.m., according to his own testimony, John awoke, asked his wife to shift over to give him more room in the bed, and discovered her insensible. He then shouted for others in the household to bring him a candle, and the Hendrickson family first tried to revive Maria, then determined that she was dead. There were six other members of the Hendrickson family in the house that night: John's mother and father, his brother and sister-in-law, and two of his sisters. John sat silently on a trunk at the foot of the bed for a prolonged period of time, while the family sent for advice and assistance from neighbors, the closest of whom were a quarter of a mile away. The neighbors corroborated the time of death and the condition of the body, lying stiff on the bed in a clean nightgown.

Monday morning the body was placed in a coffin and transported to Maria's mother's house in Clarksville. The Van Dusens and their friends, unwilling to accept the Hendricksons' story without additional inquiry, sent for Dr. Thomas Smith, one of the coroners of Albany County, who in turn asked Dr. John Swinburne and Dr. Samuel Ingraham to accompany him. They viewed the body on Monday evening, empaneled a coroner's jury on the spot, took preliminary testimony from Hendrickson himself, and ordered that a post-mortem examination be conducted. On Tuesday morning

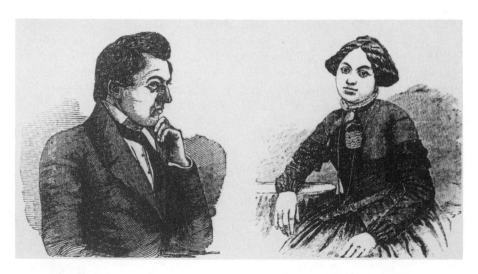

John Hendrickson, Jr., and his wife Maria. From Barnes and Hevenor, *Trial of John Hendrickson, Jr., For the Murder of His Wife Maria* (Albany, 1853).

the three of them conducted the post-mortem, laying Maria's body on some boards in her mother's front room. They made a preliminary finding of death by poisoning and removed a section of Maria's intestines to deliver to a colleague in Albany, Dr. James H. Salisbury, for further analysis. On Sunday, March 13, five days after their first autopsy, the same three officials had Maria's body exhumed, removed most of the rest of the intestines, and delivered those as well to Dr. Salisbury.[4]

After two weeks of chemical testing, Salisbury confirmed the unanimous opinion already reached by Swinburne, Ingraham, and Coroner Smith: Maria Hendrickson had been poisoned and the agent of her destruction was aconite, or more precisely aconitine, the alkaloid thought to be the active ingredient of aconite.[5] Aconitum, known also as monkshood, wolfsbane, and blue rocket (after the distinctive spike of flowers atop the plant from which it is derived), was an ancient poison mentioned in several classical texts.[6] It was also used medicinally, particularly in minute doses by homoeopathic physicians, and hence it was available in ordinary drugstores.[7] Maria, in fact, favored homoeopathic physicians herself and formerly had taken minute amounts of aconite in pill form. Druggists in Albany testified that they routinely prepared tincture of aconite by soaking the plant's roots in alcohol, that the tincture was for sale to anyone willing to pay sixpence an ounce for it, and that a man answering Hendrickson's description had inquired after and purchased some a week before Maria's demise. On the basis of this evidence the grand jury indicted Hendrickson for murder, and the local district attorney, Andrew J. Colvin, who had a reputation as a zealous prosecutor, began to prepare what would appear to be a strong case. Lest he slip, however, District Attorney Colvin induced none other than Levi S. Chatfield, attorney general of the state of New York, to join his team.

Hendrickson's trial began on Monday, June 13, 1853, a little more than three months after his wife's death. District Attorney Colvin had by this time amassed additional circumstantial evidence against the accused. He had witnesses who not only confirmed the tentative identification made by the Albany druggists but revealed that Hendrickson had earlier asked about prussic acid, then popularly regarded as the quickest and most lethal poison available. He had witnesses who testified further to Hendrickson's unsavory character. He had the chance observations of passers-by on the night of Maria's death, who opened the possibility that a candle had been alight in Hendrickson's bedroom an hour or two before he raised the alarm, thereby suggesting that the murderer cleaned up the vomit and the general disarray of his wife's death agonies before feigning alarm and calling for others. On this last point the District Attorney was even able to produce a laundress who testified that a nightgown from the Hendrickson household, later sent to her for ironing, stank so strongly that it made her nauseated.

The ultimate strength of the prosecutor's case against Hendrickson, however, continued to rest upon the conclusions of his medical experts, all of whom asserted on the basis of their various examinations and tests that Maria died after ingesting a lethal dose of aconite. None of the other peripheral circumstances, however damning, could prove beyond reasonable doubt that Maria had fallen victim to an unnatural agent of death, and an American jury—legendarily reluctant to convict in capital cases—would probably not take a man's life on the basis of sorry tales, corrupt character, and a miserable marriage. But on the crucial ground of medical evidence, District Attorney Colvin appeared secure. Dr. Ingraham was little known, a country practitioner from the Van Dusens' village, a friend of the family who happened to be available and on the scene when the coroner was sent for. But in Smith, Swinburne, and Salisbury, Colvin had a formidable lineup.

Thomas Smith had practiced medicine in Albany over eight years and was currently serving as one of the county's official coroners. He had far more experience with post-mortem examinations than typical American coroners, having attended, according to his own estimate, about forty of them during the year immediately preceding those conducted on the body of Maria Hendrickson. Smith frequently assisted Dr. Alden March, one of Albany's nationally prominent medical educators, when the latter was called upon to conduct post-mortem examinations. Smith testified proudly that "a satisfactory cause of death" had been discovered in nineteen of the twenty cases for which he had so far been legally responsible as a coroner. He had been careful and systematic in his procedures, he was a veteran witness, and he had an enviable record to preserve.

John Swinburne, who accompanied Smith to the Van Dusen home and assisted the Coroner and Dr. Ingraham with the post-mortem examinations, had never before been a witness in a case where the detection of poison was at issue. But what he lacked in courtroom experience, he made up for in credentials. Swinburne, then thirty-three years old, had graduated from the Albany Medical College, where he was thoroughly familiar with the medical jurisprudential teachings of T.R. Beck and Amos Dean. Most importantly, Swinburne had conducted the Anatomical Department of the Albany Medical College for two years after his graduation, then opened a private dissecting room in his own house, where he had been performing post-mortem examinations for the last three years. He testified that he regularly spent his leisure time dissecting bodies and that he had "performed many of the post mortem exams for the authorities of the County of Albany, for the past five years." It is doubtful whether anyone in the state was more familiar with the signs of death than Swinburne, who had already performed nine other autopsies during the three months since the death of Maria Hendrickson.

The prosecution's star witness, however, was James H. Salisbury, the person to whom Coroner Smith had delivered Maria's viscera for further analysis. Though Salisbury was only twenty-eight years old, he had a medical degree, a medical practice, and previous experience as a witness in a trial for murder involving poison. In that instance he had successfully isolated arsenic in the stomach of a woman whose husband, like Hendrickson, had also been indicted for her murder. What made Salisbury an especially powerful witness, however, was his well-certified standing as an expert medical chemist. He had been studying chemistry since he was fourteen years old, and he had attended the region's best-known schools, including Albany Medical College and Rensselaer Institute. Above all else, his "main business" in recent years had been "in the labratory *[sic]*." He had been Chemist to the State Geologic Survey, an agency that Beck had been influential in establishing, and was presently in charge of the chemical laboratory of the State Agricultural Society. In short, Salisbury was the closest thing New York had to an official state chemist, and one of relatively few individuals in the entire nation earning a living as a laboratory researcher outside academe.

Moreover, Salisbury was interested in poisons generally and in aconite specifically.[8] He had been devoting special attention to aconite for the past two years, he confirmed, both because he was interested in the substance for its medicinal potential and because aconite posed a scientific challenge. Little was known about the ways it affected living organisms, great chemists disagreed about its fundamental properties, and it was considered one of the most difficult poisons to detect once it entered the body. Salisbury had conducted numerous experiments, mostly on cats, and was convinced that he could isolate and identify the substance. He swore that he had done exactly that when his friend Dr. Swinburne, who had been aware of Salisbury's research on aconite, directed Coroner Smith to take Maria's viscera to the Agricultural Society laboratory.

Unfortunately for the prosecution, virtually no one else in the scientific world was prepared to defend Salisbury's chemical claims. Aconitine was classified as a vegetable alkaloid, and no chemist had yet devised a satisfactory method of isolating vegetable alkaloids once they entered the body, much less aconitine specifically. Indeed, the Parisian College of Pharmacy had offered a large reward for the discovery of tests that would detect the presence of vegetable alkaloids, but the prize remained unclaimed. It was on this point that the defense would ultimately concentrate its counterattack.

John Hendrickson, Sr., had retained Albany lawyers Henry G. Wheaton and William J. Hadley to defend his son. They did their best to tear away at the heavy veil of circumstantial evidence enshrouding their client by trying to create some doubt about the exact time when the passers-by thought they saw a light in the Hendrickson home; by suggesting the anti-Hendrickson prejudice of many of the witnesses who testified about John and Maria's wretched marriage; by challenging whether the soiled nightgown had even belonged to Maria; and by bringing John's kin to the stand to corroborate his version of what happened (and what did not happen; none of them claimed to have heard any struggles or vomiting) the night of Maria's death. Yet Wheaton and Hadley realized that their best chance to save John Hendrickson, Jr., from the gallows was to launch a frontal assault against the prosecution's medical experts.

Wheaton opened the counterattack by denouncing "the presumptious [*sic*] positiveness of the [prosecution's] medical witnesses." They were young and brash and wrong and displayed upon the stand "the zeal of partisans" rather than the spirit of fair-minded inquiry. Significantly, Wheaton blamed the essential nature of the medical profession itself—"the manner in which their professional business is conducted," as he put it—for the kind of testimony entered against his client. Unlike attorneys, whose positions were constantly tested and reversed in open courts, physicians had "no tribunal" where "their professional opinions" could be reviewed and corrected by "a body able and authorized to decide upon them." With unerring instinct Wheaton went directly to the French model, which had long been dear to the early champions of state-supported medical jurisprudence in the United States. "Gentlemen," he apprised the jury, "they tried the experiment several years ago in France, of executing men on the truth of chemical theories," but found it impossible to "bring the dead men to life, when the theory upon the faith of which they were executed, was found untrue and exploded." Wheaton claimed that the courts of France had "profited by the lesson" and clearly so should professionals in the United States.

Wheaton and Hadley eventually brought three medical witnesses of their own to the stand to try to counterbalance the evidence offered by Smith, Swinburne, and Salisbury. One of the most fascinating undercurrents in this highly charged and symbolic trial was the quality of those three witnesses. Two were from Albany: Barent P. Staats and Ebenezer Emmons. The third was Lawrence Reid from New York City.

Staats was an aged practitioner whose biochemical opinions had been formed in a much earlier era. He had previously tangled with the Albany medical establishment over the cause of death in another well-publicized incident in the city, and he became hopelessly confused and self-contradictory upon cross-examination. He was, in short, an extraordinarily weak witness. District Attorney Colvin had no difficulty subjecting Staats to savage and sarcastic ridicule. Emmons was a more credible witness, but he was the man whom Salisbury replaced as head of the state laboratory, and he had to be subpoenaed to take the stand. The essence of his testimony was that he doubted anyone could chemically isolate a vegetable alkaloid in the manner Salisbury described.

The third expert for the defense was Lawrence Reid from New York City. Although he identified himself as having been Professor of Medical Chemistry in the College of Pharmacy in New York for seven years, cross examination revealed that he had been dismissed from that post. He now claimed a similar professorship in the Pennsylvania Medical College of Philadelphia, but worked and lived in New York. The only thing he had ever published was a method of making his "blue pills"; he was not certain of his own age; and he could not recall the details of his brother's textbook on chemistry, though he said he assigned it in his classes and followed its procedures when doing analyses himself.[9] Worse, he was perilously close to being an early prototype of the professional expert witness, for he had testified "in most of the capital cases in New York for the last ten years." There were rumors openly referred to in court that Hendrickson, Sr., through an intermediary, had promised Reid $400 to take the stand in behalf of his son; to put that sum in perspective, the county paid its own expert witnesses no more than $25, notwithstanding the fact that the latter had also expended considerable time in conducting the post-mortem examinations.

The inference is inescapable that the established medical community of Albany would not come forward to refute Smith, Swinburne, and Salisbury. Their reluctance cannot be attributed to lack of awareness or lack of interest. On the seventh day of the trial, the day the prosecution began to call its medical witnesses, the court reporter noted that "the room was filled with spectators, including . . . many prominent members of the medical profession." On the thirteenth day, when Reid took the stand, the same reporter sensed that "the interest, excited by the difference of opinion existing between the medical and chemical profession, is accompanied with no little excitement; and among those present we noticed several well known to the medical and scientific world." At one point in the trial, when there was an outside chance that Alden March might be called from the audience, he left hurriedly on "professional business." The most charitable interpretation to place upon the behavior of the members of the Albany medical community was that they believed John Hendrickson guilty, that they believed on the basis of material and anatomical indications that his victim had been poisoned, and that they believed little would be gained in debating whether or not one of their most promising young professionals had actually isolated the specific chemical agent that killed Maria Hendrickson.

The defense, lacking any incentive for restraint and no doubt frustrated by the poor quality of the witnesses available to them, lashed out at the most vulnerable aspects of the prosecution's expert testimony. Wheaton went especially at Salisbury, whom he accused of careerist ambitions and perverted professionalism. Salisbury had made an inexcusable mistake in not saving the aconitine he claimed to have isolated from Maria's remains. He said he tasted it, tested it, and satisfied himself that he had succeeded; then inexplicably administered it to a cat in order to double check that it was the poisonous agent he was after. Even then, the cat did not die. Wheaton, in a splendid bit of nineteenth-century courtroom oratory, homed in on this sequence of events in his peroration:

> Just look at it—the confidence of this Dr. Salisbury. He, so he says has discovered this aconitine; he has solved the great problem; and yet calls no one in to see his discovery, or to confirm it. He is in too great a hurry; he cannot wait; but administers it all to a cat. He could not wait, he had such a desire to send his name abroad; he could not stop a single moment; could not bring a particle of it into court for us to see it, or taste it; but he gives it all to a cat! . . .
>
> Ambition urges him on. If the prisoner is convicted, his name goes

forth linked with this case; it goes abroad, amongst scientific men throughout the world, that he has solved the problem all others have failed in. . . . But without your verdict, all this has been in vain. . . .

To the cat again: The doctor says he gave it all the substance he discovered; and yet, after about two hours of trifling sickness, it recovered, and then it required a further dose of six drops of tincture of aconite to kill it! Now the 50th part of a grain of aconitine is sufficient to endanger human life; yet he says he obtained from a 20th to a 25th part of a grain from the viscera submitted to him for examination, gave it all to the cat, the cat did not vomit, retained it all, and in three hours was well. What a cat! What a doctor! What an opinion, founded upon such facts!

The cat should have died out of deference to the Dr.'s opinion, or the Dr. should have given up his opinion out of deference to the life of the cat.

The Honorable Levi S. Chatfield himself, attorney general of the state of New York, responded for the prosecution late in the afternoon of July 5, the trial's twentieth day. The attorney general first complimented the jurors for their patience, then began his summation with the arresting, if hyperbolic, proclamation: "This is a case, gentlemen, of more importance than has ever occurred in this country, and of as great importance as any that have ever occurred in the civilized world." And the reason for such cosmic import lay in "the medical and chemical questions which have arisen there." Chatfield did not address those questions directly that afternoon, preferring to remind the jury of the strong circumstantial case against Hendrickson and to plant in the jury's mind the likelihood that the entire Hendrickson household was involved in a cover-up. But the next day the attorney general spoke from nine o'clock in the morning until six o'clock in the evening, and the clear purpose of his oratory was the rehabilitation of the prosecution's experts. As Chatfield put it, Wheaton had "thrown down the glove" in his effort "to crush Drs. Swinburne and Salisbury" and the attorney general was ready to "take it up, and meet him on the ground of their credibility."

Chatfield mustered three overriding arguments in defense of his experts. The first was obvious and relatively easy for a lawyer of his skill and experience. It involved marshaling a combination of ridicule, insinuation, hearsay, and fact against the weak witnesses called by the defense. It produced precisely the sort of withering effect that so many physicians dreaded when they were forced to contemplate testifying in court. In considering our experts, Chatfield was suggesting to the jury, do not lose sight of the fact that those called by the other side to refute them were pathetic.

The second argument was both clever and more revealing to modern historians. Chatfield implicitly granted the anti-expert, anti-elitist bias of the general American public and turned it to his advantage. In essence, he argued that his experts were neither theoretical in their orientations nor elite in their backgrounds (both of which would have been pejorative), but were oracles instead of practical experience and first-hand knowledge. "John Swinburne was not put on that stand because he had a diploma in his pocket, not because he had been born with a silver spoon in his mouth, and been reared in the lap of luxury," but because he was "an intelligent, scientific and honest man" who embodied the "sound, practical sense" and "incorruptibility" of the nation's "middling classes." Swinburne, a veteran who had "dissected at least one hundred and fifty bodies," was "learned and intelligent in spite of colleges." Salisbury, in turn, knew "more about aconitine than any man living" because he had gone beyond theory and books to "experiments which he made for the purpose of satisfying himself." Paradoxically, Chatfield was trying to strengthen the testimony of his experts by disassociating them as individuals from the groups generally considered expert in their fields. This was to some extent necessary because they claimed to be able to do something the textbooks considered impossible, but impressive also as a method of undercutting Wheaton's attacks on their professional ambitions.

The third argument the attorney general made in defense of the prosecution's expert witnesses was the most intriguing for present purposes, and quickly turned into the most troublesome. "The physicians of Albany," Chatfield asserted, "are highly intelligent [especially in the realms of medical jurisprudence, he might have added], and willing to assume all reasonable responsibility." Yet they did not come forward to refute Swinburne or Salisbury. "I cannot for a moment believe that, watching this case with intense professional interest, they would have stood quietly by and seen a fellow being sacrificed by professional falsehood." In short, the attorney general was appealing to the implicit existence of a professional consensus; a body of persons whose collective, agreed-upon opinions acted as both a sanction and a check against the individual judgment of its members.

Presiding Judge Richard P. Marvin conferred with his associate justices, Cornelius Vanderzee and Samuel O. Schoonmaker, and decided to charge the jury the evening after Chatfield concluded. This he did, stressing the importance of the case generally and of the "medical and chemical evidence" specifically. The jury deliberated that night and most of the next day before returning a verdict of guilty. Judge Marvin denied a defense motion to delay sentence, then ordered that Hendrickson be hanged August 26, seven weeks and a day later. In his unusually lengthy remarks at the sentencing, Judge Marvin underlined his belief that "science advances—as it unfolds to the student the great storehouse of knowledge, and lets man penetrate into the very arcana of nature." In Hendrickson's case, Marvin asserted, science had made another advance, for it was science that detected a previously undetectable poison and it was science that "unerringly" pointed Hendrickson out as the guilty individual. He hoped that the trial would have a salutary effect on public opinion and cut down on the number of murders. "In this day of light" no one could commit murder "without leaving the evidence of guilt." The practitioners and processes of medical jurisprudence would find them out.

Hardly had Hendrickson been convicted, however, before his remarkable case began to elicit the attention of professionals outside Albany. But it did so in a way that must have made the champions of medical jurisprudence everywhere extremely uneasy. Two events set the stage for the national furor that followed. First, Hendrickson's defense team won a temporary stay of their client's execution pending an appeal. Second, a transcript of the testimony taken in the Hendrickson case began to circulate widely throughout the country. Ironically, this transcript had been co-published by the assistant district attorney of Albany County, who was proud of the "prominence [the Hendrickson case] must ever occupy in the criminal annals of the country," for it was the first time prosecutors had won a conviction by demonstrating the cause of death to have been one of "the POISONOUS VEGETABLE ALKALOIDS, which thus far appear to have eluded that certainty of detection which has been obtained with reference to the metallic poisons."

Among those who read the transcript was David A. Wells, who would later establish a lasting reputation as a political economist, but was then twenty-five years old, living in Cambridge, Massachusetts, and deeply immersed in the study of chemistry.[10] Wells was convinced that Salisbury had erred in his chemical testimony; that aconitine could not be detected in the manner Salisbury described on the stand. Though Wells apparently knew none of the principals in the case, he took it upon himself to help coordinate a public rebuttal of the prosecution's medical and chemical evidence. He wrote to many of the leading chemists in the country, urging them to come forward publicly against what he viewed as a wrongful conviction, and he prepared a long paper of his own in criticism of his two Albany contemporaries.

Wells eventually published his critique in the *Boston Medical and Surgical Journal* under the title "Interesting Case of Medical Jurisprudence—Poisoning by Aconite."[11] In his paper Wells reviewed the literature on the subject, including the research conducted in Paris by the three toxicological giants Orfila, Raspail, and Flaudin, the extensive investigations undertaken in Edinburgh by Fleming and in England by Christison, and the most recent contributions to the field by Stass of Brussels. On this basis Wells argued that there were many skillful chemists besides Salisbury who had looked closely at the properties of aconite, but none had obtained the results Salisbury claimed. Many, in fact, obtained results that contradicted Salisbury's conclusions. Wells assailed Salisbury's procedures as well, and agreed with Hendrickson's defense attorneys that failure to save the purported aconitine was inexplicable and unforgivable. Wells surmised that the procedures Salisbury used had produced a phosphate and lactate of lime, which would taste just as Salisbury described it, and would make the poor cat uncomfortable for awhile without killing her, which was precisely what happened. Finally, he attacked the corroborating medical evidence offered by Swinburne, who was evidently unaware of the contradictory and uncertain physiological effects of aconitine previously observed by physicians who examined the bodies of persons known to have ingested it by accident.

In the meantime Wells's letters to others began to have dramatic effect. A formal statement of protest was drafted by Wells's friend, Augustus A. Hayes, assayer to the Commonwealth of Massachusetts, who intended to send it to the governor of New York with a recommendation that the latter either order a retrial for Hendrickson or commute his sentence altogether. The substance of the protest alleged that Hendrickson had been convicted on unreliable evidence, and in support of their opinion Wells and Hayes solicited an impressive list of American chemists to join them as co-signers of their statement: Charles T. Jackson, another assayer employed by Massachusetts, and John Bacon, Jr., a physician who also served as chemist to Massachusetts General Hospital, both from the Boston area; Benjamin Silliman, Sr., Benjamin Silliman, Jr., John A. Porter, and James D. Dana, all of Yale (the last was also sitting president of the American Association for the Advancement of Science); John Torrey, professor of chemistry at the College of Physicians and Surgeons of New York, Edward N. Kent and James Chilton, also from New York, and E.H. Ellet, now living in New York but formerly professor of chemistry at South Carolina College (the institution whose medical jurisprudential tradition had been built by Thomas Cooper); James Lawrence Smith, professor of chemistry at the Louisville Medical College in Kentucky; L.D. Gale and George Schaffer, both chemical examiners for the United States Patent Office, and five other scientists from Washington, D.C., including Joseph Henry of the Smithsonian Institution, Beck's most famous student. Other toxicologists, including Emmons, who had appeared only under subpoena at the trial, preferred to write separate letters of their own to the governor, some of which detailed their repeated failure to obtain the results Salisbury claimed on the stand, even when they followed Salisbury's procedures exactly.[12] That sort of pressure was hard to ignore, and it began to bear heavily upon the previously silent professional community of Albany.

Adding to that pressure was a public letter from Alonzo Clark, sitting president of the New York State Medical Society, to the dean of the Albany professional community, T.R. Beck.[13] Clark, professor of pathological anatomy at the College of Physicians and Surgeons of New York, was less concerned about the chemical evidence that upset Wells than he was about the conclusions Swinburne and Smith deduced from the observations they made at their two post-mortem examinations. Clark put his views carefully but unambiguously: "I am fully persuaded that the inferential opinions . . . expressed by these medical witnesses are not warranted by the facts presented in their testimony." Worse, he was "pained and oppressed with the conviction that the medical witnesses for the prosecution have . . . abused the confidence with which criminal courts so often compliment the man of science."[14] When Clark's letter was made public, seven of Albany's most prominent physicians, including Alden March, the nationally famous professor of surgery at Albany Medical College and later president of the American Medical Association, Thomas W. Hun, the professor of physiology and materia medica, and James H. Armsby, the professor of anatomy, broke their silence and publicly endorsed Clark's reservations.[15]

As if to lend official sanction to Clark's letter, the New York Pathological Society assembled and resolved formally that the statements made by Swinburne "concerning the post-mortem appearances" of Maria Hendrickson "in no wise justify the opinion that death was preceded by vomiting, or was caused by the administration of aconite." More pointedly, they added, "the post-mortem examination as detailed by Dr. Swinburne is faulty." That resolution was endorsed unanimously by the association and also went to the authorities at Albany.[16]

Charles A. Lee, a prominent and influential professor of pathology and materia medica in Buffalo, and a pioneer in the field of medical statistics, brought the Hendrickson case to an even wider audience in the pages of the Philadelphia-based *American Journal of the Medical Sciences*.[17] Lee offered his opinions in the form of a lengthy review of the published transcript of the trial. Lee's detailed critique addressed both the chemical and the anatomical issues in the case with devastating effect. Lee was particularly troubled as well by the fact that the "confident and positive" manner and demeanor of Swinburne and Salisbury had apparently carried more influence with the jury than "the more careful and judicious testimony . . . of men of age, professional skill, and enlarged experience." In other words, it seemed to be superficial impression that mattered rather than scientific rigor; foolhardy confidence seemed to triumph over professional caution. That, of course, was profoundly unsettling to men like Lee, who favored systematic, objective, and state-supported medical jurisprudence. A case like Hendrickson's, lamented Lee in the last line of his review, "makes us question, at times, whether the boasted right and privilege of trial by jury, be, indeed, a blessing or a curse."[18]

By the spring of 1854 Hendrickson's case had become a national *cause célèbre* among professionals in the United States interested in medico-legal issues. George H. Tucker of the Society of Statistical Medicine published a paper in the *New York Medical Journal* in March that year surveying all known cases of aconitine poisoning in the United States and Europe. His survey was clearly occasioned by the Hendrickson furor, since the subject of aconitine poisoning had apparently never been discussed in an American medical journal prior to Hendrickson's trial.[19] It was certainly being discussed now, however, as publications like the rival *New York Medical Times* printed reports of aconite poisoning cases in 1854 and 1855 for a readership that probably never thought about such cases before 1853.[20] Professional interest on this scale heightened tensions in Albany, especially after the New York Supreme Court and the New York Court of Appeals both affirmed the verdict of the original Albany Court of Oyer and Terminer.[21] Hendrickson's revised date of execution, Friday May 5, was drawing closer and closer.

The governor to whom the nation's medico-legal experts were directing their collective protests was the Democrat Horatio Seymour. Governor Seymour was in a more difficult position than might at first appear. On the one hand, the national protest he confronted would suggest that some sort of retrial might be in order, even if he was not inclined to let the unsavory Hendrickson go free as a matter of principle. On the other hand, Seymour's own attorney general had personally taken charge of the original prosecution now being protested, the conviction had been affirmed through the state's highest appellate courts, and there was no question that popular opinion in Albany County among ordinary citizens was overwhelmingly against clemency for Hendrickson. The *Albany Evening Journal* put the last consideration baldly and defiantly in an editorial reply to the letter from Hayes and his many prominent co-signers: "No capital conviction among us was ever more in conformity with public sentiment than this of HENDRICK-SON."[22]

On May 1, the *Evening Journal* printed a long "Reply" by District Attorney Andrew J. Colvin to the professional protests flowing into the city from elsewhere around the country.[23] Colvin considered the protest letters *ex parte* statements orchestrated and pushed into print by the defense team. The other side had lost in open court, failed on appeal, and was now desperately attempting "to frame a judgment which will operate upon the Executive." The district attorney had nothing but contempt for Alden March and the other six local physicians who had publicly conceded Clark's condemnation of Swinburne's post-mortem observations; they had all been present in court at the time the testimony was taken and should have come forward then, if that is what they really believed. Their opinions on this matter were not to be trusted now, after the fact, without cross-examination.

In contrast, alleged the district attorney's "Reply," T.R. Beck was among those who all along continued to believe that Hendrickson poisoned his wife, though Beck thought the poison was something other than aconitine. In that opinion Colvin considered Beck wrong, but Beck had at least been consistent and straightforward throughout the controversy and would not contradict the ultimate conclusion that Hendrickson deserved to go to the gallows. Moreover, the district attorney could cite in support of the prosecution's evidence some outside professional opinion of his own, including a letter from T.G. Geoghegan, professor of forensic medicine at the Royal College of Surgeons in Dublin, Ireland.[24] Geoghegan considered the post-mortem indications described by Swinburne not inconsistent with four reports of aconite poisoning that had come to his attention. The case had, indeed, become internationally famous, just as the attorney general ten months before had told the jury it would.

On May 3, the *Evening Journal* carried a final letter from Wells, his fourth public epistle on the subject. Wells volunteered to come to Albany and demonstrate the chemical errors in the prosecution's case. But that same issue of the paper also carried a letter from Governor Seymour to the sheriff of Albany County. The letter was dated May 2, and it conveyed to the sheriff the governor's decision not to intervene in the course of justice mandated by the courts.[25] Governor Seymour, whose biographers identify him as an unwavering disciple of Jeffersonian and Jacksonian principles, had resolved in this instance as in so many others to leave the decision to the local population that made it and would be most directly affected by it in the short run.[26] Judge Marvin had proved correct in his admonition to Hendrickson at the time of his first sentencing: "You ought not to expect a pardon. In your case, Hendrickson, the Executive will never pardon. It is best that you should understand this now. No Governor, in your case, will interpose his pardon. You should, then, prepare for death."[27]

On Friday morning May 5, 1854, John Hendrickson, Jr., was hanged in the courtyard of the Albany County jail. A special reporter for the *New York Times* estimated the crowd around the building at between 2000 and 3000 people. Many country people had come into the city for the event, and a large press corps was present. Local militia units had been deployed that morning, but were unable to prevent a near riot as would-be viewers pushed forward for the few spots from which the actual execution could be seen. There had even been rumors that the Hendrickson family might attempt a last-minute rescue, but nothing of that sort took place. The hanging was described in detail by the popular press and subsequently remarked upon in many of the nation's medical journals as well. The latter especially mentioned that Hendrickson protested his innocence to the moment of his death.[28]

The questions raised by the Hendrickson case did not, of course, die with Hendrickson himself. For several of the principals, the case lived on as one of the most searing traumas of their professional careers. John Swinburne, for example, continued his medical practice in Albany, but labored through the rest of the decade under the weight of his testimony in the Hendrickson case. In 1860 Swinburne was prevailed upon by friends in Lewis County to help them with a difficult coroner's inquest. Though Swinburne had given up his "dissecting rooms" and private courses in pathological anatomy, he agreed to do the favor. Accompanied by Professor Charles H. Porter of Albany, Swinburne went by train to Boonville, then overland in a wagon to the even more obscure village of Greig. There they conducted a post-mortem examination which led Swinburne to conclude that what appeared to be a suicide had actually been a homicide in which a woman was first asphyxiated, then set up to look as if she had cut her own throat. During subsequent proceedings before the coroner's jury, counsel for the man who would be indicted for murder if the death was ruled a homicide first accused Swinburne of taking this otherwise improbable case for money, then attacked the Albany practitioner for his testimony in the Hendrickson case.[29] Even in tiny Greig, in a case where he was on strong ground, the Hendrickson trial thus bore down upon Swinburne, who could not have forgotten the opprobrium heaped upon him by the state's professional establishment.

Edward Hartshorne, the Philadelphia medico-legal expert, used the Hendrickson case to admonish his professional colleagues against "ignorance and indiscretion" when performing forensic post-mortem examinations. In his 1856 annotated American edition of Alfred S. Taylor's *Medical Jurisprudence*, a volume which had been published in the United Kingdom without reference to the celebrated Albany case, Hartshorne asserted that Hendrickson was "unjustly convicted of the poisoning of his wife."[30] Hartshorne repeated his attack on Swinburne's techniques in his 1861 American edition of Taylor. "The case of John Hendrickson, Jr., convicted, on altogether insufficient medical testimony, of poisoning his wife with aconite, affords a lamentable instance," Hartshorne alleged, of the "perversion of medico-legal investigation."[31] In the same fashion, David A. Wells used the Hendrickson case as an illustration of bad science for student readers in his *Wells's Principles and Applications of Chemistry*, first published in 1858, and widely republished thereafter.[32]

Swinburne let his professional wounds fester nine full years, then in 1862, with the nation itself staggered by the Civil War, Swinburne reopened the professional civil war among the nation's forensic toxicologists with an article rebutting the Hartshorne and Wells versions of the Hendrickson case. Swinburne's long, somewhat rambling essay revealed how raw his wounds remained after nearly a decade. He labeled his tormentors "false," the victims of "foolish philanthropy," "mercenary motives," and "gross ignorance." He tried once more to gainsay Alonzo Clark and the pathologists, he quoted Geoghegan in his own defense, and he rehearsed the arguments of the district attorney and the attorney general. Yet the only really new piece of evidence Swinburne had to offer resulted from a case of accidental death by aconite poisoning that had occurred since the trial. In that case, Swinburne claimed, the post-mortem appearances fully justified the conclusions he had drawn after examining the body of Maria Hendrickson.[33]

Wells, in turn, never one to avoid controversy or hide his views, reentered the lists in the following volume of the same journal. For Wells, Hendrickson was "the boy-prisoner solemnly reiterating his innocence to the very last." The case "stands unparalleled upon the records of American criminal or medical jurisprudence . . . because it involved the life of a young man who, but for evidence which has been shown to be wholly unreliable, would probably have been declared innocent." In fact, however, Wells had no fresh evidence at all, save his statement that "a majority" of the experts who signed the original Hayes protest letter would still be willing to defend their position in court. Wells also denied that any of those who protested had been induced to do so by the defense team and he asserted that no one involved received any compensation whatsoever. They had all acted, in Wells's version of the story, according to "the demands of science, of justice, and of humanity."[34]

The career most crippled by the Hendrickson case was that of the promising young state chemist, James H. Salisbury, though it is difficult to

say whether his subsequent activity was a tragic denouement or grist for
the mills of those who pegged him from the outset as a skillful but rash
young scientist willing to rush forward with grandiose claims on the basis
of flimsy evidence. In retrospect, it did not help his reputation that he had
asked even prior to Hendrickson's indictment that his scientific testimony
before the coroner's jury not be published, a point his fellow professionals
made surprisingly little of then or afterward.[35] Soon after the trial, Salisbury left New York and went west to Ohio, where he lived first in New-
ark, then in Lancaster.[36] Salisbury shifted the emphasis of his research from
chemistry to physiology and carried on microscopic observations in a Cleveland laboratory during the years of the Civil War.[37] But the Hendrickson
case would not go away. In 1862, the same year Swinburne and Wells
resumed their confrontation, Salisbury finally published the results of the
poisoning experiments he had conducted in June 1853 in connection with
his Hendrickson analyses.[38]

By 1866, Salisbury had re-established himself as professor of histology,
physiology, and pathology in Cleveland's Charity Hospital Medical College. In 1867 he announced to the medical world that he thought he had
discovered the causes of syphilis and gonorrhea, and in 1868 he published
a "Description of Two New Algoid Vegetations, One of Which Appears to
be the Specific Cause of Syphilis and the Other of Gonorrhoea."[39] Salisbury, an able technician, may have observed some previously overlooked
bacteria that needed further analyses. In that case, his findings would have
constituted a modest but solid contribution to the exciting new field of bacteriology. But it seemed all too reminiscent of the Hendrickson case that
Salisbury did not stop there, preferring instead to make more startling assertions in an area of research already associated with quack wonder cures
and unsavory practices.

Certainly the heaviest toll exacted by the Hendrickson case, however,
was not upon the career of any single individual but upon the entire field
of medical jurisprudence as pioneer professionals like T.R. Beck had conceived it. More than most people through world history, Americans by the
middle of the nineteenth century were accustomed to rehearsing the fundamental verities of their society in open court. Indeed, trials seemed both
to express and to embody many of the democratic republic's most cherished
ideals, which was one of the reasons why medical jurisprudence had seemed
so important to professionals in the new nation in the first place. But the
Hendrickson case had revealed enduring problems, notwithstanding more
than a generation of serious work on medico-legal issues and the incorporation of courses in medical jurisprudence into medical school curricula.
Experts still disagreed. Professional ambition still influenced behavior. An
expert consensus seemed impossible to determine, even in cases that attained the national notoriety of the Hendrickson case. Government authorities, elected in large part to implement their constituents' circumstantial
sense of fairness, found themselves in conflict with the opinions of their

own experts. Appropriately enough, in the face of professional doubt and confusion, those officials sided with their constituents. And all of these problems had arisen in the theoretically precise realms of forensic toxicology, where so much real progress had been made. In the far less clear-cut arena of medico-legal insanity, the situation by mid-century was even worse.

CHAPTER TEN

The Implications of Insanity:
From a Professional Asset to a Public
Embarrassment

Like forensic toxicology, which had been one of the two most visible aspects of legal medicine optimistically reviewed by Beck in 1841, the other, insanity, was also destined to encounter dramatic public reversals during the next two decades.[1] Trouble resulted chiefly from two major developments. The first was a distinct shift near mid-century in the fundamental direction of the public asylum movement.[2] The second was the effect of applying the century's new interpretations of insanity to questions of criminal culpability.[3] As those two developments unfolded, the general subject of insanity, which had originally helped propel the field of medical jurisprudence to new levels of prominence in the United States during the early decades of the nineteenth century, became after 1850 a serious stumbling block on the road to further advancement.

Despite the sunny hopes and apparently bright successes of America's early insane asylums, ominous clouds of obdurate reality hung over them by mid-century. Cure rates proved far less bullish in practice than they had once appeared to be in theory. Instead of rehabilitating and releasing substantial proportions of their patients, state-supported asylums were everywhere filling with larger and larger numbers of chronic cases. The result was all too predictable. Public officials, whose expectations had been raised, grew leery of the enterprise; paying substantial sums for top professionals to deliver cures was one thing, but paying high rates for medically suspect human holding tanks was another. Housing the unfortunate might be more effectively, even more humanely, and certainly more frugally, accomplished in some other fashion. To make matters worse, Edward Jarvis, a nationally important pioneer in both psychiatry and statistics, published an article exactly at mid-century which demonstrated, even though Jarvis was a strong advocate of state-supported asylums for the insane, that central asylums did not, and inherently could not, serve all the various regions of their states equally.[4]

As overcrowding increased, conditions worsened and the asylum movement as a whole found itself caught in a series of vicious cycles. Deteriorating conditions diminished further the likelihood of increasing cure rates, partly because the physicians inside the asylums no longer enjoyed the situations they considered essential for bringing about cures and partly because they had to spend so much of their time, energy, and resources caring for chronic, incurable cases. Deteriorating conditions also provoked legislative investigations of asylum management and asylum philosophies. Especially probing reports were debated at the state level by legislators in Massachusetts in 1849, Rhode Island in 1851, and New York in 1856 and 1857.[5] Collectively, those debates made insane asylums appear increasingly imprudent and unprofessional. At the very least, they had lost their luster as exemplars of one way state-supported legal medicine might work.

In 1854 President Franklin Pierce put an unequivocal halt to an effort by humanitarian reformer Dorothea Dix to persuade Congress to reinvigorate the asylum movement with federal sanction and federal funds. Pierce vetoed a bill that year which would have provided federal land grants for the purpose of aiding the indigent insane at the state level; indeed, the President used the occasion of that veto to lay out at length his theories about the separation of powers under the Constitution and his opposition to national involvement in matters of that sort.[6] Congress did not override the veto.

Even at the organizational level, the public asylum movement was failing for the most part to advance either American physicians generally or medical jurisprudence specifically. Though they came from the ranks of physicians oriented toward science and education, and though they were at first strongly committed to upgrading medical jurisprudence within the profession and in cooperation with the state, the men who became long-term full-time superintendents in the nation's early insane asylums quite quickly established a separate association of their own and self-consciously went their own way. As attacks upon their institutions mounted, physicians inside the asylums circled their wagons and developed a defensive attitude. The Association of Medical Superintendents of American Institutions for the Insane (the AMSAII, which later evolved into the American Psychiatric Association), founded in 1844, remained a small and narrowly defined group at least through the Civil War. The AMSAII squabbled openly with public officials over salaries, budgets, and qualifications; even over architectural plans.

More damaging still was the refusal of the AMSAII to affiliate with those scientifically and educationally oriented regular physicians who established the American Medical Association in 1847, primarily as a vehicle to oversee a reconstitution of medical professionalism following two decades of anti-professional attack and unregulated standards. The AMA tried for a while during the 1850s to maintain a standing committee of its own to deal with the issues involved in mental diseases, as distinguished from traditional physical diseases, but abandoned that awkward competitive effort after the Civil War. By then it was apparent to all concerned that the AM-

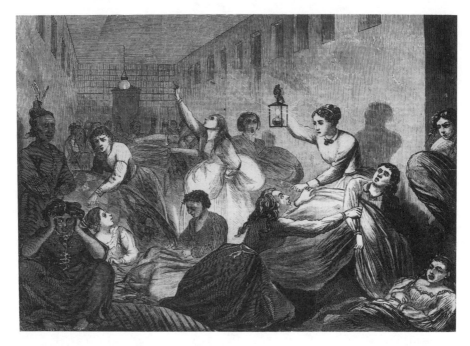

This drawing from *Frank Leslie's Illustrated Newspaper*, August 8, 1868, which purported to be a night scene in a corridor of the women's asylum on Blackwell's Island, re-enforced the negative image of such institutions that emerged after mid-century. (*Courtesy of the Enoch Pratt Free Library, Baltimore*)

SAII had become, in the apt phrase of Gerald N. Grob, "an administrative specialty" rather than a cooperative vanguard in the crusade for better medical jurisprudence.[7]

In 1855, at the direction of the Massachusetts legislature, Edward Jarvis brought forth another influential assessment of public asylums. His *Report on Insanity and Idiocy in Massachusetts* proved to be one of the most impressive and sophisticated analyses of the social patterns of insanity written during the entire nineteenth century.[8] Unfortunately for the asylum movement, however, that report seemed to confirm the increasingly common perception that publicly funded insane asylums had become places to dump those who could not or would not care for themselves and those whose families could not or would not pay to provide anything else for them. The latter was no trivial matter, since asylums housed disproportionately large numbers of poor immigrants in a decade that witnessed the greatest influx of immigrants relative to the existing population in all of United States history and a correspondingly virulent nativism among taxpayers.

Even the *Boston Medical and Surgical Journal*, a staunch advocate of more systematic medical jurisprudence and high professional standards in American medicine, largely turned its back after mid-century upon the institutions that Rush and Beck once envisioned as potential models of both.[9] The best way to relieve the situation would be to build more asylums, which key states began to do after mid-century, but public authorities were less generous with funds in the second wave of construction and staffing, since they no longer believed that the institutions they were building merited significantly larger sums of public money than alternative forms of public maintenance.[10] A great professional promise was apparently failing.

The flexible new theories about insanity that originally underlay the asylum movement had bolstered the power and prestige of physicians in other areas as well. They had allowed doctors to become champions of the living by retroactively undoing the mandates of the dead in cases of disputed wills, and they had allowed doctors to become the allies of courts (and hence of lawyers) who wished to alter apparently arbitrary, unreasonably unfair, or socially capricious arrangements of various sorts by challenging the mental soundness of those who made them. But when those same flexible ideas began to be applied to questions of individual responsibility, the result had the net long-term effect of undermining medico-legal interaction rather than continuing to advance it.

At least in theory, Anglo-American jurisprudence had long recognized in the so-called *mens rea* doctrine the abstract notion that no one should be held responsible for actions he or she could neither willfully control nor consciously understand. That basic idea had appeared in ancient Hebrew law, in Roman law, and in medieval Christian church law. Henry de Bracton articulated the idea explicitly in his thirteenth-century survey of English law. By the seventeenth century, Edward Coke was already discussing in his well-known commentaries the complex problem of "lucid intervals." Matthew Hale, another English commentator of the seventeenth century, addressed the difficulties of ascertaining various degrees of insanity and applying them to various degrees of punishment.[11] To repeat, the justice system inherited by the new American republic at the end of the eighteenth century already recognized, at least in theory, the principle that persons mentally incapable of understanding or controlling their actions should not be held accountable for them or punished for them.

Special emphasis in the foregoing, however, should be placed upon the phrase "at least in theory." Much work needs to be done on the history of American criminal law and how it was actually administered and experienced by ordinary citizens in the past. But work that has been done and extensive browsing in the original sources both leave the distinct impression that common justice in the United States through the middle of the nineteenth century leaned strongly in favor of what the community wanted done (as distinguished from what the legal technicalities might stipulate in any given case) and strongly in favor of what modern social scientists might call a strictly behavioralist approach (as distinguished from an approach that not only tried to determine whether a given person took a specific action but also tried to determine all possible reasons why the action was taken).[12]

In such a context, it is not difficult to imagine that attitudes toward the culpability of the insane were neither systematic nor systematically applied.[13] Local juries would probably excuse on grounds of insanity a well-known, prototypically obvious, and fundamentally benign village idiot who did something wrong; but most defendants otherwise appear to have been punished if they did what they were accused of doing, their mental powers, emotional controls, or psychological states notwithstanding.[14] Furthermore, as a general rule, the more heinous the crime, the less likely a jury would be to excuse the action on the basis of mental incapacity. At least one factor in this tendency to convict the most dangerous of the criminally insane resulted from a lack of acceptable alternatives: in many jurisdictions an insane murderer found innocent by reason of insanity would simply go free as a person not guilty, possibly to terrorize the community or to kill again.[15] Local juries under such circumstances tended seldom to be sympathetic to arguments of diminished capacity, as was clear in the well publicized *Birdsell* case in Cincinnati in 1829.[16] Certainly Isaac Ray believed in 1838 that American courts showed "little indulgence . . . to imbecility in criminal" cases.[17]

Despite the fact that he was one of the nation's leading experts on insanity generally and despite the fact that he devoted a great deal of attention to cataloging and explaining the new taxonomies of mental illness, T.R. Beck, when he published the first edition of the *Elements* in 1823, gave almost no attention to the ways in which the new theories of insanity he was advocating might affect questions of criminal responsibility. For Beck, as for Rush before him, the chief importance of an expanded and more flexible understanding of insanity lay in the higher probability of better treatment, more cures, and the more professional management of property, not in the realms of criminal law.[18] Beck carried over from earlier commentators the dictum that "[i]nsanity or idiotism, excuses an individual from the guilt of crimes, and he is not chargeable for his own acts, if committed when under these incapacities." And Beck pointed out that juries had a right to make the final determination as to responsibility when the sanity of an accused criminal was in doubt. But in a revealing emphasis, however, Beck italicized the observation that lunatics could have lucid intervals in which they would be answerable for their actions, thus suggesting what amounted to an inverse of the doctrine of temporary insanity. Just as an otherwise sane person could draft an unfortunate will during a short period of dementia and would deserve to have it overturned, an otherwise insane person could commit a murder that had nothing to do with their demented state and would deserve to go the gallows for it.[19] Beck was not interested in revolutionizing concepts of criminal responsibility.

But an expanded and more flexible understanding of mental illness clearly did have long-term implications for criminal law in the United States, even if they were not at first obvious or explicit even to experts in the field. The same year the *Elements* appeared in Albany, for example, a case broke in northern New York state that forced Beck and his associates at the *New-York Medical and Physical Journal* to think about some of those implications.

A man in St. Lawrence County admitted murdering his four-year-old step-son and his two-year-old daughter. The murderer's attorney decided to plead not guilty by reason of insanity. Several reliable witnesses, including the defendant's clergyman and physicians, all testified that the man had exhibited no signs of insanity; the man himself described how he deliberately planned the murders. Not surprisingly, the jury took only fifteen minutes to find him guilty. The *NYMPJ* understated the case when it observed that "the plea of insanity was unsupported."[20]

Strangely, however, both the county attorney and the presiding judge in the case were convinced under the newly expanded and more flexible definitions of insanity being advocated by professionals like Beck that the convicted murderer had to be insane. In a bizarre twist, they petitioned the governor to pardon the man whom they had respectively prosecuted and sentenced to die. Their chief argument was the fact that the act itself was manifestly irrational. Since a father naturally loved his children, their murder was a self-evidently deranged behavior and hence necessarily without malice in a legal sense. The governor was willing to pardon the man, but only if he could simultaneously commit the man for the rest of his life to the state prison. An action like that required a special act of the state legislature, since the governor could ordinarily pardon altogether but not alter sentences. Following the recommendation of a senate committee, the lawmakers authorized the governor to do what he asked in this case. The *NYMPJ*, the state's strongest public advocate for the overall cause of medical jurisprudence, found itself in the awkward position of applauding "the humane policy" of the governor and the state legislature in a capital case where there were some doubts, but ultimately disagreeing with those who shared the doubts. They were forced to face the fact that insanity had the potential to become an extremely slippery issue, which could be pushed by others much farther than they might initially have been inclined to push it themselves.

In the 1835 edition of the *Elements* Beck expanded his originally minimal discussion of criminal responsibility. True to his consistently humane vision of medical jurisprudence, he adumbrated the ways in which a better understanding of insanity might produce better judgments in the nation's criminal courts, even while he hedged his opinion of the period's most controversial extension of the new attitudes toward insanity: the doctrines known collectively as "moral insanity" or derangements of the sympathetic, emotional, and judgmental faculties as distinguished from impairment of the intellectual or reasoning capacities. But the strongest and most systematic presentation of the implications of the new and more flexible understanding of insanity in the context of criminal justice appeared three years later in Isaac Ray's *A Treatise on the Medical Jurisprudence of Insanity*.

Ray, who was thirty-one years old when he published the *Treatise* that would make him famous, epitomized in all ways but one a sort of archetype of the physicians attracted to medical jurisprudence during the first half of the nineteenth century. He was strongly influenced by French medicine and French law, deeply committed to the scientific method, and enthusiastically optimistic about the future role of medical experts in court proceedings. The one way in which this almost naively aggressive professionalizer was an exception to standard patterns was in the absence of formal coursework in medical jurisprudence during his medical school training; when Ray attended the Medical School of Maine in 1826 and 1827, the field was apparently not being taught there. But the subject of insanity, the same subject that attracted so many of his contemporaries, quickly engaged the formidable mind of this young practitioner as well.[21]

Ray's *Treatise* was a virtual manifesto in behalf of the innocent insane, a category of defendants whom Ray considered all too often the victims rather than the beneficiaries of American legal procedure. Ray believed strongly in the existence of a wide range of mental illnesses, including those that reduced the judgmental powers and emotional control of the people afflicted. Drawing upon the latest theories from France and England, Ray skillfully laid out the various imbecilities, manias, dementias, deliriums, and madnesses postulated by experts through 1837, and he described the ways in which enlightened courts should identify and deal with each. Ray was sharply critical of American courts for retaining conceptions of insanity altogether too narrow. "The little indulgence shown to imbecility in criminal courts sufficiently indicates that either the psychological nature of this condition of mind is very imperfectly understood," Ray argued in a sentence characteristic of the sort of positions he took throughout his *Treatise*, "or the true ground on which the idea of responsibility reposes is not clearly perceived."[22]

Most American physicians generally, along with most champions of medical jurisprudence specifically, hailed Ray's *Treatise* with guarded optimism when it first appeared.[23] And well they might have. Ray's *Treatise* and its subsequent revisions would shape debate in the field for almost half a century after its publication.[24] Now that medical experts knew more about the varieties and manifestations of various sorts of mental illnesses, fewer citizens would have to suffer punishments for actions they could not willfully control or reasonably understand, provided of course the courts and the public could be educated up to the levels of understanding that experts in mental illness were finally reaching. Ray and others urged American state legislators to insert language overtly tolerant of insanity pleas into their criminal codes.[25]

Within five years of Ray's *Treatise*, English courts formulated the so-called M'Naghten Rule, or "knowledge of right and wrong" test, which quickly caught on in American courts as a convenient and conveniently formulaic way to address the question of criminal responsibility in cases where insanity of various sorts was being alleged.[26] While the rule had serious drawbacks and limitations, and while several American state courts proposed alternative formulations during the 1840s and 1850s, existence of the M'Naghten Rule tended to make insanity defenses more easily and confidently initiated by attorneys after 1843.[27] The tide seemed to be flowing strongly in the direction of significant change. Experts in the medical jurisprudence of insanity might soon become crucial arbiters in the process of American justice, a process Ray himself continued to consider altogether too rigid and needlessly bound to inappropriate precedents.[28] From 1844 to 1849, under the editorial leadership of Amariah Bringham, the *American Journal of Insanity*, official organ of the AMSAII, endorsed Ray's call for the broad application even in criminal cases of flexible interpretations of insanity, including the new doctrines gathered somewhat loosely and eclectically under the rubric of moral insanity.

By mid-century, however, many people inside the medical and legal professions, not to mention many more people out among the general population, began to have grave misgivings about how far the new insanity doctrines should be pushed in the context of criminal responsibility. The chief difficulty with pushing them too far lay in the practical impossibility of distinguishing confidently between disease and depravity. Victims of disease should be treated by medical experts rather than punished, but if the only identifiable manifestation of their mental illness was their depraved action, how could they be distinguished from persons who really were depraved and richly merited punishment for what they had done to others in society? That basic question had kept T. R. Beck from fully endorsing the all-out application of moral insanity in criminal cases, but his was a benevolent neutrality toward ideas he considered potentially useful. When he succeeded Brigham for a short stint as editor of the *American Journal of Insanity* at mid-century, he tried to maintain his neutrality. Others by then were far less restrained and considered the new doctrines dangerously corrosive not only of professional credibility but even of the social order itself.

Charles R. King, a regular reviewer of medico-legal material for professional journals, had sounded a typical note of warning in 1845 in the nationally prominent *American Journal of the Medical Sciences*. Assessing the second edition of Ray's *Treatise*, which had been published at Boston in 1844, King acknowledged the book as a powerful and important summary of European and American opinions about insanity, but implied strongly that Ray was too soft on the subject generally, too ready to grant too many forms of insanity, and too reckless with the rights of society.[29] That same year the venerable Robley Dunglison, the man who had carried medical jurisprudence to the University of Virginia two decades earlier, washed his hands of the burgeoning insanity debates altogether. "It has always been the expressed conviction of the writer," he recorded in his widely circulated *Cyclopaedia of Practical Medicine*, "that medical men are no better judges of the existence of mental alienation, than well-informed and discriminating individuals not of the profession."[30] While the statement was somewhat disingenuous, the timing was significant. Here was another of the early advocates of serious medical jurisprudence now discouraged and disillusioned with what had become of a once-crucial and once-central part of the field.

Not everyone despaired, of course. Samuel White, a veteran of medico-legal battles and an asylum superintendent, devoted the annual address of the New York State Medical Society in 1844 to a reiteration of his belief that additional research would eventually uncover physiological causes and "corporeal" indications of mental diseases, even of the moral insanity that was "receiving considerable attention at the present day." It was not involvement with the issue of insanity per se that was hurting medical jurisprudence, but the pursuit of "[m]etaphysical researches to the neglect of corporeal phenomena."[31] Three years later John McCall devoted the same occasion to a direct refutation of Dunglison's opinion. McCall urged his fellow physicians to stick with Ray's approach to the subject of criminal responsibility; it would eventually allow them, he exhorted, repeating the essential promise of medical jurisprudence from the outset, "to vindicate . . . medical truth and professional standing."[32]

By the mid-1850s, however, there was little question that the professional and public tide had turned strongly back against the expansive positions associated with Ray and the rubric of moral insanity. Edward Hartshorne, one of the nation's leading experts on medical jurisprudence and editor himself of an American edition of Taylor's *Manual of Medical Jurisprudence*, observed publicly in 1856 that "no subject in the whole range of medico-legal inquiry" had become "so universally embarrassing as . . . mental aberration."[33] In 1857 John P. Gray, who had taken over editorial control of the *American Journal of Insanity*, launched from within the core of the AMSAII itself what would become a powerfully influential and relentlessly sustained frontal attack upon the general ideas associated with moral insanity. In Gray's view the rush to expand the role of physicians into the realms of criminal responsibility was both unscientific and unprofessional.[34] James Wynne of the New York Medical College agreed. In an introductory address on medical jurisprudence, which opened his school's 1859 term, Wynne stated flatly that the doctrine of moral insanity had "very materially damaged the moral weight of medico-legal testimony" in the United States.[35]

The controversy over criminal insanity also reduced physicians' effectiveness in areas where they had made earlier progress, notably in the adjudication of wills. Judge Campbell of the Court of Common Pleas in Philadelphia no doubt spoke for many of his rank-and-file judicial colleagues when he told an 1851 jury trying to decide the validity of a will in which lumber mills, rental properties, and thousands of acres of prime real estate were at stake, "I confess that my faith is not very strong in the opinion of medical witnesses, no matter how distinguished in their profession," in cases involving retroactive determinations of sanity. Do not, he counselled the jurors, "surrender your judgment to theirs."[36]

Also telling, especially as a harbinger of long-term developments within the medical profession, were efforts by the still nascent AMA to distance itself from the controversy over applying moral insanity to questions of legal responsibility. In 1858 the AMA, barely a decade old and struggling to establish credibility as the national voice of mainstream medicine in the United States, published two reports that bore upon the issue: C.B. Coventry's "Report on the Medical Jurisprudence of Insanity" and D. Meredith Reese's "Report on Moral Insanity in Its Relations to Medical Jurisprudence."[37] Near the outset of his carefully balanced survey, Coventry acknowledged the revolution wrought by Beck's generation as "one of the most brilliant achievements of the medical profession in modern times." The insane had been rescued, to use his verb, "not merely from the neglect, but from the cruelty and abuse which they were formerly made to suffer."[38]

Pushing farther, Coventry praised Ray specifically and included various forms of moral insanity among his catalogue of mental impairments. Yet he cautioned that the latter were among the most "difficult of adjudication" in questions of legal responsibility. "Much prejudice exists in the community against the plea of insanity in criminal cases and medical witnesses have been unsparingly denounced," a point certainly not lost on the AMA's general membership. In the report's most significant concession to community sentiment, Coventry urged that a heavy burden of proof be placed upon those pleading any of the various forms of moral insanity in criminal cases. "[A] mere burst of rage or passion, or excitement which he may not control" should not exonerate a defendant. To win a plea of not guilty by reason of insanity, in Coventry's view, defendants should have to demonstrate persuasively that their actions resulted "from cerebromental disease; consequently, it is necessary to show some other evidence of disease than the act itself."[39]

Reese, who had established a national reputation as a professor of medical jurisprudence, addressed moral insanity by itself and took an even harder line.[40] The controversy over that subject had disastrously worsened professional relations between lawyers and physicians over the last ten years, Reese argued. The former had long depended upon the latter to discriminate between the sane and the insane under established rules; but physicians, many of whom did not really know what they were doing, were now growing increasingly inconsistent, arbitrary, and silly in their all-too-often "*ex cathedra*" testimony about the various derangements arrayed under the heading of moral insanity. "That our brethren of the bench and bar should smile at our ludicrous assumption of infallibility, and that a common jury should ignore such incoherent testimony, and even impute 'moral insanity' to such doctors, is not at all marvelous." And as American state court decisions in the 1840s indicated, the long-settled rules that once governed legal insanity were themselves disintegrating as a consequence of the new theories being propounded. For Reese, the best course was obvious: fight for a straightforward sane or insane determination by the courts and return to a disease-based theory of insanity for which "pathognomonic signs" were evident. Where such signs were absent, or where the act itself was the only manifestation of the insanity being claimed, "it becomes the highest duty of our profession to rally to the rescue of morals and law, by protecting the administration of justice for the public security."[41] The message to the AMA in 1858 was hard to mistake. The advance of medical jurisprudence toward the frontiers of insanity, which once seemed to advance the whole profession with it, now looked increasingly like a dangerous overextension. Powerful insiders were calling for prudent retrenchment.

Within months occurred a case that made Reese seem prescient and may well have sealed the opinions of many physicians still on the fence. Daniel Sickles, a Democratic congressman from New York City, shot and killed his wife's lover in Lafayette Park across from the White House. The victim was Philip Barton Key, son of Francis Scott Key and nephew of Chief Justice Roger Taney of the United States Supreme Court. The act, which took place on a Sunday afternoon in full view of people strolling and children playing, could hardly have been more blatant. Sickles first confronted his victim, then wounded him, and finally shot him again as he lay on the sidewalk. When the incident was over, Sickles calmly turned himself in to District of Columbia authorities. Following a post-mortem examination of Key's corpse and a formal inquiry, Congressman Sickles was charged with murder.[42]

The story made sensational headlines across the United States and daily verbatim testimony from the ensuing April trial appeared on the front page of virtually every major newspaper in the nation. The attention of the general public was riveted on the intimate details of Teresa Sickles's adultery, which the congressman had forced his young wife to write out in a long, piteous, and self-condemnatory document the day before the shooting took place. What rocked the nation's medico-legalists, however, was the formal plea of the congressman's lawyers: their client was not guilty by reason of insanity. Led by the shrewd and influential Edwin M. Stanton, who would later serve in the presidential cabinets of Abraham Lincoln and Andrew Johnson, the defense attorneys had decided to press the concept of temporary insanity to the logical extremes that Reese and others feared; or at the very least they had decided to use that doctrine as a convenient and perhaps somewhat cynical excuse to let a jury acquit the man they skillfully portrayed as distraught by infidelity and a defender of American family virtue, though in truth he was neither.

In opening for the defense, one of Sickles' attorneys put the proposition plainly:

> We mean to say not that Mr. Sickles labored under insanity in consequence of an established mental permanent disease, but that *the condition of his mind at the time of the commission of the act in question was such as would render him legally unaccountable*, as much so as if the state of his mind had been produced by a mental disease. In other words, the proposition we argue to this Jury is this: It is no matter how a man becomes insane; Is he insane? that is the question. Whether it results from disease of mind or body or sudden provocation, it is perfectly immaterial, and the privileges of accountability attach as much in the one case as in the other.[43]

The defense strategy thus rested upon the premise that "the killing of Key was the result of an uncontrollable frenzy."[44] "The provocation," argued Sickles's lawyers, "was more than human nature could bear."[45] For such a purpose, lay opinion was more useful than professional opinion, and the defense spent most of the twenty-day trial building a crescendo of moral outrage in behalf of their client. Sickles's attorneys won a crucial ruling when the presiding judge declared that "the jury are to judge how far insanity exists, strengthened by evidence of acts such as usually characterize derangement of mind, if proved."[46] Consequently, the defense was not obliged to offer any serious testimony on the nature of temporary insanity, or how it might begin or end, or how it might be distinguished from ordinary rage or mere anger. The prosecutors, in turn, were in the awkward position of trying to prove a null hypothesis and offered no psychiatric experts on their side either.

Undercurrents of power and politics ran quite flagrantly through the whole astonishing situation, and most of those undercurrents flowed strongly in Sickles's direction. President James Buchanan himself, a close social friend and solid partisan ally of Congressman Sickles, apparently encouraged the flight of a witness whose knowledge might have been damaging to the congressman's defense. As a New York City congressman, Sickles controlled the disposition of huge government contracts and a great deal of public money. The powerful political associates with whom he did business in the private sector did not want him convicted and removed, so they made sure that top legal talent would be brought into the courtroom against the local District of Columbia prosecutors. The well-connected Washington insider who had been with Sickles in his home immediately before the incident, then hailed Key in Lafayette Square while Sickles fetched his guns, and finally stood beside the congressman through the actual shooting was never called to the stand. Though Sickles certainly had political enemies as well as friends, the only cloud that appeared on the horizon of speculation was fear that one of the jurors, because he once had ties to the nativist Know-Nothing party, might not be capable of sympathy for a Tammany Democrat.[47]

On April 26, 1859, after just a few minutes of discussion, the jury brought back a verdict of not guilty. Pandemonium broke out in the courtroom, as the assembled crowd paraded Sickles on their shoulders; jurors rushed to congratulate the congressman; and the usually austere Stanton danced a victory jig upon the defense table. Most people present, including the jurors, adjourned to a nearby tavern for several more hours of partying, singing, and celebrating. Editorials around the nation the next day also proved overwhelmingly favorable to the verdict. The *New York Times*, calling the trial "one of the most remarkable cases in the whole history of criminal jurisprudence," published an entire special supplement that reviewed the event with manifest approbation.[48] But it was quite clear that the general public approval represented, at least in the immediate aftermath of the trial, a sort of folk consensus that Sickles had been so wronged by Key that recourse to personal revenge was somehow justified.[49]

Those who looked closely at the exact grounds of justification, however, found the whole Sickles case unsettling. The New York *Tribune*, for example, considered the finding of not guilty "a most mistaken and mischievous verdict." The plea of temporary insanity had been used as "a sanction to the substitution of violence and vengeance for reliance on the regular and orderly redress of grievances through the instrumentality of law."[50] In Maryland, where Key's family deplored what they regarded as an illegal manslaughter, adultery or no adultery, the *Baltimore Sun* correctly pointed out that "the defense . . . resort[ed] to insanity as the plea. The jury must therefore have based their verdict upon the insanity of the prisoner, or the law has suffered violence, and twelve perjured men left the jury box upon re[n]dition of their verdict." The *Sun* conceded that the jurors were ultimately "entitled to the benefit of an opinion that the prisoner was insane," but considered it an opinion "which no other *sane* man out of the jury box will concur in."[51]

The Tammany Democrat's defense was widely regarded around the country as the first successful use of the plea of temporary insanity in a capital case. Though little-known earlier instances were actually on the record, the Sickles case certainly brought ordinary citizens and the emerging professions face to face in an especially public, dramatic, and abrupt fashion with many of the most profoundly unsettling implications of the new inter-

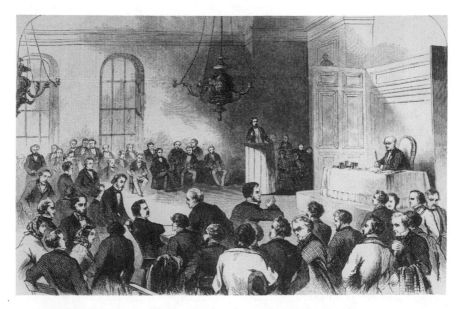

The trial of the Hon. Daniel E. Sickles for the murder of P. Barton Key, Esq., at Washington, D.C. From *Harper's Weekly*, April 9, 1859. (*Courtesy Enoch Pratt Free Library, Baltimore*)

pretations of insanity.[52] The medico-legalists had created a monster; with enough nerve and the right lawyers, a citizen with clout could use the concept of temporary insanity to quite literally get away with murder. Thus at the same time public asylums began to look increasingly expensive and ineffective, the application of flexible insanity theories to questions of criminal responsibility began to look increasingly unjust and unfair.

On the eve of the Civil War, public interactions between American physicians and their nation's legal processes were not going well. Medical jurisprudence as a separate field of study still lacked an effective economic underpinning or any state support. Physicians were being battered professionally and financially as witnesses in court. Medical malpractice cases, once rare curiosities, had exploded into a frightening phenomenon of professional life. Toxicology had been discredited in the Hendrickson trial. Insanity, a subject which had attracted many prominent physicians to legal medicine in the first place and a subject that formerly seemed to epitomize the idealistic and professional promise of medical jurisprudence, had become a public nightmare. The Civil War would do little to improve the quality of medico-legal interactions in the United States; if anything, those interactions would worsen during that conflict.

CHAPTER ELEVEN

Medical Jurisprudence
and the Civil War

During the Civil War a larger percentage of the nation's physicians worked directly and indirectly with and for governmental and quasi-governmental agencies at all levels of government than at any other time in the nineteenth century. At least 12,000 physicians served some portion of the war in the direct employ of the military. Hundreds of doctors entered the federal army's own Medical Department, which was greatly expanded during the war and eventually gained control over most medically related activities at all levels of service. Many thousands more attended the hundreds of thousands of soldiers enlisted in the state-based volunteer units, since every regiment in the Union army was supposed to have a surgeon (who was in charge of overall medical care, not just surgery) and two or more assistant surgeons. More than 5000 civilian physicians worked for the army on a contract basis, and hundreds of others were pressed into various forms of short-term or emergency service on an *ad hoc* basis.[1]

Physicians also saw direct action in the field, helped design and administer an unprecedented proliferation of military hospitals, and performed for various agencies countless numbers of examinations of many sorts, from dietary inspections to venereal disease surveys. Thousands of other doctors decided not to give up their established practices, especially with so many of their competitors away at the war, but worked regularly with quasi-public organizations: the United States Sanitary Commission, an officially recognized support group committed to maintaining the health of the troops both by supplementing and by hectoring the efforts of the military itself; the structurally independent Western Sanitary Commission, a similar and sometimes rival operation based in Missouri; the Christian Commission, which tried to elevate both the physical and the spiritual well-being of the troops; a host of less formally organized support groups of many sorts; or local draft and recruiting boards.[2]

The unprecedented mobilization of American physicians during the Civil War is sometimes considered to have paid long-term dividends for

American medicine writ large. That may have been the case in some fields. The treatment of traumatic wounds, to take an obvious example, certainly improved during the war and so did surgery in general. Thousands of young operators got more intense practice in a few years than most previous generations received during a career, and in the decades following the Civil War it was no accident that surgery became one of the few medical fields in which Americans were considered among the world's best. Civil War experience may also have refined and improved certain medical practices, including the use of hypodermic injections, the design of plaster casts, and the administration of anesthesia. Long-term health care in the United States probably benefited as well from the fact that a large number of doctors during the Civil War learned valuable practical lessons about how to manage hospitals and how to use nursing care effectively.

The Civil War also afforded many physicians the opportunity to build heroic reputations and lasting careers for themselves individually. S. Weir Mitchell, for example, did not go on to become the founding father of modern neurology completely by coincidence; during the Civil War, Surgeon General William A. Hammond let his close friend Mitchell and two other colleagues run a hospital devoted exclusively to nerve injuries and nervous afflictions. The war allowed young John Shaw Billings to stake out a spot near the top of his profession not on the basis of extraordinary medical abilities but on the basis of extraordinary administrative skills. On a wider scale, hundreds of communities had their own medical champions, whose ministrations to the local boys during the war later became legendary. Their reputations secured those physicians lasting amounts of altogether genuine public gratitude as well as handsome postwar practices. And the physicians probably deserved both, for thousands of dedicated doctors really did work heroically to save thousands of soldiers during the Civil War, often under truly miserable conditions.

In the present context, one of the best examples of a physician building such a reputation during the Civil War, or rather in this case rebuilding one, involved John Swinburne, the young Albany physician who performed the post-mortem examination of the body of Maria Hendrickson. As a result of his testimony for the prosecution in the Hendrickson case, Swinburne had been publicly rebuked by the president of the New York State Medical Society, formally censured by the New York Pathological Society, and widely castigated in the national medical press. During the war, however, he obtained an appointment with the New York volunteers and served at the front with great distinction. When General George B. McClellan retreated from the peninsula between the York River and the James River in 1862, Swinburne voluntarily stayed behind in Virginia to care for some 4000 Union soldiers too sick or too badly wounded to be evacuated. The Confederates were so impressed they permitted Swinburne safe passage to continue helping them care for the Union prisoners of war.

Following the war, New York governor Reuben Fenton appointed Swinburne to the new Metropolitan Board of Health in New York City, a highly politicized post under the circumstances. In 1870 Swinburne went to Europe and ended up at the head of the Paris-based American Ambulance Service during the Franco-Prussian War. By applying American Civil War experience, that agency revolutionized the treatment of wounded soldiers in Europe. For his efforts, the French government awarded Swinburne the Legion of Honor. Swinburne then returned to Albany, where the electorate chose "the Fighting Doctor" as their mayor. In 1888 the professionally oriented Citizens' Association of New York pushed Swinburne, a man regarded as unsound by the state's medical establishment thirty years before, seriously though unsuccessfully as a gubernatorial candidate in New York.[3]

Although the Civil War may thus have advanced some aspects of general medical practice in the United States and surely advanced the careers of several individuals, it seems not to have advanced either the public or the professional prospects of systematic interaction between physicians and their nation's legal processes. This was not from lack of activity, attention, or application. In fact, government physicians were almost constantly involved during the war in many aspects of traditional medical jurisprudence and with medico-legal issues that were crucial to the national effort. The military medicine section of Beck's *Elements* was probably read more frequently during the Civil War than at any prior time since its publication. When Surgeon General Hammond implemented a program of qualifying examinations for would-be army doctors in 1862, he included medical jurisprudence specifically among the areas in which candidates would be drilled.[4] Indeed, he was personally interested in the subject himself. The Sanitary Commission intentionally combined prominent representatives from law and medicine on its boards of directors in an effort to allow the organization to move easily and effectively across conventional professional lines. Much of what the Sanitary Commission and related groups attempted, after all, involved both fields.[5] Nonetheless, both in specific ways and in general ways, the Civil War experience on balance almost certainly did more harm than good to the fast-fading field.

The role physicians played as recruitment and screening officers provides an excellent example of a specific way in which Civil War medical activities seem to have hurt the image of traditional medical jurisprudence, both in the eyes of physicians and in the eyes of the general public. The first representatives of the army encountered by most potential soldiers was the physician commissioned to examine and certify personnel fit for service. Those citizens whose patriotism pushed them to join in the first flush of excitement usually had little trouble passing the perfunctory physicals administered to volunteers early in the war, though occasional tensions arose over young men lying about their age or eager recruits trying to conceal disabilities. The regular army at the outset did not even require formal medical exams. But serious problems surfaced soon, and the problems increased sharply as the war dragged on and both sides began to draft reluctant citizens.

Under the Union draft of 1863 the nation was divided into districts and a so-called examining surgeon was assigned to each one. Had things gone smoothly, those officers might in theory have functioned as prototypes of the health officers Beck had called for thirty-five years before. The examining surgeons, for example, were expected at least on paper to pay attention to general health conditions in their districts, since a healthy population could support the war effort more effectively in every way than a sick or struggling one could. But everyone knew that the ultimate job of each examining surgeon was to fill his district's ranks with acceptable soldiers, and that proved so tangled and troublesome a task that the district medical officers had little time to do anything else. Filling the ranks also involved them, whether they liked it or not, in a host of medico-legal problems.

Significant numbers of men hoped to avoid service altogether by means of a medical excuse; while others wanted to be certified as fit, despite genuine medical disabilities, in order to collect the bounty money offered by local communities to anyone willing to come forward and help fill the draft rolls. The former perpetrated a host of physical and legal frauds in virtually every district in the country, which the examining surgeons had to deal with. The latter, once they had their bounty money in hand, would reveal their disability to a regimental doctor and gain a medical discharge. In an effort to reduce fraud and increase vigilance, the government eventually made the individual examining surgeons personally liable for some of the costs associated with this form of medical bounty-jumping in cases where they missed a disability.[6] This, of course, put physicians in an unenviable bind they resented: on the one hand, they had to expose feigned disabilities and overlook a host of medically questionable conditions in order the keep filling the ranks; on the other, they would be fined for allowing a soldier into the army with a pre-existing condition that allowed him to get right back out.

Particularly for European immigrants, many of whom had left their homelands during the 1840s and 1850s precisely to avoid various forms of compulsory military service on the Continent, the examining surgeons smacked of old-style state medicine with an all-too-ironic vengeance. Here was medical jurisprudence of a sort they had known abroad, and they disliked it. They also tried to resist as best they could. Horace O. Crane, the examining surgeon for Wisconsin's Fifth Enrollment District during the last two years of the war, where a large proportion of the population was foreign-born and opposed to the draft, reported "frauds . . . so numerous and varied as to require the utmost vigilance" on his part. They included the frequent use of belladonna to dilate the right pupil, since a faulty right eye exempted men from service (they were thought not capable of aiming a rifle); extreme exertion before induction exams to provoke irregular and overactive heartbeats; the widespread occurrence of "bad-looking ulcers on the leg," always in the same area (Crane eventually found out that they were being "manufactured . . . by certain doctors of medicine, for which operation [the recruits] were to pay fifty dollars if exempted"); and among the Bohemians, a practice carried over from European efforts to avoid conscription in which air was inserted into the scrotum to produce inflammation and apparent hernia. To make matters worse, Crane noted with dismay in his report to the Provost Marshal General's Office after the war that he had been forced to induct many men with disabilities which should have by any reasonable standards exempted them legitimately.[7]

Frauds were by no means limited to the foreign-born, however, and presented problems for examining surgeons in every district where the draft was enforced. The belladonna-in-the-eye trick, for example, was a nationwide ruse, and so were artificially induced leg ulcers similar to those encountered by Crane. In 1862 the *Boston Medical and Surgical Journal* published an essay on how to use the new ophthalmoscope to detect simulated eye problems in draftees.[8] Induced hemorrhoids, false rheumatism, and simulated heart disease were also common.[9] Nor should a host of related issues be overlooked, including frequent collusion between would-be draft-dodgers and civilian physicians.[10] The latter granted thousands of testimonials and certificates attesting to greatly exaggerated or non-existent medical disabilities. Because so many were bogus, the examining surgeon in New York's Twenty-fourth District adopted the practice of simply dismissing all doctors' certificates presented to him after 1863, regardless of how apparently distinguished the author happened to be.[11]

Crane reported that medico-legal bribery was taken for granted in his district. As a result, "a good deal of money" was "filtched" from conscripts by people "acting as attorneys for any one able to pay them a fee," part of which the attorneys, in turn, claimed to use to persuade army surgeons to do right by their clients and grant a medical waiver. Other attorneys, for "twenty, fifty, or a hundred dollars," were willing to write out "the most glaring falsehood" in legalistic language for their clients to swear to and thereby gain exemption. "I am happy to state," added Crane, "that all attorneys are not thus dishonest; still, no man has so bad a case as not to find some one to engage for him." Some citizens did not bother with legal formalities; they were so "unscrupulous as to the means for obtaining the desired end" as to regard straightforward "bribery and corruption as legitimate."[12]

Again the problem was national and again the problem had a direct bearing on medical jurisprudence. A number of government doctors undoubtedly accepted bribes, as a dramatic investigation of the examining surgeons in Harrisburg, Pennsylvania, made evident. William W. Mayo, a founder of the Minnesota medical center that bears his last name and the examining surgeon for Minnesota's First District, was investigated for fiscal favoritism and dismissed from the army by the Provost Marshal General, though it is not clear that his indiscretions were as serious as alleged. And according to the examining surgeons themselves, unscrupulous lawyers were everywhere, complicating and undermining the efforts of the army medical officers. Kentucky examiners complained that draftees routinely presented affidavits "carefully and cunningly prepared by some pettifogging dapper case-lawyer."[13] Some attorneys tried to manipulate the system, some lied, some bribed, some merely obfuscated. As a group, the examining surgeons considered the vast majority of the lawyers they encountered contemptible. That, in turn, did little for the interprofessional relations between law and medicine, which had, of course, already begun to deteriorate at a rapid rate during the twenty years preceding the war. Ordinary citizens, moreover, felt wronged by both professions and wrote letters of personal protest on medico-legal matters to the President and the Secretary of War.[14]

In a less specific way, the overall interaction of the medical profession and the government during the Civil War served to confirm in the minds of the public and the profession alike many of the real and potential dangers involved in state medicine generally. To put it succinctly, the shotgun arrangements cobbled together in the face of a national emergency did not ripen into a fruitful or fulfilling relationship. Indeed, by the time the war was over, both sides seemed eager for a quick annulment, and the public was more than willing to grant one. The unprecedented interaction of the professions and the state during the Civil War thus ironically rendered the very concept of state-managed medical jurisprudence less attractive than ever.

The U.S. army began the Civil War with a tiny handful of second-rate doctors. Locked into a seniority system of promotion and poorly structured, the Medical Department was woefully unprepared for the scale of activity that lay ahead. The reform and expansion of military medical care took the better part of two years to achieve. During that period virtually every sort of squabble that could be imagined took place. Federal officials appointed some physicians, state officials others, and the two clashed. Regular physicians refused to serve with homoeopaths, and both refused to acknowledge the competence of other sects to do anything, even though some of the troops themselves preferred Botanics or Hydropaths.

Even after the initial waves of conflict and confusion, major disagreements broke out within the Medical Department over hospital design, ambulance services, the scope and nature of the nursing corps, and what medicines would be routinely available for dispensing. Logistic and supply problems undermined the best efforts of government physicians. Soldiers clashed with doctors over appropriate assignments, malingering, medical discharges, health-related furloughs, and battle readiness. Some field doctors apparently took bribes, and there was a substantial amount of medically related influence peddling.

Particularly corrosive for the long-term prospects of anything approaching the old republican vision of state-based medical jurisprudence was the persistent power of politics and personalities to affect the relationship between the medical profession and the government. Indeed, problems involving politics and personalities permeated the wartime Medical Department from top to bottom. The best-known and most widely publicized political battles were fought at the highest level, that of the Surgeon General. After a season of confusion, incompetence, and overall mismanagement in the army under Secretary of War Simon Cameron and in the Medical Department specifically under Surgeon General Thomas Lawson, Lincoln replaced Cameron with Edwin M. Stanton, the political lawyer from Ohio who had danced upon the table after his winning defense of Sickles in 1859. Stanton, in turn, replaced Lawson with William Alexander Hammond, a relatively young physician whose energy, intelligence, and commanding personality gave promise of being just what the Medical Department needed to effect the near-revolutionary improvement that was called for.

The new Surgeon General brought reform and reorganization to the medical services, as well as his own strong interests in medical jurisprudence, but Hammond almost immediately clashed personally with Secretary Stanton. Both men had imperious egos to go along with their considerable professional abilities, and neither could abide the other's posturing. Personal dislike escalated quickly to political intrigue, and Stanton finally dismissed Hammond, despite the latter's measurable successes, largely on the grounds that the two could not work together and did not trust one another. Hammond had lost in a battle that pitted his own arrogance and temperament against the arrogance and temperament of his boss; neither professional competence nor the good of the troops appeared to play much of a role in this dragged-out and altogether public dramatization of the politics of military medicine.

While Hammond relinquished his post to Joseph Barnes, who took over as Surgeon General late in 1863 and served through the rest of the war, Hammond did not step aside gracefully. At Hammond's own insistence Stanton placed largely trumped-up charges of mismanagement before a formal court-martial, which duly found Hammond guilty in 1864. Hammond replied by publishing evidence of influence peddling in medical affairs at the highest levels of Congress and argued that the Secretary of War not only routinely used partisan criteria to make medically related decisions that should have been determined by professional standards and assessments of the national welfare, but actively intervened to save venal or incompetent political associates in the Medical Department from the army's own internal standards and regulations.[15] Neither the public nor the rest of the profession could have found the spectacle edifying, and neither the lawyer nor the doctor in this ugly confrontation offered much hope of future cooperation between the two. Though the verdict against Hammond was ceremonially reversed fifteen years later, the damage was done. Hammond, to make matters worse, would remain involved in the medical jurisprudence of insanity long after the war, where his unfortunate personality continued to do harm to the field and bring back fresh memories of how poorly the state and the professions had interacted during the Civil War.

What was true at the top, regrettably, was true as well through many other levels of military medicine during the war. Doctors refused to obey the direct orders of commanders whose credentials they did not like.[16] Doctors who remained outside the army resented as unfair competition any treatment afforded civilians by military physicians or military hospitals, though a great deal of such treatment was rendered to otherwise grateful citizens. Physicians working under federal authorities sometimes clashed with those holding state and local appointments. One such instance with dreadful results occurred at the Elmira, New York, federal prison camp: roughly one-fourth of the Confederates interred there died of disease (about twice the death rate in other federal prison camps), while the regular army commander feuded with his chief medical assistant, who was a surgeon of volunteers, and seven contract surgeons, an assistant surgeon from a militia unit, and a New York State National Guard surgeon over what to do. A subsequent formal inquiry resolved little.[17]

Professionals working for the Sanitary Commission made such harsh criticisms of government medical care that the Commission itself declined to publicize many of them in a brief history of its own activities through 1864, lest their criticisms hurt the war effort.[18] Surgeon General Barnes had to resort to the short-term impressment of doctors during the spring offensive of 1864 in the East, and by the summer of 1864 found himself hard-pressed "to locate an adequate number of able private physicians willing to take the required examination" for contract surgeon jobs.[19] From start to finish, the forced union between the government and the medical profession was proving to be less than idyllic from almost any point of view.

A final and intriguing piece of evidence for the proposition that state medicine was in a general sense discredited during the Civil War was not something that occurred, but something that did not. Despite the unprecedented scale of interaction between physicians and the government during the conflict, there appears with a single exception to have been no serious discussion of retaining any significant aspects of the expanded wartime medical service after the war. Nor did anyone propose altering the relationship to serve peacetime or civilian needs.[20] Most state-level medical activities ceased completely with the end of hostilities, and no one questioned the operative assumption that the army's own Medical Department would return as quickly as possible to a skeletal crew primarily manning the forts of the West. During the spring of 1865, even as the principal Confederate armies were surrendering, the federal government precipitously reduced the number of its military hospitals, abruptly dismissed its contract physicians, and began to auction off its excess medicines, supplies, and equipment.[21] No one in either the public sector or the professional sector seems to have demurred.

The single exception to this process of rapid and complete dismantling of postwar public medicine involved the Bureau of Refugees, Freedmen, and Abandoned Lands, better known by its shortened title as the Freedmen's Bureau. Established in March 1865 primarily to help oversee the transition from bondage to freedom among the former slaves of the South, the Freedmen's Bureau from the outset provided emergency medical services to citizens of both races adrift in the former Confederacy. Since the Bureau operated under the War Department, the army continued to provide medical assistance to the Bureau even after Congress slashed ordinary medical funding. When large numbers of former slaves suffered a health crisis in the immediate postwar period, the Freedmen's Bureau, alone among federal and state agencies providing medical care, actually increased the scope of its health-related activities. General Oliver O. Howard, director of the Bureau, designed a separate medical department to oversee the dispensaries, hospitals, and home-visitation programs his officers were trying to administer in the District of Columbia and throughout the South.[22]

The Freedmen's Bureau also, of course, is well known for maintaining a system of courts throughout the former Confederacy during the Reconstruction years. Those courts existed as army-backed alternatives for any citizen, especially black citizens, unable to obtain justice in the local tribunals of the South. As a result, the Freedmen's Bureau was perforce involved in many of the activities associated with traditional medical jurisprudence, including quarantines, public health, and forensic medicine. While Congress never consciously intended it as such, the Freedmen's Bureau functioned inadvertently for more than a year after the end of the Civil War as the century's only large-scale example of a federal medico-legal agency, quite literally combining concerns for health and justice.

From the point of view of anyone interested in assessing models of government-managed medical jurisprudence, however, the Freedmen's Bureau proved most unfortunate. The Bureau's forays into social medicine almost certainly mitigated some miserable situations in the postwar South, possibly saved some lives, and probably ensured a measure of justice for some former slaves in the short run. In the long run, however, little was accomplished. Loathed by the majority of Southern whites as an invasive symbol of Yankee dominance during Reconstruction, the Bureau made little more than a small dent in a massive wall of resistance. The agency suffered as well from horribly inadequate funding, internal and external racism, and bitter political infighting. Even its supporters in Congress had considered the Bureau a stop-gap and a somewhat irregular experiment; its many opponents considered it anathema. In 1867 Congress all but eliminated appropriations for the Freedmen's Bureau and the agency curtailed its medical services precipitously between the autumn of 1867 and the autumn of 1868. A tiny handful of the Bureau's hospitals survived for a few more years, but the Bureau and most of what it had tried to accomplish in the South disappeared altogether in the early 1870s.[23]

It would be wrong to judge the Freedmen's Bureau primarily as a medico-legal agency, for it was both more than that and less. It would likewise be wrong to judge the probable effectiveness of federal medico-legal agencies in the nineteenth century by the history of the Freedmen's Bureau, even if it was the only one of its sort. But it would be safe to conclude that the most visible major exception to the federal government's otherwise adamantly consistent reluctance during the nineteenth century to enter the field of medical jurisprudence had the ironic net effect of strengthening the rule. Government-managed legal medicine was tarred with the unpopular brush of black rights, wrong-headed experimentation, political embarrassment, regional animosity, and lack of effectiveness. Those were not factors likely to lead to additional departures.

The overall impact of the Civil War experience on legal medicine in the United States thus proved on the whole quite chilling. The forced union between doctors and the government seemed to exacerbate more medico-legal problems than it solved. Medical veterans, to be sure, later spear-headed the public health movement of the 1870s, and their wartime experiences almost certainly impressed them with the need for and with the potential impact of large-scale public health efforts. But they were a distinct minority within their own profession through the 1890s, as most rank-and-file physicians in the decades following the war opposed any public treatment of the sick.[24] And the public itself did not really respond to the calls of public health reformers until near the end of the century, when the memory of wartime fiascos had faded, public health had become a separate field of its own, and bacteriology had finally given the field something substantial to offer.[25] The conclusion the public drew from the war was the same one most physicians drew: medicine and government did not mix as well as some earlier professionals had hoped they might, even in the enlightened (and now preserved) republic and even in the face of a national emergency.

CHAPTER TWELVE

The Insanity Issue
after the Civil War

The adjudication of sanity, already an explosive problem in several areas of American law by the end of the 1850s, continued to plague the field of medical jurisprudence after the Civil War. A national crusade against unjustified incarceration further discredited the flagging asylum movement. Through the late 1860s and into the 1870s troublesome and contentious insanity-related trials continued to make headlines all over the country. Purported experts continued to disagree openly and often about the psychological and physiological origins of mental disease, about the duration and cure rate of various mental disorders, and about the degree of individual responsibility associated with such contested and controversial doctrines as moral insanity and temporary insanity.[1] The medical jurisprudence of insanity had already produced by 1866, in the apt phrase of historian Janet Tighe, a "crisis in credibility" not only for those who claimed expertise in the subject of insanity but also for the American medical profession in general.[2]

Forced incarceration by the state had long been anathema to Americans. Citizens of the early republic considered both *habeas corpus* and trial by peers nearly sacrosanct principles of American law, in large part because they provided bulwarks for the individual against the arbitrary exercise and potential abuse of state power. From the Revolution on, Americans placed a transcendent and nearly absolute value upon personal liberty. That commitment to personal liberty remained intense in the United States right through the first half of the nineteenth century, as Tocqueville in the 1830s and many historians since have demonstrated. The concept of incarceration, even for what purported to be beneficent purposes, was therefore something many Americans in the early nineteenth century had viewed with inherent skepticism. As a result, the early champions of insane asylums not only had to persuade legendarily parsimonious lawmakers to spend public money on their costly new institutions, they also had to sell doubting citizens on the larger philosophical virtues of at least some forms of state-controlled institutionalization in the first place.[3]

Lingering fears about the potentially anti-democratic danger of asylums had remained just beneath the surface of public opinion. A few individuals launched exposés in the 1840s and early 1850s, claiming to be the victims of illegal conspiracies. Morgan Hinchman was typical of the early protesters. He alleged in court that his physicians were in league with his former friends in an effort to have him confined in an insane asylum in order to settle his property in such a way as to obtain some of it for themselves. Hinchman's attorneys neatly characterized this use of asylums as an effort "to convert benevolence into malice."[4] A handful of similar cases kept popular suspicions alive, produced temporary protests, and generated regional concerns, but failed to elicit nationally widespread public, political, or legislative responses.[5] After a decade of internal disarray and external criticism during the 1850s, however, the nation's insane asylums were more vulnerable than ever to frontal attack during the 1860s on the key subject of individual liberty.

Battles against unjustified incarceration were eventually fought at several levels in several jurisdictions, but the most important, most visible, and most lasting public confrontation of the period grew out of a series of developments that took place during the war but had nothing directly to do with the armed forces. They involved instead the private battles of a minister's wife named Elizabeth Ware Packard, who lived in Manteno, Illinois, a rural town some forty miles south of Chicago. Mrs. Packard had lost faith in her husband's rigid Calvinism in 1859 and began discussing her doubts at church and in the community. Her husband first tolerated her exploration of new ideas; then, apparently pushed by members of his embarrassed congregation, he decided that his wife must have become mentally deranged. In the summer of 1860, the Reverend Theophilus Packard had his wife committed to the Jacksonville Asylum in central Illinois. Under Illinois state law he could do that with the consent of a single physician, as long as the asylum was willing to take her.[6]

Though she maintained all along that she was perfectly sane, Mrs. Packard spent the next three years in Jacksonville Asylum under the supervision of Andrew McFarland, a domineering physician-psychiatrist whose entire career was strewn with conflict and controversy.[7] After an initial period of romantic fascination with McFarland, Mrs. Packard became his avenging fury. In the fall of 1863, Mrs. Packard nonetheless found herself in the awkward position of trying to resist an order from the Jacksonville trustees that she be discharged. Though she considered herself falsely committed, and though she denounced Superintendent McFarland, a formal discharge would return her legally to the custody of her husband, a prospect she dreaded more than life at the asylum. Given her husband's subsequent actions, her fears were altogether reasonable.

Upon Mrs. Packard's return to Manteno, the Reverend Mr. Packard locked his wife in an upstairs room while he considered the best way to have her committed to an asylum in Massachusetts. The two had both grown up in Massachusetts; they had married, lived, and worked there until 1854;

and Theophilus Packard still had strong local contacts in that state. Elizabeth Packard got word about her virtual imprisonment to her friends, who
persuaded the local Illinois authorities to draft a writ of *habeas corpus* in her
name. A tragi-comic trial ensued and as it drew to a close, Theophilus
Packard, sensing that his wife would probably win both her freedom of
movement and her claim to legal sanity, bolted the state, taking most of the
family's possessions and all of their children with him back to Massachusetts.[8] Elizabeth Packard won her legal freedom two days later, but found
herself abandoned by her family and largely without resources, legal or
otherwise.

At this juncture, Elizabeth Packard decided to take her case to the
court of public opinion. In books, pamphlets, and door-to-door appeals, she
carried her story first into Chicago, then all around the state. Especially
telling in the context of this chapter was the warm and positive reception
she received, for it indicated clearly the tremendous residue of doubt and
suspicion among vast portions of the general public about insane asylums
and how they worked. She stressed several points in her tale, including the
need to bolster the rights of married women in matters concerning property
and child custody. But both the abuse of asylum inmates at the hands of
medical authorities and the ease with which false commitment could be
accomplished, particularly the latter, stood out. As the legal historian Hendrik Hartog has rightly recognized, Mrs. Packard was tapping into the
American people's "republican obsession with the misuse of public power."
The rules governing commitment to insane asylums permitted "corrupting
and corrupted relationships" and "joint conspiracies" between influential men
with sinister agendas, like her husband, and professionals with vested interests, like McFarland and the doctor who first certified her insanity, whereby
ordinary citizens were wrongly incarcerated.[9] And once imprisoned, public
authorities, acting through the power of the state, connived with and protected those who heaped additional mistreatment on the innocent.[10]

By the end of 1864 Mrs. Packard had sold some 6000 copies of her
first published exposé, then left Illinois and headed back to Massachusetts.
There she continued her crusade against false commitment. As in Illinois,
the public seemed to respond quickly and favorably. In support of Mrs.
Packard's positions, a prominent group of reform-minded men petitioned
the Massachusetts legislature to alter their state's commitment rules. Though
their suggested amendments failed when the state's most prestigious experts
on insanity came out against them, Massachusetts lawmakers did enact a
statute designed to prevent the possibility of secret commitments. Mrs.
Packard turned next to Connecticut, where her cause was again debated in
a state legislature. In 1866 she returned to Illinois, where the legislature, as
a result of her earlier campaign, had repealed in 1865 the law under which
she had been committed. She then played a prominent part in a drawn-out
investigation of the entire Illinois insane asylum system that eventuated in
the resignation of her old adversary, Superintendent McFarland, under heavy
public and political pressure.

In 1867 Illinois lawmakers passed a bill that mandated jury trials in sanity proceedings. Other states where Mrs. Packard continued her personal efforts, including Iowa and Massachusetts, soon followed suit. Some states, including Iowa and Pennsylvania, also enacted what were called "mailbox laws" explicitly to guarantee asylum inmates unfettered communication with the outside world.[11] In 1874 the lawmakers of influential New York state, under pressure from the popular press, also tried to tighten procedures for commitment.[12] During the course of her crusade between 1864 and 1873 Elizabeth Packard became the first woman ever to address a number of the American state legislatures she targeted. Throughout New England, in New York and Pennsylvania, and across the Midwest, Mrs. Packard and her cause became well known to ordinary citizens and well regarded by them. Countless newspaper editorials and legislative debates over a ten-year period leave no doubt that she and the issues she personified had touched a surprisingly raw public nerve. When she died in 1897, some obituaries placed her impact on public opinion second only to that of Harriet Beecher Stowe among her contemporaries. Whether or not that judgment was true, the Packard phenomenon was certainly not ephemeral.

For the cause of medical jurisprudence, of course, Elizabeth Packard's political crusade was crippling. Instead of beneficent examples of the way the law, the state, and medicine might work together to help cure one of society's most troubling ailments, insane asylums appeared to be dismal places where patients were warehoused, managers wasted money, and citizens were abused.[13] Worse, they made legal medicine appear perverted,

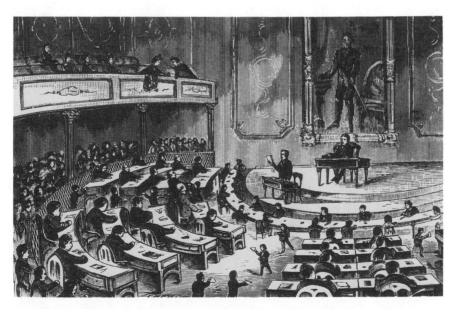

Elizabeth Packard, in the balcony, acknowledged by the Illinois legislature. From E.P.W. Packard, *Modern Persecution, or, Insane Asylums Unveiled* (Hartford, 1875).

or at least pervertible. Influential individuals could ally themselves with, or out-and-out purchase the services of, elite professionals, both doctors and lawyers, then use the power of the state to deprive ordinary citizens of their rights and remove them from society. Important property considerations were certainly at stake as well; people committed to insane asylums, after all, would be legally stripped of the right to manage their own affairs.

Ultimately more profound were the basic rights of American liberty. The popular press called the Packard-inspired legislative acts of the late 1860s and early 1870s the nation's new "Personal Liberty Laws." In the non-slave states, that label had powerful connotations to a generation which had tried only a decade earlier to counter the Fugitive Slave Act of 1850 with a prior wave of so-called Personal Liberty Laws. The implication was all too obvious: medical jurisprudence gave physicians the power to enslave American citizens. That was no trivial matter, especially in an era when almost anyone could claim to be a physician, and especially in an era when those same state legislatures were almost simultaneously debating and ratifying the Fourteenth Amendment to the federal Constitution, which was designed to guarantee civil rights and due process for all citizens, even former slaves.

Long-term advocates of asylum care fully recognized the larger implications of what had happened. Though they spent a great deal of time and effort railing against Mrs. Packard personally and against all that she rep-

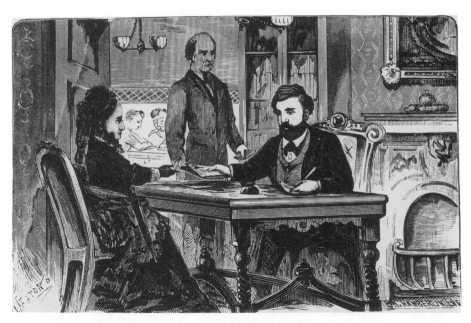

Governor Carpenter of Iowa presents a signed copy of his state's "Packard Law" to Elizabeth Packard. From E.P.W. Packard, *Modern Persecution, or, Insane Asylums Unveiled* (Hartford, 1875).

resented generally, they never fully recovered either their optimism or their momentum. Isaac Ray, whose influential *Treatise on the Medical Jurisprudence of Insanity* had best captured the optimistic spirit and forward-looking excitement of the earlier era, accurately caught the tone of the late 1860s as well. Writing in the *American Law Review* in 1869 to an audience self-evidently interested in medico-legal issues, Ray observed:

> Until a comparatively recent period . . . [the] danger of [insane asylums] being converted to the nefarious purpose of depriving sane persons of their liberty, was scarcely thought of. A crime so revolting to every sentiment of right and humanity, and requiring the co-operation of parties so unlikely to work together, seemed to be so improbable as to make any special legislation supererogatory. . . .
>
> Of late years, with little or no foundation therefor, a change of sentiment has occurred, whereby admission to hospitals for the insane has come to be regarded, to some extent, as exceedingly liable to be perverted by bad men from its proper purpose.[14]

Ray went on to rue the nation-wide burst of Packard laws as misguided and unnecessary. Those laws were misguided in his view because ordinary juries would be no better at determining sanity than experts and because jury trials over sanity would become counter-productive public spectacles. The laws were unnecessary in his view because English and American court precedents, which he rehearsed, already provided sufficient safeguards. But Ray realized that his views would not prevail in the post-Packard period. Consequently, even though he continued to favor the "old" system, "whereby friends assumed the management of the case . . . under the advice of . . . physicians," and even though he pleaded that "England and France" continued to make that system work perfectly well, Ray proposed a commission arrangement as a sort of compromise to salvage the situation in the United States. In those few exceptional cases that, in their opinion, merited special treatment local judges should be empowered to appoint a commission consisting "of not less than three nor more than four persons, one of whom, at least, shall be a physician, and another a lawyer." The commission would investigate the case and report directly to the judge, much as expert witnesses were empowered to do under the French system.

Ray asked his legal brethren a final, plaintive, and telling question at the end of his essay. As his readers well knew, "wrongful imprisonment" occurred every day in the United States in ordinary criminal cases. In many of those cases the accused really was the victim "of conspiracy or perjury." While some citizens wrongfully seized in this fashion under the powers of the state were eventually declared innocent and released, others suffered unfairly. With criminal actions of that kind "no rare, extraordinary thing," and considering "we are told very calmly that such wrongs are a part of the price we pay for public order and good government," why, pleaded Ray, had the public become so incensed about the extremely unlikely danger of false commitment to insane asylums by knowledgeable people of good intentions?

The answer was clear. The public still feared the power of the professions in league together or in league with the state, especially in matters as unsettling and uncertain as the determination of sanity. Criminal courts might sometimes make mistakes, or be misled by lies, but people accepted the standards those courts were trying to apply, even when they failed to apply them perfectly. And criminal courts had institutionalized various mechanisms and procedures designed to minimize mistakes. In the case of public asylum commitments, however, people correctly sensed the lack of acceptable standards, even among purported experts. Already questioned by legislatures during the 1850s on their effectiveness and their costs, public asylums came to be regarded as downright sinister after the Civil War. Consequently, after mid-century, many prominent champions of medical jurisprudence seemed to be on the wrong side in the great American debate over how to deal with insanity.

The attack upon asylums constituted only one of the ways in which insanity continued to be a serious problem for the champions of medical jurisprudence after the Civil War. A steady drumbeat of articles, essays, lectures, and comments reminded both professionals and lay citizens that the issue of insanity had become a nightmare in American courts at all levels and in many different types of cases. Even in cases that involved the validity of wills, medical credibility was slipping. A Chicago judge was widely quoted in the nation's legal press, for example, when he castigated two medical witnesses in 1875 "summoned by the contestants 'as experts' for the purpose of invalidating a will deliberately made by a man quite as competent as either of them to do such an act." [15] But the largest and most troubling problems continued to circle around the difficulty of determining the criminal responsibilities of the mentally impaired.

While hundreds of public statements could easily be cited, one of the most revealing indications of the profound uneasiness over those issues, even among professionals with the greatest sympathy for and the most direct interest in the dilemmas of medical jurisprudence, came not from a formal criticism or a prepared analysis but from a spontaneous outburst at a private social event. Members of the Medico-Legal Society of the City of New York decided in 1873 to celebrate the fifth anniversary of their charter by holding a gala banquet at Delmonico's. After a great deal of food and drink, the president began to call upon various luminaries for impromptu remarks. The tone of the evening was distinctly jocular and self-congratulatory, but Lewis A. Sayre, an orthopedic surgeon who had long been one of the leading professionals and professionalizers in the city, could not resist blurting out what troubled him most:

> There are certain questions of "emotional insanity" which should be wiped out of the statute book—and "transitory insanity." It is high time that we, both legal and medical men, should rise in our might and stamp with the infamy it deserves, and call moral depravity—moral depravity! (applause)—and not attempt to excuse it under the damnable garb of moral insanity! (Great applause.) [16]

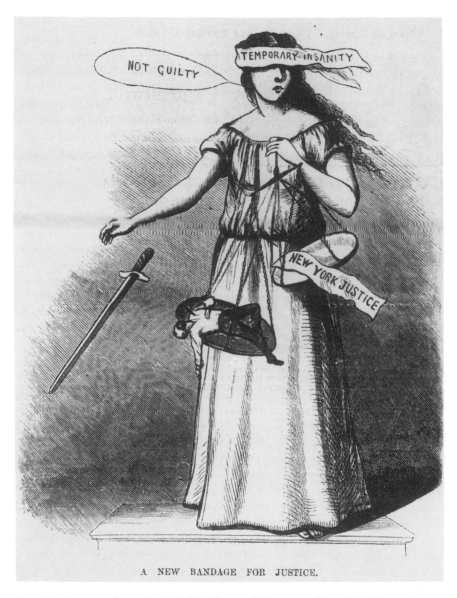

A NEW BANDAGE FOR JUSTICE.

A satirical cartoon from *Frank Leslie's Illustrated Newspaper*, May 28, 1870, condemning the plea of temporary insanity. (*Courtesy Enoch Pratt Free Library, Baltimore*)

Wine-soaked syntax aside, Sayre clearly believed that the continued application of flexible new insanity doctrines (emotional insanity was one of the latest) to questions of criminal responsibility was badly undermining the value of legal medicine in the eyes of the general public. As the applause suggested, Sayre was not alone.[17]

Later in the evening, J.K. Herbert, a lawyer who had used insanity defenses with considerable success in his own practice, defended flexible theories, and other members of the society regretted that the leading advocates of those defenses could not attend the dinner and were therefore not present to defend them. But Whitelaw Reid, a formally trained lawyer as well as the managing editor of the nationally influential *New York Tribune*, re-emphasized Sayre's fears in strong terms. He hoped the "two recognized professions" in the Medico-Legal Society might "agree to abolish forever from the face of the earth the doctrine and the practice of 'Emotional Insanity.' (Great applause. A voice—Good)."[18] Charles Woodbury, another lawyer, called for a crackdown upon crime. Let "the terrors" of the law, not the excuse of weak moral perception or inadequate education, be "brought home to every person" who behaved lawlessly.[19]

The medical profession was also accused of applying a double standard in the insanity defense. In 1873 James A. McMaster attacked some of the leading professionals of New York in the columns of the *Freeman's Journal and Catholic Register* for not mounting as vigorous a plea of insanity for a poor Catholic boy accused of murder as they would have mounted for their wealthy friends. McMaster's accusations touched off a heated debate within the legal community as well.[20] In 1876 the popular *Frank Leslie's Illustrated Newspaper* printed a satirical cartoon suggesting that emotional insanity was a convenient disease of the rich and dissolute.[21] Several years later, the *Albany Law Journal* went so far as to suggest sarcastically that homicidal mania, "like the gout," seemed to be "a gentlemanly affliction, exclusively confined to the upper classes." Pulling no punches, the *Journal* continued, "If a nigger or a low-down white man kills another, he always appears to have his senses, and this is so apparent that the community usually hang him at once to save delay and possible miscarriage of justice."[22]

The most serious and potentially far-reaching efforts to address the mounting problems associated with the medical jurisprudence of insanity took place in the state of New York. Republicans there controlled the legislature during the early years of the Reconstruction period, and they used their power in Albany to launch a number of significant institutional reforms, including the creation of a Metropolitan Board of Health for the New York City area.[23] When the Democrats returned to power at the end of the decade, they were able substantially to reverse implementation of most of the Republican initiatives, but were unable to reshape the state's infrastructure to suit themselves. The result was stalemate and corruption, which came to a dramatic head in 1871, when a citizens' revolt broke the Tweed regime in New York City while a Democratic governor watched helplessly from Albany.

With the machinery of state in disarray, the Democratic governor and the Republican legislators agreed in 1872 to create a special bi-partisan commission on reform. The thirty-two commissioners, who were supposed to act as dispassionate experts, were told to study New York's entire system of government and make suggestions for rebuilding and improving any of its aspects, up to and including the recommendation of constitutional

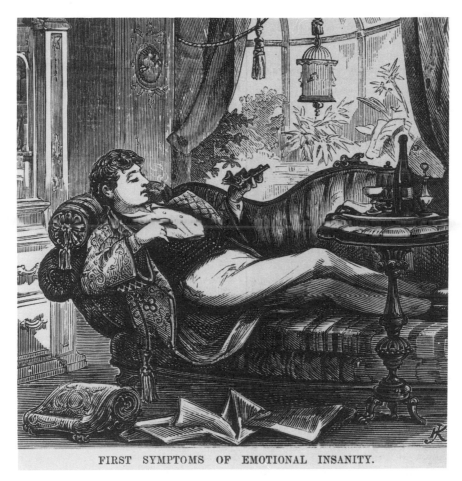

FIRST SYMPTOMS OF EMOTIONAL INSANITY.

A satirical cartoon from *Frank Leslie's Illustrated Newspaper*, July 19, 1873, suggesting that the wealthy were chief beneficiaries of the plea of emotional insanity. (*Courtesy Enoch Pratt Free Library, Baltimore*)

amendments.[24] This unusual procedure, coupled with the general crisis of government in New York, created a political climate, albeit for quite different reasons, strikingly similar to the one Beck had enjoyed half a century earlier while the first great code revision committee had been in session. Prominent professionals, especially those from law and medicine, were again in an unusually strong position to influence public policy, and again openly invited to do so.

A number of prominent physicians pressed an idea which had intrigued many medico-legal theorists for a long time: the concept of a lunacy commission, experts who would determine legal sanity in disputed cases. The French had created lunacy commissions early in the nineteenth century, and Isaac Ray, since the first edition of his *Treatise*, had been urging their adoption in the United States.[25] By mid-century several other experts had advanced their own versions of how lunacy commissions might operate. Some, including Ray himself and William Stokes of Maryland, urged commissions that would supplement normal court proceedings. Others, like Francis Wharton, co-author of the Wharton/Stille textbook and a life-long student of the medical jurisprudence of insanity, initially favored commissions that would in essence replace standard jury determinations.[26] D. Meredith Reese and C.B. Coventry, who had urged the American Medical Association to distance itself from the controversies over insanity in the late 1850s, clearly liked the commission idea as a way to get the vast majority of regular practitioners out of what they regarded as the no-win business of adjudicating sanity.[27] But no jurisdiction had adopted such a suggestion.

In the climate of structural reform associated with the New York Revision Commission, however, the concept of a lunacy commission seemed worth reconsidering. John Ordronaux, then professor of medical jurisprudence at Columbia Law School and considered one of the nation's leading authorities in what would now be called forensic psychiatry, led the resurgent effort to substitute a standing commission of experts for ordinary juries in cases that hinged on mental competence.[28] Ordronaux considered the opinion of experts far fairer and more reliable than ordinary perceptions in such matters, and some of his most persuasive essays chronicled the ways in which well-intentioned juries could reach disastrous conclusions when insanity was at issue.[29] Such prominent New York medico-legal professionals as Roger Stephens, William Hammond, James J. O'Dea, Clark Bell, and David Dudley Field all made plain their desire for some sort of reform.[30] In 1874, augmented by the Packard crusade, their combined pressure brought legislative results. New York created the nation's first state lunacy commission, and Ordronaux was appointed to its chair. On its face, this appeared to be a major development in the medical jurisprudence of insanity, especially in such a key jurisdiction.[31]

Yet beneath the surface the commission was neither as radical a departure as it appeared to be nor as likely to solve as many jurisprudential problems as its backers might have hoped it would. The commission law authorized the experts to make a determination in criminal cases only when the defendant made no other plea than insanity. Moreover, if the defense disagreed with the commission's ruling, the defendant could demand a regular jury trial to redetermine his or her status in the normal fashion. Much of Ordronaux's time as commissioner was consumed in matters of jurisdiction, asylum oversight, and battling about expenses. To make matters worse, the professionals who helped bring the commission into being could never fully agree about the sorts of rulings the commissioners should be trying to make or where next to push the reform movement.

The New York Medico-Legal Society never formally endorsed the commission and the society's members consistently failed to reach consensus on any of the thorny issues the commission might have tried to address. New York's neurologists organized a separate pressure group to goad both the commissioner and the asylum superintendents whom Ordronaux was, in turn, trying unsuccessfully to supervise.[32] The state's lawyers also began to wonder how far the commission's powers extended. In the afterglow of popular resentment over charges of false commitment and abuse within the asylums, they questioned publicly how long a person should remain in an asylum if sent there by the state lunacy commission; a day, a year, forever? Who should make that determination, and through what sort of proceeding?[33] Outside New York, the AMSAII declined to support the proposition that other states should consider lunacy commissions as well. Indeed, though a minority of superintendents considered the new lunacy commission a promising step forward, they could not persuade the majority even to wish New York well with its experiment. At the International Medical Congress held in Philadelphia in conjunction with the national centennial in 1876, the aging Isaac Ray openly opposed the New York commission as having been founded upon a bad idea, although he had been urging experiments along similar lines for almost forty years.[34]

Ordronaux soon found himself spending a great deal of time and effort defending even the limited powers his commission had on paper.[35] In 1876 a member of the state legislature introduced a bill that would mandate life imprisonment for anyone acquitted in a capital case on a plea of insanity, a clear manifestation of the popular fear that influential frauds might use the commission to get away with murder.[36] In 1877 Ordronaux was forced formally to defend conditions inside the state asylums to which his commission committed people.[37] By 1879 Ordronaux had to defend himself. State senator Dennis McCarthy published an attack upon Ordronaux in the Albany *Evening Journal* and introduced a bill to abolish the commissioner's job. After a debate in the legislature, Ordronaux's allies side-tracked the effort to oust him, but not before Ordronaux's enemies, including William A. Hammond, forced yet another official investigation and report.[38] In 1880 a physician-politician in the New York Assembly called for an investigation of the management of the state's asylums as well as an inquiry concerning the "fitness and efficiency of the State commissioner," and the speaker of the Assembly himself introduced still one more bill to get rid of Ordronaux's job and emasculate the commission he oversaw.[39]

By the end of its first decade the New York State Lunacy Commission had acted usefully in a number of cases. But virtually every professional observer conceded that this innovation, even when it worked well, was incapable of solving very many of the tortured legal problems associated with the jurisprudence of insanity. Once again, as they had done half a century earlier, elite professionals interested in medical jurisprudence had nearly, but not quite, engineered a potentially significant breakthrough in the nation's most populous and politically influential state, only to come up short, still divided and still without solid structural support for what they thought they had to contribute. Instead of a solution, American physicians continued to face what seemed to become a tougher and tougher professional dilemma.

Something of a nadir was reached in the late 1870s, when two of the country's best known experts on the various types and degrees of insanity went at each other in a vicious, intraprofessional feud that had national and interprofessional repercussions. The principals were William A. Hammond and Eugene Grissom. Hammond, the domineering personality removed as Surgeon General of the Union army during the Civil War, had returned to New York City at the end of that conflict. There he focused his professional energy on the emerging field of neurology, which he had helped nourish during the war. Through the late 1860s and into the 1870s, he wrote frequently on the subject of insanity and its relation to the law, and he became an active member in several organizations that explored the medico-legal problems of insanity in great detail.

Hammond combined an unusually expansive and inclusive definition of insanity with a belief that society, at least most of the time, still had to punish the insane, especially those who killed. The former made Hammond a popular witness for parties wishing to break wills, since his expansive and inclusive theories could be made to apply to almost anyone. Whitelaw Reid quipped that Hammond's theories about neurology allowed Hammond to testify as an expert that everyone was insane. Hammond's other contention, however, that most demented persons most of the time had to be held to the standards of the law, made him an attractive ally of prosecutors, especially in homicide cases where the defense was hard pressed to demonstrate a manifestly obvious degree of gross mental incompetence. The latter theory also put Hammond frequently at odds with the increasingly separate and professionally defensive association of asylum superintendents, who believed, of course, that the insane should be spared punishment and sent instead to their asylums for correction and cure.[40]

By the early 1870s Hammond and the neurologists, on the one hand, and the New York asylum superintendents, on the other, were at each other's throats in the legislature at Albany, rehashing many of the issues that had arisen earlier in the case of Elizabeth Packard. Hammond also got more and more heavily involved in more and more cases of medico-legal insanity, almost to the point of becoming a professional witness. In two of those cases, the McFarland case and the Reynolds case, Hammond took embarrassingly inconsistent positions, which allowed those who retained him to win acquittal for McFarland and execution for Reynolds. In a third instance, the Montgomery case, Hammond took two contradictory positions on consecutive days after conferring with the interested counsel between sessions. In one of Hammond's best-known will cases, the famous neurologist gave scientifically slippery testimony that helped break an apparently air-tight testament; his enemies learned later that he had insisted on a fee of $500 up front in that case and an additional contingent fee of $2500 more if his clients won on the basis of his testimony.

In 1878 Hammond's opponents could stand it no longer and launched a frontal attack against him and what they thought he stood for. The salvo was fired, appropriately enough, from a podium at the national convention of the Association of American Superintendents, meeting that year in Washington, D.C.. It took the form of a paper entitled "True and False Experts," written and delivered by Eugene Grissom, superintendent of the North Carolina Insane Asylum at Raleigh. Grissom was no narrow partisan; he held degrees in medicine and in law, and he sat on the AMA's Judicial Council, notwithstanding the increasing professional distance between the AMA and the superintendents.

Later published in the *American Journal of Insanity*, the essay reviewed Hammond's testimony in several key cases and pulled no punches about what the superintendents thought of him. "[H]e is the type of a reckless class of men who are attempting to control the medical and even the secular press of the country [the New York *Herald* had earlier been castigated for serving as an editorial outlet for Hammond's views], and to poison the public mind until they shall have worked upon popular ignorance and passion, as they hope, to the destruction of the present system of providing for the insane in the United States." Hammond himself epitomized all those "false experts, who impose upon the courts and the public mind their *presumption* for learning and their *ignorance* for discovery." He was "a moral monster, whose baleful eyes glare with delusive light; whose bowels are but bags of gold, to feed which, spider-like, he casts his loathsome arms about a helpless prey."[41]

Hammond replied in two public letters. His astonishing language did little to elevate this extraordinarily nasty intraprofessional debate: "A distempered and snarling cur has nobler mental and moral qualities than you; the vibrio that wriggles in decomposing filth is higher in the scale of existence; the foul bird that defecates in its own nest is less odious. . . ."[42] More importantly, the letters did little to convince neutral observers that many of the allegations against Hammond, and by implication against a host of other expert witnesses in the tangled world of medico-legal insanity, were not justified. Indeed, when three nervous members of the Superintendents' Society unwisely pushed a resolution of criticism against Grissom for "stir[ring] up strife and confusion" to the detriment of the profession, a subsequent meeting of the association defeated the resolution "by an overwhelming majority."[43]

By 1884 Hammond had resolved personally never to testify again as an expert witness in a trial that involved insanity, but that did not prevent him from offering newspaper interviews castigating those physicians who continued to do so. Hammond told the public that physicians who continued to testify were seekers of notoriety (because insanity cases seemed to be receiving more and more popular attention); second-rate physicians (because top doctors could usually make more money per day in their office than they could in court); lazy (because offering expert testimony of that sort was "the least laborious" professional duty he could imagine); and panderers for public approval (because expert witnesses who "failed to suit the popular mind" were "execrated"). Though he had testified himself for many years, he now confidently informed the general public that most of the expert opinions offered in American courtrooms on the subject of insanity were "farcical" and "ridiculous" and of no legal or medical value.[44]

Since the intraprofessional chaos swirling around the medical jurisprudence of insanity surfaced repeatedly during the 1870s in state legislatures, local newspapers, highly visible court cases, professional journals, and standard textbooks, by the end of the decade most members of the informed public realized that the field was riddled with serious, apparently unresolvable problems. Suffice it here to quote the assessment of John B. Chapin, superintendent of New York's Willard Asylum (the one that would have been named for Beck), who had reason to wish the 1870s had been kinder than they were to those professionals involved with the treatment of insanity. Looking back over the contentious litigation of the previous ten years from the vantage point of 1880, Chapin acknowledged in the United States "a growing distrust of the value, and we may say, the honesty, of expert testimony." And "the want of confidence and distrust are confined not wholly to judges and jurors, but, to a certain extent, prevade [sic] the community."[45]

Any citizens still in doubt had their attentions directed to the issues in 1881 in a dramatic fashion, when Charles Guiteau, the man who shot President James Garfield, pleaded not guilty by reason of insanity when indicted for the murder. Popular media of the day made much of the events surrounding the President's death and Guiteau's trial, which in turn forced ordinary people to wrestle with the questions of mental competence that had been plaguing doctors and lawyers for decades. Even the Congress at Washington debated bills designed to clarify the plea of insanity in criminal trials.[46] As Charles Rosenberg and others have made clear, the execution of Guiteau in 1882 reflected a sense of national trauma and outrage, rather than a consensus concerning degrees of mental incompetence and legal responsibility.[47] The nation was far from the latter.

On the one hand, the medico-legal aspects of insanity remained as close to the center of medical jurisprudence in 1881 as they had been in 1811, the year Rush used insanity as his example of the promise inherent in the field and Beck defended his dissertation on the subject. On the other hand, the medico-legal aspects of insanity were no longer a source of optimism and potential for people interested in the interaction of physicians and the law. The problems associated with insanity still intrigued a number of professionals interested in medico-legal theory, to be sure, particularly judges who had to make actual decisions about them in specific cases.[48] But for most physicians the subject of insanity had become a professional morass in the seventy years between 1811 and 1881, between Rush's lecture on the medical jurisprudence of insanity and the trial of Charles Guiteau. It no longer uplifted the medical profession; it appeared to degrade those involved with the subject. It no longer united doctors and lawyers; it further divided them, even in societies whose members committed themselves to improving the interactions of law and medicine. The only fresh institutional response after the Civil War, the New York State Lunacy Commission, fell under withering public, political, and professional fire and accomplished almost nothing of substance. No consensus emerged on how to deal with the many vexing questions involved in the issue of legal sanity. Indeed, most of those questions would remain unresolved through the next century.[49]

CHAPTER THIRTEEN

The Schoeppe Trials
and the Wharton Case

In the field of toxicology, the United States undoubtedly had more physicians capable of performing more forensic assays for more types of substances with more reliable results in 1870 than it had in 1850. New discoveries had been made and, perhaps just as important, several significant new textbooks had been published in the United States to disseminate the advances. Indeed, the work published during that period dominated toxicology into the twentieth century.[1] Yet contrary to the hopes and assumptions of many professionals then and since, two wonderfully absorbing and widely publicized cases demonstrated to a national audience after the Civil War that advances in science would not by themselves eliminate the sorts of difficulties revealed in the Hendrickson case at mid-century. Both situations involved trials for murder by poison and both involved women from Baltimore.

The first case broke in 1869 after Maria Stennecke, an unmarried Baltimore woman nearly seventy years of age, died in a hotel during a visit to Carlisle, Pennsylvania, her home town. She had gone to Carlisle to see Paul Schoeppe, a local physician. Twenty-seven years old, Schoeppe had grown up in Germany and claimed a degree in medicine from the University of Berlin. He had come to the United States just two years before Stennecke's death. Though the relationship between the smooth young German and the elderly Baltimore spinster began and continued as doctor and patient, the two had grown increasingly close during Stennecke's frequent trips up to Carlisle in the winter of 1868–69. Notwithstanding local gossip about this odd couple, and notwithstanding some uncertainty about the exact cause of Stennecke's death, her passing did not arouse immediate suspicion. Stennecke was, after all, getting on in years, and she had suffered from various ailments, including dizziness, for some time. Indeed, that was why she had started consulting Schoeppe in the first place.[2]

When Stennecke's extraordinarily long, unusually detailed, and previously drafted will was submitted for probate, however, Schoeppe came for-

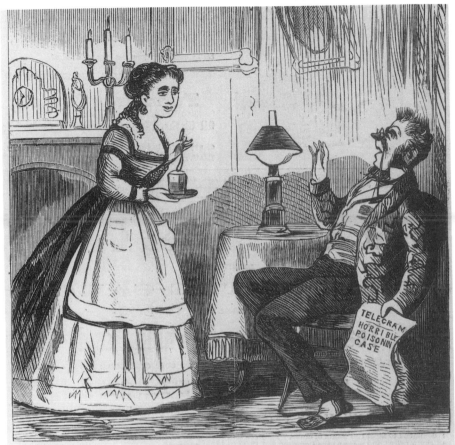

THE STRYCHNINE MANIA.

LOVING WIFE--"*Take some of this cool lemonade, Charlie; you do look so hot. I've put a stick in it.*"

SUSPICIOUS HUSBAND—(Who has been reading an account of a husband poisoned by his wife)—"*Strychnine! Oh, horror!*"

A cartoon from *Frank Leslie's Illustrated Newspaper*, August 22, 1868, playing upon the popular awareness of poisoning, even before the Schoeppe and Wharton trials. (*Courtesy Enoch Pratt Free Library, Baltimore*)

ward to challenge it with a short, blunt, and clumsily drafted substitute document supposedly executed just days before Stennecke died. While the former parceled Stennecke's considerable estate, valued at approximately $45,000, piece by piece to many relatives, friends, and good causes, the latter summarily made Schoeppe sole heir to everything. Rumors raced through Cumberland County that the doctor had first taken emotional advantage of his vulnerable patient, even promising to marry her; then duped her into making him her beneficiary (though many observers believed the will to be an out-and-out forgery since none of it, including the purported signature, appeared to be in Stennecke's handwriting); and finally killed her in order to collect. The doctor's friends urged him to have Stennecke's remains publicly analyzed at his own expense to squelch the rumors, but a nervous and defensive Schoeppe declined, inquiring instead about how long after burial various substances might still be detected. That was enough for the local authorities, who indicted the doctor and ordered an exhumation themselves.

An initial post-mortem assessment by a Carlisle physician led him to believe that physical indications consistent with death by poisoning were present, so parts of Stennecke's viscera were sent to Baltimore in an effort to obtain a more sophisticated chemical analysis than any of the local physicians could perform. Besides, most of the local doctors were already involved in the case one way or another and might not be viewed as neutral investigators. The stomach was turned over to Professor William E.A. Aiken, a veteran physician who had taught medical chemistry at the University of Maryland Medical School in Baltimore for thirty-two years.[3] Aiken was told that he should test for indications of poisoning and that local observers had reason to suspect the murderer may have administered morphine first and possibly some other poison afterward. Schoeppe was alleged to have purchased two separate batches of prussic acid shortly before Stennecke's demise, one in Carlisle and one in Harrisburg. Aiken was also told that he would receive $250 for his analysis, regardless of what he found.

Aiken was unable to identify any morphine, but that did not surprise him. Morphine was considered nearly impossible to detect with certainty unless investigations were done almost immediately after death, and in this case two full weeks had passed. Far more important, Aiken "satisfied [him]self" through chemical tests that Stennecke's stomach did still contain significant amounts of the deadly prussic acid. The prosecutor in Carlisle was delighted with that information, and he decided to rest his otherwise somewhat puzzling and altogether circumstantial case on Aiken's testimony and the purported presence of prussic acid.

During the trial Schoeppe's lawyers concentrated their counterattack on that same evidence. Aiken was a veteran, no doubt, argued the defense, a practitioner who had been left behind. He had employed old-fashioned chemical tests and conducted them sloppily. Indeed, the defense implied, Aiken's procedures might inadvertently have created an indication of prussic acid where none was present. To defend their contentions, Schoeppe's attorneys retained T. G. Wormley, who journeyed to Carlisle from his post at Starling Medical College in Columbus, Ohio. The author of several important papers on forensic toxicology, Wormley was one of the nation's two or three top experts in the detection and medical chemistry of poisons. He performed well on the stand, claimed that he was being paid a flat fee of $200 without contingencies or bonuses tied to the outcome of the trial, and suggested that he would be glad to have his arguments and conclusions tested and retested by experts around the nation.

When the trial ended, the Cumberland County jurors believed their local prosecutor and the testimony of Professor Aiken, the prosecutor's expert from Baltimore, rather than the defense and their expert from Ohio. The jury found Schoeppe guilty of first-degree murder. The judge, in turn, sentenced him to death, and Schoeppe's lawyers appealed to the Pennsylvania Supreme Court for review under a writ of error. When the high court balked, Schoeppe's lawyers orchestrated a remarkable appeal to the governor, John White Geary, former adventurer, former territorial governor of Kansas, former Democratic boss of California, military hero, and now Radical Republican chief executive of Pennsylvania.[4] The appeal neatly illustrated once again the sorts of political and professional cross-currents within which the apparent scientific neutrality of medical jurisprudence actually operated, and it evoked haunting memories of Hendrickson's appeal to Governor Seymour fifteen years before.

Though Schoeppe's case had begun as little more than a local scandal, the verdict attracted the close attention of two influential groups: prominent regular doctors interested in the professional implications of medical jurisprudence, on the one hand, and German politicians, on the other. The former had good reason for being uneasy about the verdict. For obvious reasons, physicians were reluctant to support murder charges associated with the loss of a patient unless the evidence was absolutely iron-clad.[5] Malpractice was already bad enough. Physicians could ill afford a wave of criminal indictments in cases where the death, as distinguished from Schoeppe's probably criminal attempt to cash in on it, could have resulted from the patient's own mistaken overdose or from unrelated natural causes. In any event, the evidence in this case was far from iron-clad, whether Schoeppe was a physician or not. Wormley's criticisms carried great weight when Schoeppe's defenders began to circulate transcripts of the trial. Medicolegal experts near and far began to come forward in opposition to the scientific testimony proffered by Professor Aiken.

Frederick Genth of Philadelphia, who had studied medical chemistry in Germany a generation before Schoeppe, led an early charge upon Aiken's evidence of prussic acid. Several of Genth's Philadelphia associates quickly followed. John J. Reese, certainly one of the leading forensic physicians in the United States, agreed with Genth and attacked the conclusions of the local post-mortem as well.[6] They were joined, in turn, by Henry Morton and Andrew Nebinger, two other prominent medical jurisprudents of Philadelphia.[7] A committee of the German physicians of Philadelphia protested the verdict, as did a special committee of the Pennsylvania Medical Society.[8] The College of Physicians of Philadelphia unanimously adopted a report condemning the medical conclusions upon which Schoeppe had been convicted; the committee that drafted the report had Edward Hartshorne, Taylor's American editor, in the chair, and included Isaac Ray among its other members.[9] The county medical societies of Cumberland, Luzerne, and Allegheny counties also weighed in against the verdict.[10]

Beyond Pennsylvania, the Medico-Legal Society of New York City discussed the case and published conclusions critical of the prosecution's medical evidence.[11] The faculty of the Yale Medical School, organized as the New Haven Medical Association, formally demurred as well.[12] K.N. Horsford, Rumford Professor at Harvard, joined B. Ogden Doremus, the professor of chemistry and toxicology at New York's Bellevue Hospital Medical College in a letter defending Schoeppe.[13] Additional protests arrived from physicians in Chicago, New York, and St. Louis.[14] Even in Aiken's Baltimore, "several practitioners of high repute and scientific ability," particularly among the city's German physicians, believed "that the evidence did not clearly establish the existence of prussic acid" in Stennecke's stomach; ten of them formed a delegation to convey that opinion to Governor Geary in person.[15] By any standards, that was an impressive outpouring. In defense of the positions taken by Aiken and the Carlisle doctor who performed the post-mortem stood a handful of other Carlisle physicians and some of Aiken's colleagues at the University of Maryland.[16]

Governor Geary, however, probably felt more acutely the pressure from German politicians than he did the concern of America's medico-legalists. Those politicians, along with what would now be termed German-American community activists, feared prejudice against a recent immigrant, and by extension, against the large German minority in Pennsylvania. Their fears were well founded. Local spectators in Carlisle, a town with many Germans and overt ethnic tensions, had shouted to the jurors to "hang the d—d dutchman," and the presiding judge had charged the jury that anyone unable to accept the circumstantial evidence before the court was a fit subject for the lunatic asylum.[17] In his formal plea to the governor, Schoeppe consciously characterized himself as "a poor foreigner" and argued that "an immense prejudice was raised against me."[18] The German-language press in the United States, still a potent force during this period, rallied to Schoeppe's defense. The *Staats Zeitung* of New York and the *Demokrat* of Philadelphia led that rally and sought review of the medical evidence by official medico-legal officers back in Prussia, where the case also made prominent news.[19] Frederick Dittman, chief counsel for an umbrella pressure group known as the Society for the Relief of Distressed Germans, took command of the gubernatorial lobbying process. Eventually the Prussian ambassador himself journeyed up from Washington to have a private interview with Governor Geary in Harrisburg.[20]

With pressure building and Schoeppe still under a death sentence, Geary granted a public hearing in November 1869 on Schoeppe's petition for a pardon or a retrial. As the *Philadelphia Inquirer* noted, it was "the first example in the history of the Commonwealth of an Executive having a formal argument in public in the case of a man convicted of murder, and will, doubtless, form a very important precedent."[21] Dittman, the German community's national activist, led the defense and pointedly pleaded from his "German heart" for justice to a German.[22] He also presented a list of Cumberland County signatures "several yards long" in favor of a pardon for Schoeppe, along with the impressive list of medical protests pouring into Harrisburg.[23] Outside the governor's residence, German politicians pressed their allies in the Pennsylvania legislature to pass quickly a bill that would require the state Supreme Court to review all capital cases, whether the court found technical errors or not; the bill had been drafted with Schoeppe's predicament overtly in mind.[24]

All of this put Geary, a politician struggling for his political life in the churning party realignments of postwar Pennsylvania, in a difficult spot. Geary was in the process of slipping out of the Republican party as he had the Democratic party and positioning himself for a run at the presidential nomination of what became the Labor Reform party. His inclination, according to a correspondent of the *Philadelphia Inquirer* who interviewed him on the subject, was to take a hard line against what he regarded as increasing rates of crime and let the sentence stand.[25] But even if Geary were prepared to ignore the cries of outside experts and to defend local justice as Governor Seymour of New York had done in the Hendrickson case fifteen years before, he had to take seriously the power of the German community in a state where Germans constituted an enormously influential bloc, especially in the region where the trial took place. Moreover, the state legislature itself, under pressure from German politicians all over the country, was now fully determined to try to force a review for Schoeppe. If Geary did what Seymour had done, he would be in the position of heartless executioner, killing a citizen in the face of grave public and professional doubts.

Geary tried to wriggle out of the situation by sending his attorney general, F. Carroll Brewster, to Philadelphia to urge members of the Pennsylvania Supreme Court to accept political necessity. But that court was unwilling to overrule itself and inclined to consider the legislature's new capital-case-review law *ex post facto*. Nonetheless, the justices agreed to take the whole matter under consideration, which was enough for the governor. On December 14, 1869, a greatly relieved Geary was able to lift Schoeppe's death warrant pending judicial clarification.

When the Pennsylvania Supreme Court balked again and sustained Schoeppe's conviction, the Pennsylvania legislature responded with a second Schoeppe-inspired bill. The special act that emerged had the procedural effect of authorizing the court in Cumberland County to reconsider its own case, which it eventually did in the summer of 1872 under a new local judge. Feelings ran high in Carlisle and the court had difficulty seating an impartial jury. As in the first trial, the key battles pitted outside experts against each other on the subject of forensic toxicology and post-mortem appearances: Aiken and his Baltimore-based allies for the prosecution against Reese, Genth, Wormley, and several others for the defense. With a national spotlight now fixed upon the trial, the Baltimore *Sun* braced itself for a "protracted and tedious" confrontation over the medical and chemical facts of the case. The new judge tipped his hand by ruling that Aiken could testify as a chemist, but not as a medical expert. This severely undercut the prosecutor's chief witness and the jury returned a verdict of not guilty after two weeks of medico-legal disputation. The scene immediately following the verdict was remarkable. Jurors weeping for joy rushed to embrace the polished young immigrant doctor they had saved from the gallows; professional journals around the country breathed a collective editorial sigh of relief.[26]

For American physicians interested in medical jurisprudence, the Schoeppe affair thus appeared to be something of a victory. A national outcry by medical experts had been influential in forcing the reconsideration of possibly flawed medical testimony. Outside expertise from Philadelphia and New York had overcome local prejudice in the Pennsylvania countryside. A physician had been acquitted in a case that might have set ominous malpractice precedents. Schoeppe himself certainly treated the outcome as a victory and promptly tried to capitalize upon it by taking to the lecture circuit. Addressing audiences in Philadelphia on "Science in Law and Its Abuses," Schoeppe talked about the dangers of American justice in general and the weaknesses of American medical jurisprudence in particular.[27]

But the victory was hollow, embarrassing, and less professionally significant than it may have seemed at first glance. It was hollow because the beneficiary subsequently turned out to have feet of clay. By 1874 Schoeppe was in prison in Illinois over another forgery swindle and wanted in Maryland in connection with the disputed Stennecke will, which he had foolishly insisted upon pressing to probate. Further investigation revealed that he had fled Prussia after a conviction for forgery in that country and that he did not have the medical training he claimed to have when he set himself up as a doctor in Carlisle, which probably explained why he had known so curiously little about the medical chemistry that saved his life.[28] In retrospect, Schoeppe was almost certainly guilty of trying to extort Stennecke's estate. Whether he intentionally killed Stennecke to do so or merely tried to make the most of her death can never be determined.

The case was also embarrassing because the two intraprofessional battles in Carlisle had revealed once again the ways in which medical experts could disagree with one another diametrically, even on a subject as theoretically scientific as forensic toxicology and even when the life of a fellow practitioner was at stake. Medical witnesses seemed to confuse as much as they clarified, and the trial revealed flagrantly obvious geographical and ethnic divisions within the medical establishment. Baltimore physicians fought Philadelphia physicians; German doctors fought Anglo-American doctors; organized experts in medical jurisprudence fought everyday healers and local practitioners.

Finally, the case was far less professionally satisfying than it may have seemed, since it was probably won for the wrong reasons. The lifting of Schoeppe's death warrant almost certainly had more to do with ethnic politics in Pennsylvania than it did with the official recognition and fair-minded assessment of medico-legal expertise in the nation as a whole. German-generated protests had reached Governor Geary from as far away as Chicago and Berlin. The Pennsylvania legislature had responded to German-

American political pressure, not to the force of medico-legal arguments from Philadelphia and New York; the legislators, after all, could easily have sustained the medical arguments from Baltimore and Carlisle, not to mention the rulings of their own state Supreme Court, had they wished to duck the whole business. Aiken, though he may have been right about Schoeppe, could not stand scientific scrutiny from those at the top of the medical profession. Reese and the medico-legal societies, on the other hand, even though they held the scientific high ground, ended up after the fact looking like obfuscators and defenders of one of their own rather than champions of justice.

Many of the principals involved in the two Schoeppe trials were simultaneously engaged as well in another capital case also involving allegations of murder by poison. This case had broken in Baltimore after Schoeppe's initial conviction but before his retrial. By the time it was over, this second case, the case of Elizabeth Nugent Wharton, would prove to be even more spectacular than the Schoeppe case, and from the point of view of medico-legal interaction, even more damaging.

In the summer of 1871, Elizabeth Wharton of Baltimore was accused of murdering General W. Scott Ketchum and attempting to murder a young clerk named Eugene Van Ness. The case had all the elements appropriate to a public spectacle and quickly became one. Both the accused and the deceased had moved among the nation's highest social and military elites. Elizabeth Wharton's husband, a West Point graduate who died in 1867, was the son of a prominent Philadelphia judge and a member of one of that city's most powerful and influential families. Elizabeth herself had also grown up in Philadelphia's high society and her brother was a leading physician in Norristown, Pennsylvania. Ketchum, a well-connected fifty-eight-year-old veteran of War Department politics, lived in Washington but served the Baltimore widow as long-time family friend, confidant, and financial adviser. Van Ness, an employee of the venerable Baltimore investment house of Alexander Brown and Sons, kept Mrs. Wharton's accounts.[29]

On a visit to Baltimore in June 1871, the general fell gravely ill in Wharton's home and died after three days of agony. During Ketchum's illness, the widow had summoned Van Ness for a financial consultation, and Van Ness, too, came down with the same near-critical symptoms, though the younger man would eventually survive. The coincidence excited suspicion from Van Ness's wife, from the attending physicians (at least one of whom had suspected poison from the outset), and from the general's formidable friends and relatives in Washington. Testimony subsequently indicated that General Ketchum had been pressing Wharton for several thousand dollars he had advanced her and that Van Ness had been keeping a secret set of double books for the widow. Some Baltimoreans remembered that Wharton's only son had died suddenly a year earlier and that his mother had been the beneficiary of unusually large life insurance policies. When the deputy state's attorney for Baltimore City learned from Jacob Frey, a deputy police marshal sent to watch the widow, that Wharton and her grown daughter were leaving for New York City, where they had previously booked tickets for Europe, he issued a warrant for the widow's arrest.

Philip C. Williams, the physician who attended Ketchum at his death, had suspected poisoning from the beginning. Aided by Samuel Claggett Chew and F.T. Miles, both of whom were professors at the University of Maryland Medical School in Baltimore, Williams conducted an autopsy to try to determine what killed his patient. Ketchum's stomach was removed and delivered for chemical analysis to William E.A. Aiken, the same Maryland professor who had conducted the examination of Maria Stennecke's stomach. Aiken once again "satisfied himself" that the deceased had been poisoned, this time not with prussic acid but with tartar emetic. An antimonial poison used in tiny doses to induce vomiting and purging, tartar emetic could be purchased commercially in nineteenth-century pharmacies. Aiken claimed that General Ketchum's stomach contained at least twenty grains of the substance, which would certainly have been enough to kill him. About fifteen grains of the same substance were recovered from the glass of punch Wharton had given Van Ness, and witnesses testified that Wharton had purchased sixty grains of tartar emetic from a store near her home some days before these coincidental events. Amid much public furor, a grand jury indicted the widow Wharton for the murder of General Ketchum.

Opinion in Baltimore turned sharply against Wharton, even though she had formerly been among the city's most socially prominent figures and one of Baltimore's leading Episcopal churchwomen. Citing the hostile climate there, Wharton's defense team, led by J. Nevitt Steele, succeeded in having the trial postponed until December and transferred to Annapolis. But nothing could damp a burgeoning public interest in this case of murder and money among the rich and famous. From the trial's first day, December 4, 1871, the largest courtroom in Annapolis was full of spectators for every one of what would eventually total fifty-two sessions. Special trains brought people down from Baltimore, an unusual proportion of whom were women. Maryland aristocrats, including James Howard, J. Harman Brown, and General Shriver, jostled for seats with Naval Academy dignitaries, several state judges, members of the Maryland legislature, and visiting congressmen over from Washington. Both outgoing Governor Oden Bowie and Governor-elect William P. Whyte attended sessions, and they sometimes had to pull rank to gain admission to the crowded scene.

The Baltimore *Gazette*, which later published its transcript of the trial in book form, covered the proceedings in detail, as did the Baltimore *Sun*, the *Baltimore American*, and the Baltimore *German Correspondent*. For obvious reasons, the Philadelphia and Washington papers also proved attentive, and so did those of New York City, where Ketchum and Wharton both had strong ties. Indeed, the Baltimore papers engaged their counterparts in Philadelphia and New York in heated editorial exchanges over Wharton's probable guilt or innocence. Commentators in Maryland openly damned her; those in Pennsylvania and New York generally gave her the benefit of the doubt. No wonder the presiding judge of the three-judge panel hearing the case promptly sequestered the jury for the duration of the trial. By the fourth day, Frank Leslie's "special artist" arrived to begin sketching the principals, and the *Gazette* observed accurately that the Wharton trial was "attracting much attention throughout the country."

Wharton's defense attorneys decided that their best chance to win acquittal was to undermine the credibility of the prosecution's medical and chemical evidence. Accordingly, they made virtually no effort to find holes in the tight circumstantial net surrounding their client but launched instead a frontal assault upon the expert testimony of the physicians who performed the Ketchum autopsy and especially upon Aiken, the medical chemist at the University of Maryland Medical School who claimed to have found the antimonial poison in Ketchum's stomach. Aided by the substantial resources available to Mrs. Wharton, Steele brought in many of the top forensic toxicologists in the United States to cast doubt upon the knowledge and the procedures of the prosecution's leading medical witnesses. This strategy would eventually prove effective in defense of Wharton, but further crippling for the cause of medical jurisprudence.

The prosecutor's experts were, in fact, a bit shaky. The post-mortem had been performed by the three doctors who already harbored suspicions, without neutral observers present and without calling the coroner. Aiken's conclusions, if not actually wrong, resulted from laboratory techniques fairly portrayed by big-time national experts as unacceptably sloppy and old-fashioned in cases where people's lives were at stake. Nor did Aiken present any actual antimony, which was customarily considered conclusive evidence in analyses like this. Steele's team tore Aiken to shreds on cross-examination for the latter's lack of record-keeping, outdated scientific expertise, and idiosyncratic methods. One of the defense attorneys eventually bellowed to the jury that he "would not buy a jar of pickles or a wheelbarrow of guano upon [Aiken's] analysis." Steele also made much of the fact that the prosecution's experts were all colleagues at the University of Maryland Medical School. He suggested strongly, and with some reason, that the faculty had closed ranks to defend one another's findings, right or wrong. If any one of them looked bad, the whole medical school would look bad. In the words of the defense, the prosecution's experts feared "that the University of Maryland was on trial, and that blood [i.e. Mrs. Wharton's execution] was demanded to support it."[30]

The chief prosecutor, Maryland's recently installed Attorney General Andrew K. Syester, was a veteran of more than twenty-five murder trials. Always in the past, however, he had represented the defense. He certainly now realized the vulnerability of the state's experts and, even as the trial proceeded, he took an unusual step in order to try to close with a flourish. He had Williams, Miles, and Chew re-exhume General Ketchum's remains and re-examine what they could still work with after six months. They, in turn, gave the general's liver and kidneys to William P. Tonry. Though a

Baltimore resident and professional friend of the University of Maryland group, Tonry was not on the faculty and had functioned since 1863 as analytical chemist in the Surgeon General's office in Washington. Tonry's powerful testimony in behalf of the poisoning theory, based upon what he had isolated in the general's liver and kidneys, constituted the prosecution's high point.

The defense moved quickly, however, to neutralize Tonry with one of their own first witnesses, R. S. McCulloch. McCulloch, who had also worked as a government expert in medical chemistry, had taught at Princeton and at Jefferson Medical College before going to Washington and Lee. A superb witness, McCulloch translated French toxicological texts for the jury, performed chemical experiments in the courtroom, and handled cross-examination beautifully. He dismissed Tonry's results as too little, too late, and too inconclusive (though they were not), then renewed the relentless attack against the original examinations performed by Aiken and his associates. Steele followed by calling Frederick A. Genth of Philadelphia, who by now must have been growing accustomed to confronting Aiken. Jovial and outgoing this time, Genth nonetheless continued the attack.

Steele's strongest expert was yet another veteran of the Schoeppe case, the University of Pennsylvania's John J. Reese. Though Reese criticized many aspects of the prosecution's evidence, including the autopsy methods employed by Williams, Miles, and Chew, he leveled his heaviest guns, as he had in Carlisle a year before, at Aiken's toxicological testimony. On the stand for three days, one of which included ten hours of cross-examination, Reese performed magnificently. The press hailed the presentation of this "strikingly handsome" expert "with a Bismarck cast of features . . . calm and dignified." Reese clearly "impressed everyone," including the governor, who had come especially to hear him.

The battle of the experts became especially bitter as three physicians from Washington Medical School successively took the stand for the defense. Washington Medical School, also located in Baltimore, was an arch rival of the University of Maryland, competing across town for students, patients, and patronage. The first of the three Washington witnesses, Edward Warren, had been professor of materia medica at the University of Maryland before the Civil War, but resigned to become Medical Inspector-in-Chief of Robert E. Lee's army and Surgeon General of Confederate North Carolina. Denied his old chair after the war, Warren became instead professor of surgery at Washington, and he now had a chance to operate upon the reputations of the faculty who refused to take him back.

Warren not only continued the defense effort to undermine the credibility of his old colleagues but introduced an alternative possible cause of death: cerebro-spinal meningitis. Since that disease had confusing symptoms and since the original post-mortem examiners had not checked the spinal column while they still could, meningitis served neatly as a theoretically possible alternative cause of death. Warren's associates on the Washington medical faculty, John Morris and Harvey Byrd, then took the stand to reinforce the plausibility of Warren's hypotheses. Attorney General Syester tried to counter with the imputation that these and other defense experts were grasping for straws they would never take seriously in the absence of the handsome fees that the Whartons were capable of paying. The defense shot back that Williams was said to have been a paid volunteer for the prosecutor, and Syester found himself in the awkward position of apologizing publicly to Warren and Morris and having to write an open letter declaring that Williams' participation in the case against Wharton was *"compulsory, under the State's process, and not voluntary."*[31]

Steele's list of defense witnesses continued with physicians from Baltimore and Pennsylvania, who continued the attacks upon the evidence presented by Aiken, Williams, Miles, and Chew and continued also to support the plausibility of the meningitis theory. Local medical experts from St. John's College in Annapolis testified for the defense in an obvious effort to win the confidence of the local jurors.[32] The defense then concluded with an impressive string of character witnesses willing to speak in Wharton's behalf. To offset the effect of General Ketchum's lofty place in the army, the character witnesses included a colonel who came all the way from San Francisco with special permission of the Secretary of War in order to testify in behalf of the widow; U.S. Army Assistant Adjutant General Richard C. Drum; U.S. Army Inspector General Delos B. Sackett; and General Winfield S. Hancock, the nationally known Pennsylvania Civil War commander, who would shortly run for the presidency of the United States.

In rebuttal, the prosecution could do little. Baltimore area physicians testified that meningitis had not been epidemic at the time of Ketchum's demise, but the most impressive of those who testified, including Nathan R. Smith, Christopher Johnston, and William T. Howard, were other University of Maryland faculty members who could be made to look like friends defending their professional associates. When Aiken himself was recalled to rebut McCulloch's damaging testimony, the word "fraud" was bandied about on all sides and the courtroom dissolved into a nasty "spirit and temper of recrimination."

Summing up for the defense, Steele and the members of his defense team painted a picture of overzealous professionals either trying to cover for one another or trying to get ahead. In their scenario Williams had embarrassingly lost one of his most prominent patients, General Ketchum, and decided that his "professional reputation" was at stake. He easily enlisted the aid of Marshal Frey, the Baltimore law enforcement officer "who, like all of his class, was eager to bag his game," in a hasty indictment of Elizabeth Wharton. Aiken's evidence was laughable. He asked the court to believe his assertions and his memory, but he had no tangible results to present and a wretched recollection of scientific detail. In one of his lowest blows, Steele offered the opinion that if Aiken had been after "ten grains of gold, instead of antimony" in Ketchum's stomach, the professor would have found them and retained them; but since it was only antimony and a woman's life at stake, he did neither. The Maryland faculty, in turn, rallied for professional self-defense behind the otherwise shaky case and shoddy job of their fellows. Tonry, the toughest prosecution witness to controvert, was pictured as the victim of professional temptation: he had "been afforded an opportunity of making a world-wide reputation by discovering antimony in General K's remains" six months after the fact and in organs where it would be difficult to detect under those circumstances. He said he did find evidence, but in the face of such temptation, the jury should "regard his testimony with extreme caution."

The case finally went to the jury on January 23, 1872. Restive jurors had been sequestered through the holidays and even made to attend two funerals *en masse*, when one of their number lost a pair of relatives. Local and national wagering odds favored acquittal, and those who bet that way won their money the following day. Originally divided eight for acquittal and four undecided, the jurors first resolved not to return as a hung jury, then reached a unanimous verdict of not guilty on a fifth ballot. The three presiding judges admonished sharply against any public outbursts, and the trial ended amid congratulations to the defense.

For champions of medical jurisprudence writ large, however, the Wharton case had been anything but a source of congratulations. From one perspective, a woman regarded by her local community as almost certainly guilty of murder went free not as a consequence of demonstrated innocence but as a consequence of apparent professional incompetence and manifest professional infighting. From another perspective, a woman would almost certainly have hanged had she not had available to her the influence of an enormously powerful family and the resources required to bring to her defense the likes of John J. Reese. And the whole business was conducted in a national spotlight of intense publicity. In addition to its articles about the trial, *Frank Leslie's Illustrated Newspaper* had printed a half-page drawing of the courtroom scene with Professor Williams in the witness box, a portrait of Warren, and a full-page drawing of the courtroom scene as the verdict was announced. *Leslie's* popular format had helped to assure the accuracy of its own summary observation: "This case will be remembered as one of the most important criminal prosecutions of the country."[33]

Whether the details of the case itself were remembered or not, the unsettling and unflattering medico-legal lessons it seemed to epitomize were drawn explicitly by the national press and would not soon be forgotten. As the New York *Tribune* remarked, "justly or unjustly, most people will consider that science has not been cut a dignified figure in the trial that has just been finished. Those who followed the case may not have had all their suspicions allayed, but they will not have them strengthened by the evidence of chemical experts." The New York *Evening Express* agreed: "The case, we suppose, has scarcely a parallel as a doctors' war, chemical experts having been arrayed for weeks in hostile squadrons, though after all nothing seems certain about their conflicting tests, unless it is their uncertainty." Nor did the *Philadelphia Telegraph* mince words: "This trial has been the grave of reputations of medical experts whose opinions previously were es-

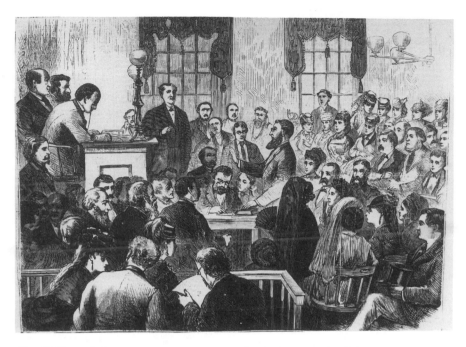

Dr. Williams being sworn as an expert medical witness at the Wharton trial. From *Frank Leslie's Illustrated Newspaper*, December 23, 1871. (*Courtesy Enoch Pratt Free Library*)

teemed to be as good as other men's facts. The counsel for the defence made the doctors contradict each other and themselves in a manner that was in the highest degree edifying to the public at large."[34] Scores of other national and local publications made similar observations following the verdict at Annapolis.

Recrimination reverberated in the nation's professional press as well. Virtually all of the principals in the Wharton case published their own self-serving post-mortems of what they thought had taken place. Because the trial had "excited so much interest throughout the country," John J. Reese decided to review the medical and chemical disputes as he saw them. He offered his retrospective analyses in the nationally circulated *AJMS*, which was published in his home city and managed editorially by professional friends of his.[35] Horatio C. Wood, another of the expert witnesses for the defense, offered an analytical overview of his own in the prominent New York-based *Medical Record*.[36] To illustrate the extent of the coverage of this professional dispute, Wood's analysis of the case, which was just one among many and by no means the most prominent, was promptly reprinted for a general audience in *Lippincott's Magazine* and discussed for a legal audience in the *Albany Law Journal*.[37] Both Reese and Wood, of course, cast the prosecutor's witnesses in extremely unflattering light. In behalf of the latter, Chew and Williams both replied, the former in separate articles in the *Richmond and Louisville Medical Journal* and the *Medical Record;* the latter in separate articles in the *Richmond and Louisville Medical Journal* and the *Medical and Surgical Reporter* of Philadelphia, a rival of the *AJMS*, which had refused to print Williams's reply to Reese.[38] Reese rebutted briefly in the *Medical Record*, characterizing Chew as a blunderer.[39]

Aiken, the University of Maryland professor whose conduct of the original chemical investigation had drawn the most withering fire from the beginning, tried to defend his actions in a pamphlet. Procedures like the ones he performed had been perfectly acceptable in the judgment of other courts in other cases, he claimed. The prosecution failed to convict Wharton not because she was innocent and not because Aiken himself had erred, but because her unscrupulous lawyers had used lucrative fees to entice famous outsiders and professional rivals to cast essentially irrelevant and ultimately false doubts upon his findings. "Every one knows to what lengths a mere lawyer, especially if he is wanting in gentlemanly instincts, will go," Aiken complained. "No one is, therefore, surprised if such a one perverts the meaning of testimony to suit his own purposes."[40] Aiken was by no means alone in this line of defense, incidentally. The editors of the *Indiana Journal of Medicine*, for example, after rehearsing all of the testimony in the Wharton case and attempting to replicate all of the chemical analyses done on all sides, concluded that Aiken was probably right and that his tormentors were largely obfuscators.[41]

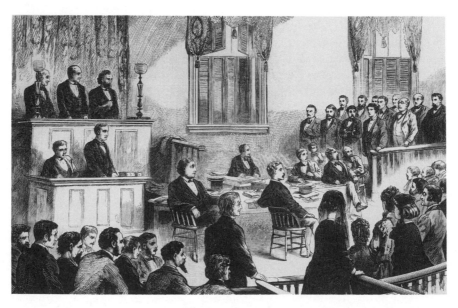

Jury foreman declaring Elizabeth Wharton not guilty. The defendant is standing in the foreground with her back to the viewer. From *Frank Leslie's Illustrated Newspaper*, February 10, 1872. (*Courtesy Enoch Pratt Free Library, Baltimore*)

John Thomas, one of the defense lawyers, shot back at the University of Maryland group in a pamphlet of his own: "It is singular they have not intelligence enough to recognize the fact, that it is their profession—not mine—that is responsible for the differences of scientific opinion which were expressed at the trials and which they seem determined to discuss anew, whenever they desire to advertise themselves." The defense attorneys were not the least bit unscrupulous or unprofessional in their use of the best experts they could find, argued Thomas. "Lawyers cannot be expected to know everything. They are entitled to have the aid of experts, and to pay for it."[42] Under the nation's current judicial system, they would have been remiss not to have done what they did.

Thomas went on, however, albeit from his own perspective, to raise a point that had troubled many of the nation's newspaper editors as well, not to mention the editors of the nation's medical journals.

> The want of official and impartial experts is a sad defect in our system of criminal procedure. If we had had them, we might have been spared the disgraceful exhibition of the two witnesses by whom the prosecution was started and sustained, officiously combining in themselves the functions of State's Attorney, Coroner and expert. We would have been spared the discreditable battles of the doctors, which have done so much to shake public confidence in their profession. We should perhaps have felt less indignant than we do at the moral superiority over our own profession, which Dr. Chew claims for his as a class.[43]

In its lead editorial the day Wharton was declared not guilty, the *Baltimore American* had opined that "the trial itself has been one of the most remarkable that ever took place in this country, and will no doubt pass into the books on medical jurisprudence as a leading case." The editors were right. Along with a handful of less well-publicized cases from the postwar period, the Schoeppe and Wharton trials helped confirm the awkward truth that many of the problems raised in the Hendrickson case just after mid-century still remained as troublesome as ever after the Civil War, perhaps more troublesome than ever, notwithstanding scientific advances. Professionals would continue to refer to the Schoeppe and Wharton cases repeatedly through the remainder of the century as a sort of metaphor for the problems surrounding the subject of expert testimony.[44] Only now those problems were fast becoming more obvious to ordinary citizens than they had been at mid-century. Expert judgment seemed potentially as vulnerable to the influence of money, greed, ambition, political pressure, interprofessional power plays, intraprofessional rivalries, friendship, error, and obstinacy as any other kind of judgment; all of which boded ill for the field of medical jurisprudence in the United States.

In Maryland itself, both the *Baltimore American* and the Baltimore *Sun* had expressed in no uncertain terms their disgust with the performance of the state's medical experts, and both called for action from the legislature in Annapolis. The former thought a neutral commission of experts should be appointed by the courts in cases of this nature.[45] The latter agreed and also endorsed a bill already introduced by an irate state senator that would systematize all future post-mortem examinations in Maryland and require both certified tests and more careful record-keeping.[46] Nor was Maryland by any means the only state where legislators turned their attention to the tangled issues involved in expert testimony. Indeed, the Schoeppe and Wharton trials took place at a time when American physicians were re-engaging what would shortly become an intense, nation-wide concern about the declining fortunes and mounting problems of the expert medical witness in American courts.

CHAPTER FOURTEEN

The Crisis of the Expert Witness

Issues associated with insanity hurt the image of the medical profession, rent the fabric of medical cooperation, and damaged the public image of medical jurisprudence, but probably affected the vast majority of American physicians only indirectly. So, too, the great confrontations over forensic chemistry, like the Schoeppe and Wharton trials. The number of cases in American courts that involved medical testimony of a more routine or traditional sort, however, was already great and apparently growing after the Civil War. Stanford Chaillé, extrapolating from figures he collected for New Orleans during 1875, estimated in 1876 that nearly 9000 criminal trials resulted from autopsies and coroners' inquests alone each year in the United States. Added to those would be the many criminal cases that did not stem from deaths but involved medical evidence nonetheless (such as rapes, assaults, batteries, wounds of all sorts) and a huge variety of civil suits in which medical testimony was needed (compensation for injuries, accidents, disputes over wills, and the like). Consequently Chaillé estimated, conservatively it would appear, that at least 20,000 trials each year involved medical testimony.[1] For twenty years following the Civil War, physicians throughout the country simply took as given, in the words of a Brooklyn doctor in 1879, that "most physicians in active practice are frequently called to testify" in court.[2]

The frustrations associated with being an expert witness were thus experienced personally by a large percentage of American physicians, a fact repeatedly attested to during the 1870s in their local medical journals. Little wonder, then, that the plight of the expert witness became the most widespread and most intense subject of medical jurisprudential discussion within the medical profession as a whole during the postwar decades. Medical societies from coast to coast debated with great frequency and emotion the problems associated with medical testimony. Four principal issues commanded their attention.

First, physicians risked their personal reputations each time they took

the witness stand as an expert, whether they did so voluntarily for remuneration or under order from public authorities. A lapse at any point in the
process, an emotional outburst during cross-examination, a line of question-
ing that revealed gaps of knowledge, much less an actual mistake, could all
ruin a promising career almost instantly. And growing commercial interests
increased the pressure on individual physicians, who sometimes found
themselves under withering personal attack even when they were right. To
cite a single example from the postwar period, a doctor in Blacksburg, Virginia, testified in a capital case that he had found arsenic in a preparation
of subnitrate of bismuth. When the manufacturers of the bismuth, Rosen-
garten and Sons of Philadelphia, heard about the case, they launched a
smear campaign against the doctor, alleging incompetence and perjury, because the testimony threatened their firm's future sales. The fact that the
physician turned out to be entirely correct in this case, where another person's life was at stake, did not lessen the damage done to the physician's
own standing by the chemical company.[3]

Second, the process of eliciting medical evidence continued to make
physicians look scientifically weak, internally divided, and dangerously unprofessional. In the words of S. H. Tewksbury, a physician who prepared
a formal presentation on medico-legal evidence for the Maine Medical Association in 1869, "medical testimony generally, in a court of law, is one of
the most unsatisfactory exhibitions of medical science." And the process
affected not just the "standing and prospects" of each physician who got
involved, "but the character of his profession" as a whole. Trials involving
physician-witnesses had become "a direct injury to the profession."[4] Courts
remained reluctant to distinguish among physicians, and the profession itself, as a Boston lawyer painfully reminded the nation's physicians in 1869,
had "no tribunal which can expose and punish quacks and pretenders, whose
misdeeds are often attributed to regular practitioners."[5] The *Boston Medical
and Surgical Journal* was convinced by 1872 that "scarcely a trial in the civil
or the criminal courts occurs, requiring the assistance of a medical expert,
that does not bring into unenviable notoriety, not the medical witness alone,
but the medical profession which he represents."[6]

The third principal issue was the increasingly obvious fact, even among
regular doctors, that handsome private fees were creating something of a
marketplace for medical witnesses willing to tailor their testimony to the
requirements of whoever retained them. Since the 1840s, to be sure, A. S.
Taylor's widely used treatise on medical jurisprudence had assumed that
expert opinions purchased in the marketplace would inevitably "correspond
with the wishes or the interests of the parties who call them," and hints of
trouble had surfaced during the 1850s in cases like that of Hendrickson.
But after the Civil War the problem seemed to be growing more flagrant,
and it was openly acknowledged at high levels. In 1868, even before the
Schoeppe and Wharton trials, Chief Justice Reuben A. Chapman of the
Supreme Court of Massachusetts declared that "the opinions of experts are
not so highly regarded as they formerly were." In a case that hung upon

medical testimony, Chief Justice Chapman told the jury, "Many experts can be hired for the occasion. You must judge yourselves of the evidence offered you."[7] The chief justice of Vermont concluded that "experience has shown . . . [that] medical experts differ quite as widely in their inferences and opinions, as do the other witnesses. This has become so uniform a result with medical experts of late, that they are beginning to be regarded much in the light of hired advocates." A member of the Supreme Court of Maine had made similar remarks from the bench.[8]

During the 1870s, regular physicians grew deeply fearful that the adversarial legal system might eventually corrupt a number of their colleagues and render meaningless, or even suspect and sinister, anything the medical profession or the field of medical jurisprudence had to contribute to the cause of justice. The doctors' fears were real: the nation's daily newspapers during the 1870s often questioned the value of "outside experts" brought at great expense for a particular trial, and courtroom lawyers routinely began their cross-examination of expert witnesses by asking about any compensation the expert had been promised. The Boston Bar Association even claimed to detect a trend toward "the formation of expert witnesses into a profession" of their own, a trend that raised "a grave question of public policy."[9] According to a prominent member of the Philadelphia bar who published a treatise on expert testimony in 1879, the general American public seemed to regard most expert testimony as "rather pernicious than beneficial."[10]

The fourth principal issue associated with the postwar crisis of the expert witness was a less well-known and somewhat paradoxical inverse of the third. If handsome private fees undermined credibility and risked corruption, the continuing lack of professional compensation for physicians acting in the public interest seemed to be undermining what might be called the civic morale of the medical profession. During the 1870s American physicians grew more openly and more universally resentful than they had been prior to the Civil War of the fact that their knowledge and experience could be impressed without professional compensation by public authorities in virtually every American jurisdiction. Sometimes the impressment seemed fairly reasonable. When lawyers in court were themselves quasi-impressed public defenders, for example, or when their clients had essentially no resources, lawyers had little choice but to ask the court to subpoena any medical experts their cases required. But most of the time the unwillingness of public authorities to pay more than ordinary expenses amounted to a levy upon the medical profession by the state, a levy made particularly odious because it fell unequally upon the profession's individual members.

To compound difficulties, the power to subpoena medical experts without special compensation was open to serious abuse. If a lawyer simply did not wish to pay top fees to top experts, or needed to establish otherwise straightforward medical points with as little expense as possible to his clients, he could ask the bench to subpoena at public rates of compensation those physicians whom he wanted to put on the witness stand. In some courts, lawyers used their powers to conduct what amounted to fishing expeditions in an effort to find doctors whose views might bolster their position.[11] Especially in malpractice cases, those fishing expeditions had already proved enormously galling and more than a little costly in time and money to subpoenaed physicians.[12]

During the late 1860s frustration over both the process and the lack of compensation for publicly mandated testimony provoked isolated incidents of rebellion among physicians. Once in a while friendly magistrates might even support their protests. In 1868, for example, a United States District Court in Chicago sustained a physician who refused to testify as an expert "without having first received honorary fees therefor."[13] But a physician in a Sacramento, California, police court was arrested for contempt a month later when he took the same position.[14] The latter was certainly the norm nationally. But physicians were beginning to elaborate the legal concept that would become their chief counter-argument during the postwar period. As the *BMSJ* phrased that argument in 1868, physicians' "professional knowledge, which forms their capital in business, is personal property," and the courts had no right arbitrarily to seize citizens' personal property.[15]

Physicians in Massachusetts launched concerted efforts to do something about the plight of the expert medical witness. In the winter of 1868–69, following Chief Justice Chapman's blast from the state's highest bench, the Suffolk District (i.e. greater Boston) Medical Society, one of the most professionally oriented and policy-minded medical organizations in the country, appointed a committee to consider legislative remedy. The Suffolk District physicians also persuaded the Boston-based American Academy of Arts and Sciences, an organization then dominated by prominent lawyers, likewise to appoint a committee and join them. The combined group drafted a bill for legislative consideration that would permit the courts themselves, not just the contending sides, to call expert witnesses and let the experts function, where appropriate, as a special commission advisory to the courts. The court, in turn, would pay the specially-chosen medical experts "reasonable and proper" fees. Emory Washburn, perhaps the state's most prominent law professor and certainly the state's most respected authority on the problems involved in legal medicine from the legal side, appeared before the judiciary committee of the legislature to support the bill.[16] But the judiciary committee never acted upon the proposed law. The disgruntled doctors and lawyers of the Suffolk District Medical Society and the American Academy of Arts and Sciences could do no more than lay out their arguments publicly, offer practical advice to physicians about how to behave if called under the present system (advice that differed little from Beck's half a century earlier), and "hope much from the future."[17]

Four years later they tried again. A coalition of the Suffolk District Medical Society, the American Academy of Arts and Sciences, the Boston Society for Medical Observation, and the Boston Society for Medical Sciences mounted another major effort to persuade the Massachusetts legislature to let judges appoint court experts in cases where medical testimony was germane, and to pay the experts at professional rates. Emory Washburn, who again led the fight, had long believed that the courts could safely be given such powers, which he considered akin to the appointment of accountants in settlement disputes or receivers in bankruptcy. Yet his own comments must have chilled many citizens.

> And though cases may occur where, by selection or exclusion of one or another who may be named an expert, injustice may be done to a party, the great cause of justice will, on the whole, be vindicated, and the confidence of the public in the purity of its administration, as well as their respect for its ministers [i.e. lawyers] and instrumentalities [i.e. expert physicians], strengthened and confirmed.[18]

If that was the best the plan's chief advocate could muster, no wonder the legislature again refused to alter the state's longstanding judicial procedures.[19]

In 1879 the Massachusetts Medico-Legal Society organized a third major push to secure reform of the state's methods of obtaining medical evidence. This time they had the active support of Attorney General George Marston. That officer helped draft a bill designed to permit Massachusetts courts to call neutral medical experts while still conforming to the rigid fair-trial guarantees of the state constitution.[20] Like the others before it, however, this effort also failed. Moreover, Marston himself, in his official capacity as attorney general, believed that physician-witnesses at autopsies should be paid "fit and proper" fees rather than the standard *per diem*, but then undermined the probability of that happening by ruling formally that the state could not be held responsible for those fees. Fees would have to be assessed against county authorities, who were free to, and almost always did, refuse to pay them.[21] After more than a decade of effort, Massachusetts physicians found themselves in 1880 where they had been in 1865, or indeed in 1825: subject to subpoena and without any binding legal claim to professional rates of compensation from the courts.

In Missouri, Thomas Kennard, vice president of the Medical Association of Missouri and of the St. Louis Medical Society, complained bitterly in 1872 that there were "few amongst us who have been long engaged in practice, who have not been repeatedly summoned before our courts of justice to testify as experts . . . yet the idea of compensating us for our time, trouble and opinion never seems to have been entertained by the parties who saw fit to demand such services of us." Kennard emphasized the physicians' property argument: "professional knowledge is our own capital . . . and no court or citizen has any legal right to demand it of us without" compensation. He identified three chief sources of difficulty: "unscrupulous lawyers"; a legal system that continued perversely to refuse to distinguish either a regular witness from an expert witness or the qualifications of one expert witness from those of another; and a tendency among physicians to curry favor from "rich and wealthy corporations" by providing unpaid service to those who could easily pay. That practice, he believed, undercut arguments in favor of compensating physicians for public service in behalf of the many who could not afford to pay.[22]

From influential New York state came several suggestions for reform, some of which made their way into the legislature in the form of bills. The *Albany Law Journal*, citing the Schoeppe and Wharton cases, endorsed a system of state-supported medico-legal toxicologists, who would be appointed by the governor upon the recommendation of the state medical society.[23] Along with several members of the New York Medico-Legal Society, John Ordronaux favored the creation of expert panels to determine disputed points of medical science.[24] Others raised the possibility of appointing what might be called science judges to sit with regular judges. The former would adjudicate the medical aspects of a case while the latter adjudicated the law of the same case.[25] Still others favored *ad hoc* commissions of three physicians, one chosen by each side in any given confrontation and one chosen by the court.[26] Clark Bell called again for implementation of the French system in New York and offered a report from Paris that it was working well in France.[27] But no changes cleared the legislature.

In the meantime, New York experts continued to go uncompensated when impressed into public service. In 1875, for example, a New York City coroner called the distinguished Robert O. Doremus to examine the bodies of some people the coroner suspected of having died from poisons. Doremus, professor of chemistry, toxicology, and medical jurisprudence at Bellevue Hospital Medical College, was one of the best-known analytical and experimental chemists in the United States.[28] When Doremus later submitted a bill for the examinations he performed, the coroner refused to pay. Doremus thereupon brought suit in the city's Court of Common Pleas for compensation at expert rates. After losing at that level, Doremus appealed. Judge Larremore, who heard the appeal, cited New York statutes of 1868 and 1871 to sustain the coroner. "Fully recognizing the utility and necessity of chemical analysis in furtherance of justice and the detection and punishment of crime," ruled Larremore, "I am forced to the conclusion that plaintiff's services, however meritorious, were unauthorized." The judge told Doremus that "his appeal should be addressed to the legislature and not to the court."[29]

The 1875 meeting of the American Public Health Association resolved formally against the nation's system of soliciting medical evidence in court cases and appointed a committee to inquire about alternatives, especially those that seemed to work in other countries.[30] In Maryland, where popular outrage over the Wharton verdict had prompted the legislature to debate changes in the system of obtaining expert medical testimony, Christopher Johnson, president of the Medical and Chirurgical Faculty of Maryland, shared the same concerns. Even after the Wharton furor subsided, debate over expert testimony had continued to be "extensive and so full of interest" to physicians in his region because "medical and other expert witnesses [were] continually subjected to great inconvenience and injustice."[31] Johnson deplored the fact that Maryland's doctors were being "compelled to give away knowledge which has cost them years of toil and research."[32] He hoped his state might adopt the French system of court-appointed medical experts, who could be both appropriately paid and legally neutral, but he was not optimistic; in fact, he feared Maryland might more likely ignore those few rulings in other American states that had allowed for professional rates of compensation in some cases.

One of the states Johnson was referring to was Indiana. Physicians there had been aggressively pressing for court-ordered compensation since the late 1860s, and in 1870 they had won minor local victories in Indianapolis that emboldened them to continue their efforts.[33] The *Indiana Journal of Medicine* directed considerable attention to the issue in 1873 and 1874, and in doing so helped fuel a national firestorm of activity. The editors considered the possibility of expert commissions an attractive idea, but unrealistic in the United States as things actually stood. Instead, physicians would have to make the best of the situation by bringing countersuits against impressed service and by refusing to perform jurisprudential tasks without full professional fees at a generous level.[34]

When Wilson Hobbs, a physician from Knightstown, raised the issue before the Indiana State Medical Society in 1877, doctors all around the country paid attention. Most of Hobbs's long address rehearsed the standard litany of abuses suffered by medical witnesses when called into court and added an extensive discussion of the problem of privileged information, a subject with a long history in the legal profession as well. Like Beck half a century earlier and countless others since, Hobbs also cautioned strongly against using a summons to court as "the occasion to show off . . . by ponderous words and learned looks, to the amusement of fools, the disgust of court and jury, and the disgrace of the profession."

Hobbs had more to offer than lamentations and free advice, however, for he thought the time had come to launch a professional offensive on the question of compensation. He had done substantial homework on the legal issues involved in court payments, and he had solicited an opinion from John Ordronaux. As a result, Hobbs counseled his fellow physicians to respond to subpoenas, as required by the law, but not to testify as an expert unless paid in advance, a distinction he believed was technically legal under previous Indiana rulings. At the very least, this procedure would force the hands of the courts.[35]

Hobbs's paper generated considerable interest not only in Indiana but elsewhere as well. By his own account, the question of money "claimed most notice from the profession." Many of the physicians who wrote privately to him from around the country fully supported his goals but feared they had no right under the laws of their own states to proceed as he suggested. In at least three states, however, doctors emboldened by Hobbs's plan decided systematically to test the procedure he prescribed. The first test took place in West Virginia and was sustained, according to the physician involved, by "the profession throughout the state." But the end proved quickly anticlimactic. The circuit court judge of Wetzel County, where the issue was forced, decided not to demand the doctor to testify as an expert without compensation. Though this constituted a technical victory at the local level, the doctor could not press a petition to the West Virginia Supreme Court, as he and his allies in the state medical society had planned. The question remained unsettled in West Virginia.[36]

In Alabama, by contrast, where the second Hobbs-inspired test was launched, a local judge held J.J. Dement, a physician from Huntsville, for contempt when Dement refused to testify as a medical expert unless promised compensation in advance at professional rates. Dement, as planned, then appealed to the Alabama Supreme Court. In *Ex parte Dement*, however, those jurists admonished physicians in blunt terms to testify or suffer the consequences. The decision went on at length because the Alabama Supreme Court recognized explicitly "the interest taken in the question by gentlemen of the medical fraternity," who had, in the opinion of the justices, "been led into some error on the subject by the misconceptions of writers" like Hobbs. A doctor was not entitled "to be paid for his testimony as for *professional services.*" The Alabama Supreme Court was willing to see physicians paid for what they did, such as post-mortem examinations and laboratory tests, which was some advance over the situation that prevailed in most jurisdictions at mid-century, but not for sharing their opinions in the cause of justice or for their time as witnesses, expert or otherwise.[37]

The third case, in Hobbs's own state, proved most intriguing. Several physicians in Fort Wayne, when subpoenaed to offer medical opinions in an otherwise obscure rape case, decided to act upon the proposal Hobbs had given them a few months earlier at their state convention. Thomas J. Dills, a graduate of the University of Michigan Medical School, was the first physician subpoenaed. He took the stand, answered routine questions of identification, then refused to respond to the first medical question posed. Instead, he made a series of statements to the effect that "my time and my skill are my capital" and that "a distinction" existed between ordinary witnesses and expert witnesses. "I respectfully decline to give the opinion of an expert in the case now pending," Dills concluded, "except upon the payment of my fees in advance."[38]

On a motion from the defense attorney, who had the medical witnesses called in the first place, the presiding judge ordered Dills held for contempt. The sheriff whisked the physician abruptly from the hall of justice to the Allen County jail, while the judge made it clear that he took a dim view of the doctors' demonstration under way in his courtroom. Alpheus P. Buchman nonetheless repeated Dills's performance and was, in turn, unceremoniously incarcerated with his professional associate. A third physician, Joseph R. Beck, began the same ritual, whereupon the presiding judge, now "sick of the business," adjourned his court.

Local papers throughout Indiana and lower Michigan picked up the story over the weekend, and so did the papers of Cincinnati, where Buchman had graduated from medical school and still had many friends. A practitioner from Union City, Indiana, alerted Hobbs: "you have got two men at least in jail." Hobbs did not know either of the two doctors, but he knew Beck, through whom he tracked subsequent events. The Allen County Medical Society staged an emergency session "to espouse this cause in behalf of the profession of the State" and resolved to cover the cost of "the ablest counsel attainable" for their incarcerated brethren. "From every part of Indiana, and from almost every State in the Union, there came messages of encouragement . . . and promises of . . . cooperation." Medical journals throughout the nation watched the case, as Dills and Buchman found themselves professional *causes célèbres*. The defense attorneys, headed by former judge John Morris, persuaded the Indiana Supreme Court to hear their clients' appeals before the end of its November term.

The Indiana Supreme Court rendered its decision February 22, 1878. In a relatively long argument that cited a good deal of medical jurisprudential literature and featured the works of John Ordronaux, Justice James L. Worden gave an opinion that delighted the Indiana Medical Society. "When a physician testifies as an expert, by giving his opinion," argued Justice Worden, "he is performing a strictly professional service." Even better, Worden asserted that "the position of a medical witness testifying as an expert, is much more like that of a lawyer than that of an ordinary witness testifying to facts. The purpose . . . is not to prove facts . . . but to aid the court."[39] Though the Indiana Chief Justice and one of his colleagues dissented, two other justices joined Worden to sustain his opinion, 3–2.

"The medical journals in every part of the land, . . . editors . . . , professors in medical colleges, and men of all grades of prominence and respectability in the profession, east, west, north, and south," as Hobbs put it, sent letters, wrote articles, and paid close attention to the Indiana case.[40] That victory, however, had to be seen in context. The West Virginia test had fizzled, the Alabama test had backfired, and the Indiana test, as Hobbs recognized, was "law only in Indiana." Even there, the medical society feared that "the people will scout class favoritism" and object to "the increased expense of such litigation as needs the aid of medicine and surgery." Indeed, Hobbs's correspondents predicted that "the next legislature will, by statute, [try to] undo the whole business."[41]

For most ordinary practitioners, all those "men of all grades of prominence and respectability in the profession" referred to by Hobbs, service as an expert witness promised to remain a costly and professionally damaging proposition that few would relish. Even after the *Buchman* decision, Hobbs himself believed that the ultimate solution still lay in calling a professional before the court as a neutral "*expert, adviser,* or something else, but never a witness."[42] And J. W. Gordon, a physician from Indianapolis who also held a law degree, stressed in the *American Practitioner* not grounds for optimism in his own state, but continuing problems in the wake of *Buchman*. Since courts still lacked any definition of a medical expert, Indiana might find itself in the absurd position of paying blatantly incompetent posers brought in from elsewhere, as had actually happened in a recent Indianapolis malpractice case, to swear to anatomical lies. Gordon, too, thought the ultimate answer lay in some version of the "continental Europe" system of designated experts.[43]

The Indiana uproar reverberated loudly in neighboring Ohio. William Protzman, in behalf of Ohio's regular physicians, acted as a medical cheerleader for Dills and Buchman even as their case was pending. Fed up with what he considered to be the outrageously inconsistent and hypocritical posture of lawyers on the question of medical compensation, Protzman noted that attorneys charged plenty for their own opinions. Doctors, on the other hand, were relieved of their knowledge, their "capital stock," without pay; forced to become "a conspicuous mark for the legal profession to shoot at"; and placed at the mercy of "strutting" young lawyers who knew nothing of medicine and little of professional behavior. Worse, the current system of eliciting medical evidence "often loses [the physician] his best patronage, because the court-room is often filled to overflowing; a half dozen or more of his best patrons witness his confusion, and get the contagion of the lawyer's argument which means ruin, and ruin it is." Dills and Buchman, according to Protzman, had the full sympathy of "every regular in Ohio."[44]

The *Ohio Medical Recorder* noted the absence of any law or ruling about medical court fees in their state. The editors proposed a bill that would compensate an expert "called from home, and at manifest pecuniary loss to himself, or where the case requires special preparation." In return, local physicians, as a gesture of good will and civic responsibility, would agree to testify for free in their own towns. The *Recorder* claimed to have the support of a key justice of the Ohio Supreme Court for this compromise proposal and the tacit approval of several leading lawyers.[45]

The Ohio State Medical Society also got involved in the mounting controversy. That organization established a special committee to explore the subject of compensating medical experts in court, and placed its sitting president, W. H. Philips, in the chair of the special committee. Philips, in turn, used the occasion of his retirement address in 1878 to share the views of his task force. During its century of existence, Philips believed, the American republic had made overall progress in judicial science unprecedented in world history. "The matter of medical testimony furnishes, however, an exception." The inexplicable "conservatism" manifest on that subject seemed "utterly at variance with the radical and reformatory ideas of the nation." The foolish and antiquated office of coroner persisted. Doctors pressed into service remained uncompensated for the "private property" they were forced to provide the state. The "quack, equipped with brazen impudence and ever ready to advertise," continued to thrive in the witness stand, while "the highest physician [often got] injured."[46]

For Philips and the special committee of the Ohio State Medical Society the answer lay in state action. As long-range solutions, they urged creation of a Department of State Medicine in Ohio and adoption of the Prussian model of medical officers in place of the existing coroner system.[47] Those officers "should be well compensated, that men of ability may be induced to accept the position." To that end, the society hoped to build a grass-roots network of physicians at the county level to begin lobbying members of the next state legislature. In the short run, since such "radical reforms cannot be accomplished by a single spasmodic effort," all physicians should submit professional bills for every service rendered to any legal authority. Philips and his special committee believed that most of those bills would be paid, and in cases where they were refused, Philips hoped for a ruling by the Ohio Supreme Court along the lines of that by the Indiana Supreme Court.[48] But he never got one.

In concert with the state society, W. J. Conklin, professor of physiology at Starling Medical College in Columbus, observed in 1878 that "the subject of expert testimony has been lately receiving considerable attention from both the legal and medical professions." Citing Hobbs, Conklin agreed that "a man's professional knowledge" was "*his capital . . . his own private property.*" That property should not be appropriated by the state except in the most dire public emergencies, just as the government did not appropriate the service of potential soldiers except in the face of war. State governments should follow the examples of France and Prussia, where designated public experts played roles filled in the United States either by impressment or by outright partisan purchase from what Conklin labeled a "witness market," which was emerging as a semi-permanent part of the American system of medical testimony.

In the *Ohio Medical and Surgical Journal* Conklin urged his fellow professionals in law and medicine to go to the state legislature for redress, and he hoped something like the Iowa law might work elsewhere even if it was not working well in Iowa.[49] When the Ohio legislature failed to act, two practitioners in Toledo staged another Hobbsian refusal to testify as experts unless paid to do so. Their statements in the criminal murder case of *State v. Hakeos* were transcribed by the Toledo *Telegram* and endorsed by the *Toledo Medical and Surgical Journal* in 1880. Though the judge did not hold them for contempt, he made clear that he was ruling narrowly in the context of the specific case before him, where the medical opinions were not essential. As the *Toledo Medical and Surgical Journal* observed hopefully, this left the status of the medical expert in Ohio "an open question."[50] But subsequent decisions closed it firmly: "Physicians," according to the courts of Ohio, were "not entitled to extra compensation for testifying as to their professional opinions, and [would be] found guilty of contempt for refusing to testify as experts."[51]

Physicians in Michigan also formed a special committee to consider the issue of expert testimony. Edward Cox, who had practiced medicine for forty years and maintained an active interest in medico-legal issues, chaired the group. He resented bitterly the fact that he had spent, by his own estimation, about six months of those forty years attending court proceedings at seventy-five cents a day or less, rather than attending his patients at professional fees. In the celebrated Haviland murder trial Cox spent eight days before the coroner's jury in Detroit and seventeen days in circuit court. When he refused to give his professional opinion on the grounds that the state could not appropriate his property, the presiding judge agreed in principle, but ordered him to testify first and submit a bill later. Cox was instructed to direct his bill to the local Board of Supervisors, since the state government itself had no funds for such a purpose. Detroit's Supervisors promptly rejected Cox's bill "upon the advice of one of their number, a lawyer."[52] In Cox's view, that confirmed the determination of lawyers to preserve their unlimited power over expert witnesses without having to answer to the public for any of the costs involved.

Thoroughly disgusted, Cox urged the physicians of Michigan in 1879 to adopt formally an experiment tried earlier in New York. The Medical Association and the Bar Association would be charged formally to establish jointly a commission of medico-legal experts. That commission would, in turn, be recognized by the state through incorporation. Members of both the Medical Association and the Bar Association, as well as any judicial authority in the state, would then be empowered and encouraged to put before the commission any medico-legal issues that required expert investigation.[53] Unless the courts recognized the commission's reports as binding, and unless the state legislature voted funds to the commissioners, neither of which was going to happen, this scheme was doomed to fail in Michigan as surely as it already had in New York.

Whether symptom or cause, Hobbs and the test cases his paper helped provoke struck a broad and sensitive nerve in the medical profession. Even as the Indiana test cases were pending, John J. Reese, the University of Pennsylvania professor of medical jurisprudence who had been so prominent in the Wharton case, called their importance to the attention of physicians in his state. He developed the knowledge-as-capital-property argument and called for public compensation of expert witnesses. Those who could pay would be assessed costs, while the poor would pay for expert medical witnesses from a set-aside state fund. "The question of adequate compensation," declared Reese in the *Medical and Surgical Reporter* of Philadelphia, "demands the serious consideration of the profession. . . . further, . . . it is the duty of the medical profession to agitate this question until a healthy public opinion shall compel . . . a change in our statutes."[54]

The editors of the *Philadelphia Medical Times* took a similar position. If their spelling of names in the "Dill and Buchanan" case left something to be desired, their frustration with the law was unambiguous. Despite sanctimonious obeisance to fairness and consistency, judges routinely permitted lawyers, but not doctors, to be paid for court services of various sorts. When dealing with the former, they thought "sympathy with a colleague" prevailed among judges; when dealing with the latter, "jealousy of a rival profession, to say nothing of the antagonism of opinion which so often arises in the court-room between judge and doctor" seemed to rule. The best hope for physicians, therefore, lay not with the courts but with the legislature. If they failed to make headway there, the vast majority of physicians would do well to deny their own expertise when called to court and thus avoid testimony altogether.[55]

The Centennial Medical Society of Southern Illinois formally petitioned the Illinois State Medical Society in 1878 to try to do something
about the problem "of calling physicians as experts, and requiring them to
sit during the trial of cases and hear the examination of witnesses, and then
give a professional opinion in regard to the testimony, often consuming
much of their time without proper compensation." The parent society, in
turn, found in 1879 "hardly two of the legal profession" in Illinois who
agreed upon the legal rights of physicians as expert witnesses. The chairman of the special committee was reduced to rehearsing Hobbs's reports
and urging that Illinois physicians monitor future developments elsewhere.[56] The medical societies of Missouri and Kentucky were told by otherwise sympathetic legal scholars and judges that physicians in those states
remained subject to subpoena as experts without special compensation. To
alter that situation, physicians would have to win state-by-state legislative
redress.[57]

Debate had broken out among California physicians as well. W. S.
Thorne, who practiced in the San Jose area, decried the sorry status of
medical experts in California courts, where outdated knowledge, sectarian
rivalries, wide-open definitions of expertise, and personal bias were prosti-
tuting principle and undermining the profession. To remedy the situation,
Thorne called for more cooperation among medical societies, a chair in "State
Medicine" at the University of California, and above all else, a concerted
push in the legislature for proper compensation to expert witnesses. Like so
many other doctors during the 1870s, Thorne stressed the rhetoric of private property in arguing the case for compensation: "a physician's time is
practically his capital, his stock in trade, if you please. Is not, therefore,
this exercise of judicial authority, in effect, the appropriation of private
property to public uses without just compensation?"[58]

A.W. Saxe, a founding member of the Santa Clara Medical Society,
countered that the worst problems occurred in cases that involved insanity,
and in most of those cases, Saxe argued, physicians were no more competent to judge than "any person of common sense and common experience."
Harking back to California's gold-rush traditions of communal consensus,
Saxe took a position faintly reminiscent of the republican tradition half a
century earlier: physicians owed society any sacrifices they might be called
upon to make because "*justice should not only be speedy, but cheap,* so that the
humblest citizen may as readily and conveniently demand it as the more
wealthy and influential."[59] In an argument rarely expressed by American
physicians in professional publications after the Civil War, Saxe went on to
argue that special fees were logically unjustifiable as well. Ultimately, the
learned professions should serve society in their fashion as other groups did
in other ways.

But Saxe was in a distinct minority, as a later speaker tried to make
clear. J. Bradford Cox could live with euphemisms: expert fees could be
considered legal honoraria if outright pay seemed sordid. But proper compensation under some guise was essential, and the physicians of California

were right to be intensely interested in the "money value of professional and other services." In a revealing rebuttal to the veteran Saxe, Cox also pointed out that what might have been appropriate to the rough-and-tumble egalitarianism of the 'forty-niners was no longer appropriate to a maturing society three decades later. The "facts of political history" demonstrated that governments paid those who served them differential rates for different levels of skill and responsibility, and the medical society should now demand better than it was receiving from the courts in the evolving professional marketplace.[60] The Santa Clara Medical Society as a whole clearly agreed with Thorne and Cox, and the delegates resolved to press the California legislature for a law that would compensate subpoenaed physicians at professional rates. The doctors managed to introduce a bill to accomplish that object, but in the laconic report of the society's secretary for 1879, their bill "failed to become a law."[61]

In Nueces County, Texas, a physician refused to testify in a murder trial about a post-mortem he had previously performed on the body of the purported victim unless paid for the knowledge he was now being asked to divulge. The doctor argued that any knowledge he had of the case "was obtained by professional skill and from the deductions of experience, which I consider my own property." The local judge sustained the physician, but the Texas Court of Appeals, citing the *Dement* decision in Alabama, ruled in 1879 that the physician had to testify without compensation or suffer punishment. "Dr. Spohn has doubtless been misled, in taking the position he did," declared the court in *Summer v. State*, "by the misconception of certain writers on medical jurisprudence."[62]

From western New York came further evidence of the widespread professional concern. George Cothan, a professor at the College of Physicians and Surgeons of Buffalo, who had taught medical jurisprudence for more than twenty-five years, published a pair of articles on the crisis of the expert witness in the inaugural volume of the new *Physicians and Surgeons' Investigator* in 1880. In the first article, he faced up to the fact that "physicians, as a general rule, are not good witnesses," despite half a century of instruction in the nation's medical schools. Doctors were still too easily trapped and battered by lawyers, too anxious to show off, and too easily led into areas of knowledge where they were weak.[63] In the second article, he addressed the question of compensation, making yet again the case for expert knowledge as a property right and reviewing the results of the Alabama and Indiana test cases. He hoped physicians would continue to press the doctrines propounded by Hobbs until they became, if not law, at least legal practice.[64]

Cothan's colleagues in the Buffalo Medical Association invited Superior Court Judge Charles Beckwith to comment in April 1880. Judge Beckwith expressed displeasure at the way lawyers so often bullied doctors, but told the doctors, in essence, to hang on, since in the judge's opinion things were getting better than they had been just a few years ago. The New York Bar Association had recently taken up complaints about the treatment of witnesses and declared members "cowardly" who attacked "unfairly" those in the stand. Beckwith also tried to assure the Buffalo physicians that "public opinion, which controls every thing, is working a change in the manners and modes of courts and lawyers." But on the key subject of compensation, Judge Beckwith offered little hope for the physicians of his district. He rejected the property theory of knowledge, the special status of professionals, and the decision of the Indiana Supreme Court in the *Buchman* case; he commended the Alabama decision in *Dement* and undercut the possibility of legislative redress for expert witnesses as akin to the old Elizabethan system of compensating "witnesses according to their 'countenance and calling.' " "Since the trial of Dr. Schoeppe, in Pennsylvania, Mrs. Wharton in Maryland, and other equally notorious cases, one may well feel apprehensive," Beckwith conceded, about the value of experts paid by the parties themselves. But he would go no farther than a cautious commendation of the possible value of court-appointed commissions, "*quasi* officers of the court," who would make expert determinations, provided the parties adversely affected would be free to challenge them. From the point of view of the ordinary practitioner in western New York, Judge Beckwith's remarks offered little reason to look forward to future involvement with the courts.[65]

In 1880, F. W. Draper called upon the Boston Society for Medical Improvement to lobby the Massachusetts legislature one more time in favor of a bill that would create just the sort of medical commissions that Beckwith in New York had been willing to consider. In Draper's view, the general public had come to regard the typical American medical expert in court as partisan and mercenary, which not only impeded justice but hurt the profession as a whole, because "the expert is in a peculiar sense the public exponent and representative of his profession." Draper claimed the support of the Attorney-General for his bill, and hoped that Massachusetts would lead the way on this issue as it had with state boards of health and vital statistics. The members of Draper's commissions would, of course, be paid professional rates by the government. Yet even Draper conceded grave constitutional problems in legislation of the sort he proposed, and the scheme failed yet again, as it had repeatedly done there and elsewhere through the previous decade.[66]

On the opposite coast, United States District Judge Matthew P. Deady, who also taught medical jurisprudence in the medical department of Willamette University, called upon the Oregon State Medical Society in 1881 to push for reform. Undaunted by its relentless rebuffing at home, Deady hoped to implement another refurbished version of the old 1870 Massachusetts proposal for court-appointed medical experts. Deady thought that Oregon county governments could be persuaded, or forced by the state legislature, to pay for medical experts.[67] He was wrong. Halfway between Massachusetts and Oregon, the Minnesota State Medical Society's Committee on Medical Jurisprudence in 1882 recommended a shift to court-appointed experts. Though the committee also acknowledged constitutional problems with their proposal, they took the bold position that "reform is sometimes the truest conservatism" and essentially argued that the system could hardly be worse than it already was.[68]

Thus, back and forth across the nation into the early 1880s, American physicians contemplated with less and less enthusiasm their place as experts in court. And no solutions seemed readily at hand. State legislatures had consistently refused to alter the American adversarial system, and efforts to improve the lot of medical witnesses within that system were making little headway. By 1883, notwithstanding the intense agitation of the 1870s, only three states had statutes allowing even for the possibility of special compensation for medical experts: Iowa, under the state code of 1873, where a subsequent court case had thrown the operation of the law into doubt; Rhode Island, as the result of a law passed in 1882, where a justice of the Supreme Court had to approve any extra compensation as "just and reasonable"; and North Carolina, where local judges were permitted, but not required, by the terms of an 1871 statute to offer expert compensation.[69] The *Buchman* decision in Indiana stood in stark and vulnerable contrast to high court decisions everywhere else. In a judicial era generally characterized by historians as unusually friendly to private property, to capital of all sorts, and to the sophisticated classes of society, American physicians made little progress in state courts with their arguments in favor of professional knowledge as private property.

CHAPTER FIFTEEN

Medical Examiners
and Medico-Legal Societies

Though largely rebuffed by the courts, physicians interested in medico-legal involvement did appear to enjoy two major successes by the end of the century. First, those physicians who continued to look to the state for the improvement of medico-legal interactions finally succeeded in helping to bring about the substitution of official medical examiners for traditional coroners in a few jurisdictions. Second, those physicians who preferred to work within the professions to bolster the field of medical jurisprudence succeeded in establishing formal medico-legal societies to address the professional problems that concerned them. Though the former seemed to be the culmination of efforts that went back to the 1820s and was generally regarded then and since as a progressive step, the way in which the office of medical examiner came into being proved ultimately undercutting. Worse, it established structural precedents that kept anything like the sort of state medicine Beck had once envisioned in a distinctly second-rate position within the American medical profession through the entire twentieth century. Though the latter seemed to embody a new spirit of professionalism for medical jurisprudence, the medico-legal societies ironically ended up affirming instead the fact that few physicians retained the high hopes or sense of professional excitement once associated with the field.

Massachusetts physicians led the post-Civil War efforts to substitute medical examiners for coroners. Physicians there, as in New York and elsewhere, had long been critical of the office of coroner. Indeed, from mid-century on, Massachusetts commentators had regularly peppered their medical, legal, and popular publications with negative comments about what they regarded as their state's corrupt and outmoded coroner system.[1] But their reiterated calls for reform of various sorts had gone unheeded. Massachusetts lawmakers showed no more inclination to alter a political arrangement that favored those in power than did their counterparts in other states.

The public activity of Massachusetts professionals accelerated after the

Civil War, as the decade-long Washburn-led efforts to replace adversarial medical witnesses with court-appointed experts have already attested. The Massachusetts Medical Society took advantage of the spirit of elite professional cooperation engendered by that effort to mount a more or less simultaneous and concerted attack against the old coroner system as well. While the Washburn coalition labored to an ultimately futile denouement, the Massachusetts Medical Society, after decades of frustration, suddenly began in the political turmoil of the 1870s to make what appeared to be near-revolutionary headway on the subject of coroner reform.

In the early years of the decade the Medical Society exploited a series of well-publicized financial scandals and apparent miscarriages of justice linked to coroners in Boston. The *Boston Pilot* and the *Boston Daily Advertiser* joined the *BMSJ* in 1871 in attacking irregularities in a number of inquests conducted that summer in the city.[2] A "respectable class of our citizens, which includes several of the best known and most respected physicians of our city," petitioned the next session of the legislature to investigate the coroners of Suffolk County. Some of the coroners were apparently padding their expense reports with never-performed post-mortems and altering death certificates in exchange for financial and political favors.

The politicization of those positions had produced in Boston a situation which the "respected physicians" found frustrating. Under Massachusetts law, local coroners were appointed by the governor and, once appointed, they were virtually impossible to remove. Partly for those reasons, the number of coroners in Boston had risen in 1872 to twenty-five; more than six times as many as New York City, even though Boston had little more than a quarter of New York's population. Philadelphia, New Orleans, and Chicago, in comparison, each had two coroners; Baltimore, San Francisco, Cincinnati, and Washington each had one. Boston physicians hoped that the time would soon be right for "a modification of the statutes," but in the short run the politically effective coroners held the physicians at bay in the legislature.[3] Moreover, though the medical society never mentioned it, the gubernatorial appointment of coroners had long provided ruling Republican factions at the state level with valuable local leverage in the closely contested battles their allies were fighting against a strong Democratic organization at the city level.

Through the middle of the decade, Massachusetts regular physicians continued to complain about what they regarded as the embarrassment of the Boston coroners. Several of the latter claimed to be doctors, but were not recognized by the state or local medical societies; one coroner had been tried in Superior Criminal Court for performing illegal abortions.[4] What annoyed the regular physicians most was the continuing recognition and financial patronage afforded "many of the quacks of Boston" by friendly local coroners.[5] This was particularly the case after election of a Democratic governor in 1875, who began to augment the existing corps of coroners with appointees of his own. To put it differently, the Massachusetts Medical Society was not upset that too few physicians were involved with coroners' inquests, as Beck had been in New York half a century before, but irked that too many of the wrong types were involved for the wrong reasons. Justice was being administered poorly, they argued, public money was being squandered, and the regulars' rivals were being sanctioned in their neighborhoods both as and by public officials.[6] An editorial blasting one of the irregulars appointed coroner in 1875 provoked a libel suit against the *Boston Medical and Surgical Journal.*[7]

The regulars renewed their campaign at the end of 1876 at a meeting of the American Social Science Association.[8] In a major paper, Theodore H. Tyndale, a Boston lawyer who became interested in coroner reform after noting that the British Social Science Association was seeking similar reform in England, summarized the standard arguments against the existing structure. As a solution, he favored division of the coroner's separate judicial and medical functions, with the appointment of medical examiners to perform the latter. His two most telling points, however, had less to do with professional standards or governmental theory than they did with political and fiscal reality: the number of coroners in Boston had grown to forty-three and their demands upon the treasury continued to escalate.[9] Nor was it a coincidence that this effort took place just as a new Republican administration was taking over from the outgoing Democratic governor.[10]

In the state legislative session of 1877, Tyndale coordinated his testimony before the judiciary sub-committee with that of a delegation from the Massachusetts Medical Society. The attorney general of Massachusetts, Charles Russell Train, threw his prestige behind the reform movement as well, thus signaling an important shift on the part of the state's political leaders. A handful of the old-line Boston coroners, including some of the better ones, tried to defend their system, but failed. The legislature abolished the office of coroner throughout Massachusetts and provided instead for the appointment of medical examiners to investigate all future cases of persons found dead. The fact that neither house of the Massachusetts legislature seriously debated the measure before passing it hinted strongly that consensual arrangements had been struck in advance.[11] Under the terms of the bill, Suffolk County was limited to two medical examiners, who would have fixed salaries.

On July 1, 1877, when the new law went into effect, Massachusetts became the first state in the Union to abolish the ancient Anglo-American office of coroner. The two new gubernatorially appointed medical examiners in Suffolk County, moreover, who would henceforth conduct the state's autopsies in Boston, initially had the full support of the state medical society.[12] On the surface at least, this appeared to be a major breakthrough. Medical officers acceptable in the eyes of the most elite regulars were being paid by the state to perform quasi-legal tasks on a more or less full-time basis. The medical press hailed the result as a triumph of professional cooperation, an example of what could be accomplished when the legal and medical professions worked together openly.[13]

What really took place in Massachusetts in 1877, however, was the

elimination of a traditional political instrument by the state's dominant political factions after they saw how easily their opponents could use it and
how flagrant its abuses had become in contrast to other jurisdictions around
the country. Though the state's regular physicians congratulated themselves
for pressing the politicians to do the right thing, shifting political circumstances, not professional pressure, had produced results. The state's regular
physicians, after all, had been making most of the same basic arguments
against the coroner system for decades. What changed was the willingness
of the politicians, for their own reasons, to consider altering the system, to
give in to the professional pressures that had been there all along. Even
then, the politicians did not create a system that did much to advance either
professional medicine or medical jurisprudence.

The law was less revolutionary than it appeared to be and was further
from the old republican ideals of medical jurisprudence than a number of
hopeful editorials in Massachusetts and around the country tried to suggest.
The new medical examiners were still going to be political appointees, and
politicians continued to wrangle over how and by whom those appointments should be made.[14] Though the governor was now required to appoint "men, learned in the science of medicine," the statute attempted no
definition of "learned" and did not require the governor to consult any professional organizations, much less the regular Massachusetts Medical Society which had pushed for the bill.[15] When the new medical examiners called
other physicians in to help them, as they frequently had to do, they could
not pay fees any larger than could the old coroners.

Most important, the new medical examiners had distinctly limited powers
that restricted their activities to what would today be termed forensic pathology of a narrow sort. The medical examiners were in no sense the broad-
gauged and proactive medico-legal officers of the sort Beck had envisioned;
they held no policy-making power, no special judicial standing, and little
professional authority. Indeed, before the century ended, the Massachusetts
medical examiners would find themselves under attack for their methods of
proceeding and entangled in disputes over their right to "view" certain types
of cases at all and over their standing as expert witnesses in courts.[16] In a
word more telling than he might have realized, the editor of the *BMSJ* styled
the examiners' field "necropsy."[17] Indeed, the Massachusetts medical examiners themselves continued through the end of the nineteenth century to
call for European-style medico-legal officers who could perform genuinely
jurisprudential functions, as distinguished from routine autopsy chores.[18]

Following their initial appointments in 1877, a number of the new
medical examiners formed a professional organization, which they called
the Massachusetts Medico-Legal Society.[19] The first president in his presidential address of 1878 hoped that the 1877 law which created their jobs
would soon be followed by three more crucial developments: the emergence
of forensic medicine as a specialty on a par with surgery and other prestigious specialties; the reform of medical testimony and medical evidence in
court; and the reinvigoration of medical jurisprudence in American medical

schools.[20] None of those three developments took place. The examiners eventually fell to justifying themselves primarily in fiscal terms: for the taxpayers, they did a more effective job of investigating deaths for less public money than the old coroner system; for physicians, they greatly reduced the state's need to impress the uncompensated services of ordinary doctors.[21]

What happened in Massachusetts in 1877 was unique to that state at that time. Despite pressure from regular physicians elsewhere, no other jurisdiction in the nation actually eliminated the ancient post of coroner before the beginning of the present century, when both the political and the professional circumstances of the nation had changed.[22] Developments in New York proved more typical of the country as a whole. There the state's powerful regulars campaigned just as steadily through the 1870s against the coroner system as their counterparts in Massachusetts. Beginning in 1869, with the active support of the *New York Times* and the Medico-Legal Society of New York, New York physicians helped expose and publicize a "jury ring" in the New York City coroner's office. Coroners were routinely listing their political allies as inquest jurors, whether those allies were actually present or not, and the coroners were holding phantom inquiries in order to increase on their records the number of jurors for whom they could claim expenses and *per diem* fees. Taken one at a time, the jurors' fees were not large. But they could mount up. One man in 1875, for example, was credited with sitting in on two hundred inquests in three months; that would be more than two a day, seven days a week.[23] Still, physician protests notwithstanding, legislative initiatives consistently made no headway in Albany, particularly since the coroner remained a constitutional officer.

The Municipal Society, a good-government group headed by veteran public health reformer Stephen Smith, hoped after 1877 to take advantage in New York of the momentum seemingly generated in Massachusetts. In January 1878, Smith placed a coroner reform bill before the New York state legislature, only to have Tammany Democrats from New York City amend it into a pay raise for the coroners already serving.[24] The Medico-Legal Society of New York mounted another effort in the early 1880s, but again failed to alter the system.[25] New York, in fact, would not substantially change its coroner system until the eve of World War I, following a great deal of agitation during the so-called Progressive Era.[26] And even then, as historian Julie Johnson has made clear for the case of Philadelphia as well, the changes once again advanced neither the professional interests of physicians nor the general prospects of the field of medical jurisprudence.[27]

While no other state followed Massachusetts in eliminating coroners altogether, two of its neighbors adopted versions of the medical examiner concept. In Connecticut, prominent regular physicians had worked without success during the 1870s to replace or reform the coroners of their state. Not until 1883, however, did the Connecticut legislature finally respond to the renewed efforts of yet another special committee of the Connecticut Medical Society. But the physicians were far from unanimously pleased

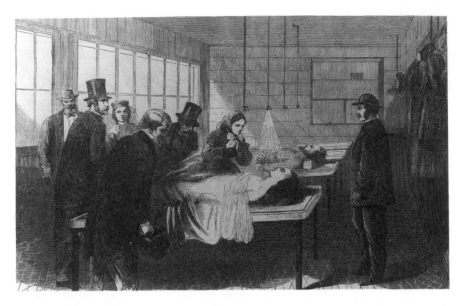

Identifying the unknown dead in the New York City morgue. From *Harper's Weekly*,
July 7, 1866. *(Courtesy of the National Library of Medicine)*

with the end result, since the Connecticut legislature made explicit the least
attractive part of the Massachusetts system: the medical duties associated
with the office of coroner, which devolved upon doctors designated as medical examiners, were made distinctly subservient to the legal duties associated with the office of coroner, which were specifically reserved to trained
lawyers. Even on such basic decisions as whether to conduct an autopsy,
the designated doctors were "directly subordinate" to the county prosecutors. As Gustavus Eliot of New Haven reported to the AMA, Connecticut's
new medical examiners occupied an "exceedingly insignificant position."[28]

In 1884 the state legislature of Rhode Island, in a somewhat similar
fashion, also created a board of medical examiners. The lawmakers were
responding at least in part to pleas for change coming from the regular
Newport Medical Society and the regular Rhode Island Medical Society.
As the law emerged, however, the new examiners were charged only with
conducting the state's investigations of death, and Rhode Island retained
locally elected coroners to oversee those investigations. This relieved the
medical rank-and-file from impressment for that purpose, but did more to
denigrate the actual work than elevate it. To make matters worse, only
twenty of the twenty-four Rhode Island doctors subsequently designated as
examiners were "regular physicians in good standing."[29]

In short, the early harbingers of the twentieth-century movement toward
medical examiners did little to enhance the power, prestige, or attractiveness of medical jurisprudence in the eyes of American physicians during
the last three decades of the nineteenth century. Indeed, by separating out

the investigation of death, and by turning the investigation of death into an altogether subordinate service explicitly under the supervision of legal and political authorities, the New England laws of the late nineteenth century, which set the tone and established the precedents for similar laws throughout the country in the early twentieth century, further dismembered the concept of medical jurisprudence and rendered forensic medicine even less attractive to most physicians than it already was. To be sure, some of the problems that exercised Beck half a century before were resolved in these new arrangements, including most importantly the substantial elimination of impressed public service for ordinary practitioners. But the price of resolving those problems in this fashion was high, for the resolution was premised upon a formal separation between medicine and law, and it was embodied in a structure that made the former something of a handmaiden to the latter. Physicians had pushed for change, and they got it; but on less than ideal terms. In many ways, the widespread institutionalization of similar structures throughout the United States in the twentieth century merely ratified the death of a dream never realized in the nineteenth century.

Attempts to meet the problems of medical jurisprudence from within the professions themselves fared little better in the last third of the nineteenth century than efforts to adjust external governmental structures. By far the best known and most successful effort to institutionalize professional support for the field involved the Medico-Legal Society of the City of New York. According to one of its founders, the society grew out of informal sessions of information-sharing among a handful of young physicians who served as working deputies to the city's coroners in the late 1850s. One of those doctors, Wooster Beach, had organized the sessions just before the outbreak of the Civil War. Through the mid-1860s, the group continued to hold their small informal meetings in the coroners' office. In 1866 the doctors decided to make their sessions formal; in 1867 they approved official statements of purpose and plans of organization; in 1868 they secured a charter from the New York state legislature.[30] This was an era of professional society-building among the elite regular physicians of New York City, as Charles Rosenberg has demonstrated. The nascent Medico-Legal Society seemed very much a part of that process and relatively insignificant at the time of its founding.[31]

Despite its modest beginnings, the Medico-Legal Society's stated purpose was grand: "advancement of the science of Medical Jurisprudence." That goal, of course, had existed more or less continuously among at least some of the city's physicians since the days of James Stringham at the beginning of the century, but this was the first time a separate professional society had been organized with the specific and exclusive purpose of advancing the field. The group hoped to achieve its ends by amassing a library on the subject, holding regular meetings, sponsoring periodic publications, serving as a clearinghouse for others elsewhere interested in the field, and "assisting courts when requested in eliciting the truth in questions arising in Medical Jurisprudence."[32]

At the time of its founding, the Society seemed to embody long-standing ideals. Four of the ten honorary memberships open to physicians went (unsolicited, of course) to Parisians, clear indication of the continuing hope that something approximating the French system might still be made to work in the United States. No British or German medico-legalist was named to the honorary roll.[33] Moreover, the New York society was delighted to learn a few months later that a similar organization had been independently established in Paris itself shortly after the New Yorkers had made their own society formal. T.C. Finnel, the first president of the New York society, was promptly made an honorary member of the Medico-Legal Society of Paris, and the two organizations exchanged an initial flurry of mutually congratulatory recognitions.[34] The archives of the Medico-Legal Society of Paris still contain a mint copy of Ordronaux's *Jurisprudence of Medicine* inscribed to his French colleagues by the proud author in 1869; Ordronaux was one of the founding members of the New York society.[35]

Both organizations marveled at the coincidence of their establishment, and both hoped that the spirit of traditional medical jurisprudence was on the brink of resuscitation after being near death, for somewhat different reasons, in both countries. Both hoped that their organizations would be able to bridge an increasingly large chasm between law and medicine. The charter of the New York society explicitly stated its desire for an evenly divided membership, half physicians and half attorneys.[36]

Through the early 1870s the New York Medico-Legal Society seemed to prosper. Its opinion in the much-publicized Schoeppe trial was well received and widely circulated. Clark Bell, a corporate attorney who had become deeply interested in medical jurisprudence through his involvement in the lunacy hearing of the Union Pacific Railroad's George Francis Train, took over the presidency of the society in 1872 and began what eventually became more than forty years of tireless activity in its behalf. Membership had risen dramatically enough by 1873 to make the Medico-Legal Society of New York the city's fifth largest medical organization.[37]

Also exciting to the principals of the New York Medico-Legal Society was the apparent emulation of their efforts in other American cities. In 1874, for example, President Bell reported an effort in Cleveland to form a medico-legal society there and expressed "honorable pride in receiving from this young and vigorous society the credit of having inspired its organization."[38] That same year United States Surgeon General John Shaw Billings wanted information about the group for his nascent national library of medicine.[39] In the meantime, many of the nation's leading authorities on medical jurisprudence had come to New York to offer papers. The society seemed to be functioning as a clearinghouse for serious research into medico-legal problems, and the membership rolls actually did include nearly equal numbers of doctors and lawyers. Paeans to the traditional ideals of integrated medical jurisprudence conceived of as a separate professional field continued to float in near-lyrical tones above the society's meetings.

Beneath the surface, however, the New York Medico-Legal Society, even in its salad days, was having little positive impact on the relationship between medicine and law. Though the society looked strong on paper through the 1870s, many of its members were inactive. In 1883 President Bell finally admitted publicly that a "considerable number of members have been so only in name, and have taken little interest in our work."[40] As the record of its celebratory dinner at Delmonico's in 1873 made clear, the society also seemed as much an elite social club as a working professional society. Indeed, the society came increasingly to look like Clark Bell's personal coterie. That was not altogether bad: voluntary organizations have always needed dedicated principals like Bell, and Bell's contributions both to the society and to the field of medical jurisprudence were certainly significant. But Bell functioned in all but name as president-for-life, thereby blocking the upward rotation of younger leaders.

Perhaps more crippling still was Bell's own obsession with the medical jurisprudence of insanity, which almost certainly proved counterproductive for the society in the long run. Nineteen of the society's first forty-seven papers dealt directly with various aspects of that subject.[41] When the *Albany Law Journal* congratulated Bell on his presidential address of 1874, it noted that his focus on legal insanity dominated his society's discussions.[42] Bell's near-fixation on that subject minimized efforts to address other issues, where progress might have been made, and maximized a relentless emphasis on what was probably the single most frustrating, most divisive, and least solvable of the professional problems the group faced.[43] Indeed, debate over that issue provoked so many "unpleasant dissensions" that a subgroup associated with William Hammond established a rival, though short-lived, New York Society of Medical Jurisprudence primarily to press its own views on insanity and the law.[44]

The contrasting progress of the Medico-Legal Society of Paris and that of New York was telling. The French organization, which is still actively in existence, won funding from its government to host an international medico-legal congress in the summer of 1878, which Bell characterized as an assembly of "great importance to Forensic Science." Delegations from all over Europe attended, but the New York Medico-Legal Society, "was not represented." Bell hosted what he billed as international congresses of his own in 1889, 1893, and 1895; but the New York Medico-Legal Society itself was limping by then, the sessions were only superficially international, and there is no evidence that the American congresses had any impact on the field of medical jurisprudence in this country or elsewhere. The tenth anniversary of the great celebration at Delmonico's in 1873 saw the New York Medico-Legal Society already dropping names from its membership roles and pleading with those who remained to pay their dues and support the library. That was also the year when the Hammond group seceded from the parent organization. The original New York Medico-Legal Society's publishing efforts ironically and somewhat misleadingly increased after 1883, when the *Medico-Legal Journal* first appeared, but that too proved to be an essentially personal vehicle for its editor, none other than Clark

Bell. He finally relinquished the *Journal* in 1915, because of his failing health, and publication promptly stopped.[45] The society itself essentially ceased to function when Bell died in 1918.

If the New York Medico-Legal Society, the largest, most prestigious, and best publicized of America's medico-legal societies of period 1870–90, proved to be a somewhat superficial organization, parallel societies elsewhere around the nation proved downright ephemeral. The Massachusetts Medico-Legal Society, founded in 1877, was not in fact an open professional society at all, but the restricted and official association of the Massachusetts medical examiners.[46] Even then, many of the state's examiners never joined. By 1888 the principal officers publicly "deplored the inactivity of members in the matter of presenting papers."[47] The association did nevertheless publish its *Transactions* through the early years of the twentieth century. Though the *Transactions* contained for the most part a dreary series of eminently practical case reports, their appearance in any form put the Massachusetts Medico-Legal Society ahead of all others in the country except New York.

Bell had hailed the formation of a medico-legal society in Cleveland in 1883, but no record of what it did seems to have survived. He and others have identified medico-legal societies founded in 1884 in Philadelphia, in 1885 in Rhode Island, in 1886 in Chicago, and in 1890 in Denver.[48] Scattered allusions suggested the possibility of similar, less formal organizations in other locations as well during this period.[49] But the plain fact was that none of them amounted to much.

On the face of it, to take the most prominent example from this list, formation of the Medical Jurisprudence Society of Philadelphia might have been a significant event. That city had long been one of the chief centers of nineteenth-century American medicine and an influential leader in law as well. Evidence that the society was established in 1884 and formally incorporated by the state of Pennsylvania in 1888, moreover, gave the impression of a lasting structure of some substance. But better perspective can be gained by a quick glance at the constitution and by-laws of that organization. Though membership was open to "any person in good standing in the regular medical or legal profession," a quorum consisted of five active members. Any three active members could call a special meeting.[50] Given the fact that roughly 2000 doctors and 1700 lawyers practiced in Philadelphia, that was a tiny society indeed.[51]

The key to understanding the Medical Jurisprudence Society of Philadelphia, and by implication most of the others as well, including the New York Medico-Legal Society during its early years of success, lay in committee structure. The Philadelphia Society's most important group was its standing committee on legislation, charged with superintending "the preparation and presentation of any bills or laws that the Society may deem necessary to frame, and [taking] proper measures to secure the enactment of same."[52] In essence, these late nineteenth-century medico-legal societies were attempting to incorporate formally the long-standing informal arrangements that had existed on an *ad hoc* basis between elite physicians and elite lawyers at least since Beck and Spencer worked together on the New York code in the 1820s.

The New York Medico-Legal Society probably had more impact on the social policies of its state legislature than it did on the professional orientation of its constituent professions or the long-term development of the field of medical jurisprudence. In its early years, for example, it helped draft and push for legislation that made abortion a felony in New York, the law that created New York's Lunacy Commission, and statutes designed to improve health and sanitation in public schools.[53] Members were also deeply involved in the New York code revisions of the early 1870s. The greatest of all New York legal codifiers, David Dudley Field, encouraged those activities in 1873. "No code, no system of law for any place or people," he told the members of the society at Delmonico's, "can be administered without the light of medical jurisprudence."[54] Major-General William W. Averell aptly suggested that the New York Medico-Legal Society had "the State for a patient."[55] And one of the society's principal leaders, James J. O'Dea, explicitly characterized it as a body concerned first and foremost with influencing public policy.[56]

Through the late 1870s and mid-1880s the society tried to alter the coroner system, further refine the laws applying to insanity, and change the methods of giving expert medical testimony. In all cases, however, they were rebuffed. The failure of those later ventures no doubt contributed to the society's transformation from a temporarily vibrant organization after the Civil War into Clark Bell's inter-professional club at the end of the century. In other localities elite doctors and lawyers either saw little reason to incorporate their *ad hoc* arrangements in the first place or decided quite quickly that formal organizations offered few additional benefits over the informal channels of influence that already existed; indeed, to organize themselves might arouse public suspicion and provoke potential rivals on any given policy.

One final, yet theoretically intriguing, observation about these medico-legal and medical jurisprudential societies needs to be made. In virtually all of the standard models of professionalization used implicitly or explicitly by American historians and sociologists, the appearance of formal organizations and societies is taken as a significant step in the solidification and advancement of professional fields. But the same cannot be said for medical jurisprudence. The appearance of the medico-legal and medical jurisprudential societies in the late nineteenth century, especially in their constitutionally overt desire to include equal numbers of doctors and lawyers, paradoxically recognized the emergence of a deep division between those two professions. These societies were designed to enhance dialogue and cooperation, particularly in matters of public policy, between the otherwise isolated members of two separately established fields; they were not designed to give form and voice to professionals who conceived of themselves as a new and different group, separate from medicine and law, operating between them. In fact, their most frequently recurring rhetorical theme was the lament that no mediating profession had ever evolved in the United States. And in a sense, they institutionalized the increasingly obdurate professional reality that one never would.[57]

In his remarks following the Delmonico dinner of 1873, Major-General Averell had cited Tocqueville's observation that "it seemed necessary to do everything in this country through associations," and then speculated about why "a century was permitted to elapse. . . . since the establishment of the Republic" before associations like the New York Medico-Legal Society finally emerged. The general surmised that America's "efforts toward material development ha[d] been too vehement, the current of capital and labor too swift and strong to permit that leisure which is essential to investigation."[58] Whether or not he was right about capital and labor, he may have sensed correctly what had happened in the profession of medicine. It had developed swiftly and strongly in channels that maximized the influence and the income actually available in the circumstances of marketplace professionalism that already prevailed; physicians interested in medical jurisprudence thus found themselves farther and farther from the professional mainstream.

The general went wrong in equating the New York Medico-Legal Society with prototypical Tocquevillean associations. The New York Medico-Legal Society and the others like it did not signal the emergence of a new field, as Tocqueville and many modern social scientists might assume, but instead ratified a realization that the old republican ideal would not be attained in the professional marketplace of the late nineteenth century. The fact that most of the late nineteenth-century medico-legal and medical jurisprudential societies were so small, so superficial, so internally splintered, and so short-lived, moreover, suggested that those few physicians still interested in cross-professional medical jurisprudence on any terms would have a tough time simply making the best of what had developed. Their failures, in turn, were perfectly consistent with the sputtering medico-legal activities of the larger American Medical Association itself during the second half of the nineteenth century.

CHAPTER SIXTEEN

Medical Jurisprudence and the AMA

A handful of prominent physicians had organized the American Medical Association in 1847. The fact that the AMA came into existence at roughly the same time that the fortunes of medical jurisprudence began to fall was no coincidence. Both developments were related to the same large shifts under way in the history of American professions. The anti-professional outbursts of the Jacksonian era that precluded state support for medical jurisprudence also unsettled the social position of law and medicine, especially medicine. Marketplace professionalism combined with essentially open access to the professions to affect both fields in similar ways. By 1850, per capita, there were many more practitioners trying to earn money as doctors and lawyers than there had been in 1800; many of the newer practitioners in both fields were poorly or irregularly trained; and the elite members of both professions feared dissolution and decline. In both professions elite leaders counterattacked during the middle decades of the nineteenth century in an effort to reverse the trends of the 1830s and 1840s. From the medical side, the founding of the AMA was part of that larger effort to find a stable structural base for America's professions.

Although the AMA subsequently grew into the quintessential historical example of a full-scale, broad-front professional association in the United States, the group functioned at first with relatively limited goals. Chief among them was an effort to persuade America's proliferating, democratizing, and sharply competing medical schools to insist upon stiffer standards in the awarding of degrees. Indeed, the most important impetus behind the initial meetings of the AMA was a growing fear that medical degrees were becoming altogether too easy to acquire. Bad enough that anyone who wished to try could compete in the medical marketplace; the nation's proliferating medical schools were allowing superficial competitors to display M.D. diplomas. Stiffer requirements for that degree, the founders hoped, would simultaneously reduce the number of practitioners able to present profes-

sional credentials to the public and strengthen the real educational base of
American medicine as a learned profession.

Most of the founders of the AMA had come to professional maturity
during the period when medical jurisprudence was a booming and exciting
field, and most of them remained committed to its long-term importance
for professional life. Nathan S. Davis, the prime mover in the organizational efforts that led to the initial AMA convention in 1847, though earlier
disgusted with the public's careless and indifferent attitudes toward the field
and what it might accomplish, had nonetheless agreed to teach medical jurisprudence in New York City in the spring term of 1848. T.R. Beck's old
friend John W. Francis, who had secured European books on the subject
and taught medical jurisprudence himself for many years, also took a leading part in the new association. Alfred Stillé of New Orleans, another whose
fascination with medical jurisprudence would never recede, was a third key
figure in the establishment of the AMA.[1]

Given both the circumstances and the individuals involved, it should
come as no surprise that the National Medical Convention of 1847 (the
organization did not style itself the American Medical Association until 1848)
included medical jurisprudence specifically among the subjects considered
mandatory in the upgraded and nationally prescribed medical curricula of
the future. Every medical school in the United States, resolved the delegates, should maintain that subject among the core offerings required of
every M.D. graduate. That commitment, present from the beginning and
a formal part of the AMA's first national policy statement, could hardly
have been stronger.[2] At the 1849 meeting, moreover, the national delegates
established committees on Forensic Medicine and on Public Hygiene, the
two pillars upon which the field of medical jurisprudence had traditionally
rested.[3]

Rhetorical commitment to the field never wavered through the 1850s,
and the annual conventions of the AMA heard occasional lectures on aspects of medical jurisprudence. In 1852, for example, the Committee on
Public Hygiene helped sponsor a report on the danger of lead poisoning in
the nation's growing systems of piped water.[4] In 1857 the AMA pronounced officially in favor of medical training for coroners and joined the
mounting protest against unpaid public service. Though "members of the
profession of medicine, everywhere, are, as a class, beneficent and self-
sacrificing, laboring always cheerfully and gratuitously in the cause of humanity," as the AMA report put it, "they, too, must live while they thus
labor."[5] But the early resolutions of the AMA proved to be largely exhortation without implementation; they had little immediate impact on American medical education and virtually no impact on the declining fortunes of
medical jurisprudence. The AMA itself was unable to coerce the medical
schools, few medical school faculties took seriously the suggestions proffered by the national reformers, and no school dared embrace the educational edicts unilaterally for fear of losing students. As David Meredith
Reese remarked to Nathan S. Davis in the mid-1850s: "Notwithstanding

the numerous reforms attempted, recommended and resolved on, by re-peated 'whereases' and reiterated at every successive meeting by high-sounding resolutions and in each volume of the Transactions, yet, in effectuating any one of these, after seven years' trial, the efforts of the Association in this respect have resulted in signal and utter failure."[6]

When Samuel D. Gross assumed the presidency of the AMA in 1868, two decades after passage of the original resolutions that included the asso-ciation's strong endorsement of medical jurisprudence, he called at the na-tional level for the sort of structural reform that T.R. Beck had proposed four decades earlier at the state level in New York and that Gross himself had called for in Kentucky when he was president of the Kentucky State Medical Society in the 1840s: the appointment of a "commissioner" in every judicial district in the land to act as an impartial medical expert in court cases, or in other words, yet another version of what Beck and his contem-poraries thought the early nineteenth-century French system had been.

Gross's medico-legal officer "should receive his appointment from the judges of the Supreme Court of the State; a fixed salary should be attached to the office; and he should have at least two assistants, to make all post-mortem examinations, as well as to inspect the living, in all cases of sus-pected crime, as abortion, infanticide, rape, and similar offenses." More-over, argued Gross in his presidential address, the commissioner "should have the privilege of summing up the medical testimony, not orally but in writing, for the benefit of the judge and jury, the latter of whom are always ignorant of the meaning of technical terms, and therefore incapable of drawing a proper distinction between points of difference on the part of the scientific witness." Gross, who had made his own national reputation in the Goetter case more than thirty years before, considered his proposal for medical commissioners the centerpiece of a program that would "advance the honor and glory of the profession, the good of our race, and the dignity and im-portance of this Association," not to mention the republic itself, whose standing virtues and grand potentials Gross extolled in purple prose.[7]

The convention appointed a special committee to act upon President Gross's proposals. Charles A. Lee, who chaired the special committee, re-sponded for the group that "no cause . . . has done more to lessen the confidence of the community in the medical profession than the manner in which physicians often give testimony before our courts. As our profession is constituted, and with the present views in regard to their duties to their clients entertained by the legal profession, we know of no remedy to meet the case except by the adoption of the plan recommended by our Presi-dent."[8] The AMA thereupon resolved itself officially in favor of Gross's call to create a vast system of publicly supported medical commissioners throughout the nation. That same year the AMA Committee on Medical Education continued to prescribe mandatory medical jurisprudence as part of the ideal curriculum, placing it in the second of two categories, "the more advanced and practical branches," where it was a theoretical co-equal of surgery, obstetrics, and "clinical medicine."[9]

The momentum generated by Gross's call carried into the following year and culminated at the AMA's annual convention of 1869. There John Ordronaux reported on behalf of another special committee in favor of "the appointment of a commissioner in each judicial district or circuit to aid in the examination of witnesses in every trial involving medico-legal testimony." The Ordronaux report also urged a system of arbitration panels in civil suits involving medical questions. The panels would have three experts, "one to be selected by each party litigant, and the third by the court." The committee somewhat blithely asserted that a "simple clause introduced into existing codes of procedure, or a special statute, where such codes are not to be found, would meet the required necessity."[10] That last statement revealed more about medical professionals' familiarity with and continued use of state codes than it did about the reality of the committee's proposal.

The AMA committee may have thought the time was right for their proposal because so many states had been experimenting with institutional and structural reforms of various sorts in the turbulent and dramatic years of readjustment and reconstruction immediately following the Civil War.[11] Or perhaps the AMA believed that its constituent medical societies in the separate states had enough power over the code-making and code-changing process to effect an alteration of the sort Gross had proposed the previous year. The Reconstruction era of the late 1860s did, after all, appear to be the first time since the late 1820s, when Beck had proposed a similar scheme for the state of New York, that the public influence of the medical profession seemed once again to be rising. Or perhaps the AMA hoped to do for the troublesome issue of medical jurisprudence what the Republican party was doing at the same time for the troublesome issue of black suffrage at the state level: resolve it with a national policy. Or perhaps the leaders of the AMA after the Civil War knew all along that their efforts to institutionalize state support for the revival and implementation of an altered and upgraded form of medico-legal interaction in the United States were unrealistic from the outset. In any event, little came of the AMA offensive.

For one thing, American legal processes themselves had begun to harden after the Civil War; any major change, much less a change with as many implications as the AMA proposal, would have been difficult to bring about by the 1870s. Historians of the legal profession in the United States make clear the fact that lawyers had responded to the anti-professional ethos of the 1830s by solidifying and formalizing their control over the machinery of the law. Judges began to give juries less interpretive flexibility than juries had exercised in the early decades of the nineteenth century, and lawyers began to monitor assiduously a host of processes formerly handled in the ordinary course of business dealings, or by the weight of community consensus, or through the political process. As a consolidating profession itself, also involved in an accommodation to the marketplace professionalism of the United States, the legal profession was in the process of creating a degree of formalism and predictability that left little room for fundamental changes of the sort that Gross and Ordronaux were calling for.

Moreover, the legal profession, like the medical profession, was far from a cohesive unit. Even if famous legal theorists like Emory Washburn and Dudley Field, at the top of their profession, were upset about the way medical jurisprudence worked in the United States and still willing to recast some of the medico-legal parts of the American justice system in a fashion suggested by their predecessors half a century before, thousands of common legal practitioners in the crowded lower ranks of the profession were surely less ready than ever to do so. The latter had no incentive to create a small army of state-compensated quasi-legal officers who would solve many of the problems ordinary attorneys were now being paid to resolve.

Yet another reason for the AMA failure lay within the medical profession itself, whose circumstances in the 1860s and 1870s differed sharply from those of regular physicians in the 1820s and 1830s. Despite the chronic frustration of prominent physicians earlier in the century with large numbers of untrained, part-time healers of many sorts, the regular medical societies of the 1820s and 1830s, notwithstanding their legendary intramural and extramural bickering, probably spoke for the direct interests of a larger percentage of the regular healers of their era than did the AMA forty years later. During the intervening decades large numbers of practitioners had obtained some formal training, however superficial, and entered the medical marketplace with the intention of deriving their primary incomes as full-time doctors.[12] Most of those new doctors probably considered themselves regular physicians in some vague or general sense, but they were not passionately concerned with organizational questions and practiced near the margins of the profession, wherever they could find a niche. The result, as Charles Rosenberg has pointed out in an excellent sketch of the medical profession in New York City immediately after the Civil War, was steep stratification within the universe of formally trained, full-time physicians themselves, not to mention the many irregular healers who still practiced outside the regular medical profession. Wealthy elite practitioners and emerging specialists could indulge their interests in science and debate the future of their profession in idealistic and theoretical terms; they organized and supported the New York Pathological Society and the New York Medical Journal Society, in fact, to do just those things. But for the vast majority, in Rosenberg's apt summary, the "acquisition of 'business' was still the physician's primary concern."[13]

The majority of American physicians probably paid little attention generally to the initiatives of the AMA, a national organization of elite professionals twice removed from them. President Samuel Gross himself, one of the nation's leading surgeons, epitomized the wealthy elite specialist. And the vast majority of American physicians had little inclination to push for an increased emphasis on medical jurisprudence specifically. For twenty years they had listened to debate over whether publicly employed experts should be paid at all, heard horror stories of physicians ruining their reputations in courtrooms, and experienced a popular backlash against the medical approach to insanity. Coupled with a steady rise in the number of malpractice indictments, most ordinary practitioners after the Civil War began to consider medical jurisprudence a subject to avoid, quite literally, at all costs.

Even within the AMA itself, enthusiasm for interaction with legal processes appeared much more limited than Gross's presidential address and Ordronaux's committee report might suggest. In 1859 the AMA had combined its initially separate sections on medical jurisprudence and public hygiene, probably as a result of insufficient activity in either to justify two different units within the organization. After a postwar shuffle in 1865, this combined section also inherited the orphaned subject of physiology to create the Section on Medical Jurisprudence, Physiology, and Hygiene. Most of their discussions focused on the old question of whether to push states to require compulsory vaccinations.[14] Following later reorganizations in 1873, medical jurisprudence found itself part of a new Section on Medical Jurisprudence, Chemistry, and Psychology.[15] This combining and recombining suggested not only that the subject had insufficient support to stand alone but also that the AMA really did not know what to do with it. More telling still, the Association's *Transactions* for the years 1870–75 revealed plainly that sectional meetings devoted to medical jurisprudence were poorly attended and often disbanded without conducting any business or hearing any papers.[16]

The AMA vented its frustrations over medical jurisprudence with surprising candor during the nation's centennial celebration in 1876. In 1874 the AMA had agreed to work with the Philadelphia County Medical Society to host an international medical congress in conjunction with the centennial.[17] The congress would feature ten special sessions, each devoted to papers that would survey "the different branches of medical sciences, illustrative of the advances made in them during the last hundred years in the United States."[18] Sixth on the list of ten special presentations, a list strongly influenced by Samuel Gross, were the linked subjects of medical jurisprudence and toxicology. Stanford Chaillé of New Orleans agreed to prepare the presentation on those topics.[19]

Unlike most of the other papers presented at the centennial medical congress, Chaillé's survey of medical jurisprudence and toxicology was from the outset an attempt to explain failure rather than to celebrate success. The advancement of medical jurisprudence, he argued,

> varies with the appreciation of medical knowledge by the rulers of a nation; and (since an adequate appreciation is limited to the educated few, and is not yet disseminated among the mass of any people), it results, that laws more favorable to the culture of legal medicine are to be found in nations ruled by the educated few, than in those governed by the people.[20]

Combined with the incentives of entrepreneurial capitalism, American democracy had stifled during its first century, in Chaillé's view, the very sorts of professional advancement that might best help the republic. "The

States of this Union have, for the most part, left the culture of medical science to individual enterprise," he stated explicitly, "which supplies solely that which the private citizen demands—practitioners of medicine to heal the sick." In the field of toxicology specifically, Chaillé conceded that real progress had been made in the last hundred years. Largely because of advances in forensic toxicology, "criminal poisoning has become . . . one of the most certainly detected, relatively infrequent, and least dreaded modes of death."[21] But the structure of "Anglo-Saxon law" inherited by the Americans after the Revolution continued a hundred years later to retard progress in other key areas. "The States have as yet made no demand for competent medical experts to aid the administration of justice, and have done nothing designedly for the culture of Medical Jurisprudence."[22]

In Chaillé's opinion, and no doubt in the opinion of most of the other unabashedly elite leaders of the AMA, the status of medical jurisprudence in the United States was deplorable. Most of the post-mortem examinations in the nation as a whole were wretchedly overseen by coroners who "owe their position wholly to political popularity, a qualification which a competent expert is most unlikely to possess," and conducted under laws that left to "accident" or "chance" the summoning of competent experts to assist the coroner. And the courts gave all sides in a dispute "full license to summon such medical witnesses as each has already found reason to believe entertain opinions the most contradictory." Indeed, Chaillé agreed with many others that "a good search and good pay can always find, in abundance, the witnesses needed on either side of any medico-legal issue."[23]

For Chaillé, and by implication for the AMA hierarchy he represented, the long-term antidote to this American illness was out-and-out "State Medicine." The old dream that every medical graduate would be competent in medico-legal situations was growing more and more patently absurd; special juries and expert commissions were unworkable for a host of ideological and structural reasons; and judicial appointments, as the French were beginning to acknowledge themselves, tended to be unreliable and uneven. Chaillé's public endorsement of state medicine represented a departure from Gross's 1868 AMA presidential plan, as Chaillé himself recognized in paying lip service to the ideals that lay behind his friend's earlier proposal. Nonetheless, in Chaillé's opinion, only a dramatic shift to the recently appreciated Prussian model, with its base of local medico-legal officers, its Medical Courts of Appeal, its Scientific Deputation of Final Arbitration, and its Ministry of Medical Affairs, might salvage the situation in the United States.[24]

Two observations are germane here. First, by no coincidence, many American medical professionals were beginning at this time to be attracted to German medicine generally; Chaillé was adding German medical jurisprudence to the attractions. While the great burst of French medical progress seemed to be flagging, the power of German science was building. The influence of German-born and German-trained physicians was palpable in New York City and elsewhere after the Civil War and a long period of

admiration and emulation in the United States for German university training, which would last through World War I, was just beginning.[25] This is
not to imply that Chaillé's latest suggestions about how to handle medical
jurisprudence in America were faddish, but they were certainly in keeping
with the larger professional trends of his day, as Beck's had been in his.

Second, there was much in Chaillé's tone that suggested grumbling,
petulance, and annoyance. While Beck in the 1820s had considered medical
jurisprudence an exciting field that might be made to blossom gloriously in
the American republic, Chaillé was more than mildly disgusted with the
actual developments of the last half century and was clearly espousing positions whose implementation he considered remote at best. "If the democratizing political principle, 'to the victors belong the spoils,' is to continue
its mastery over the virtue and intelligence of a great people," he complained in the context of ridding the nation of the coroner system, "then all
hope of efficiency in any system of State Medicine, as well as in every
public service which requires special skill and experience, must be abandoned." State medicine would come to the United States only after the
country passed "through stages of evolution." In the meantime, and for the
foreseeable future, medical jurisprudence in the United States would continue to be characterized by "the expediency . . . of mere make-shifts."[26]
In short, Chaillé and the leaders of the AMA, despite their rhetoric, no
longer considered the battle to upgrade medical jurisprudence a winnable
fight. They preferred instead to grouse about what ought to have been if
the American people had only trusted their professional experts. Against
that background, no wonder their organization ceased in the decades after
the centennial to place much emphasis on the subject, especially as the
AMA moved to win over the rank-and-file of the nation's practitioners rather
than float above them.

In 1879 the AMA merged its concerns once again to create the un-
wieldy Section on Medical Jurisprudence, Chemistry, Psychology, State
Medicine and Public Hygiene. The following year the section's title was
shortened simply to State Medicine.[27] When the AMA passed a grand revision of its Code of Ethics in 1884, medical jurisprudence received only
token acknowledgment. In the first section of Article I, for example, which
spelled out the "Duties of the profession to the public," physicians were
urged "As good citizens . . . to be ever vigilant for the welfare of the community . . . especially . . . on subjects of medical police, public hygiene,
and legal medicine." But the opening three words betrayed the attitude of
the drafters; physicians' responsibilities followed from their citizenship, not
their membership in the profession, and the drafters knew full well that no
mechanisms existed for the public vigilance they were exhorting. Section
Two of the same article stipulated that "Medical men should also be always
ready, when called on by the legally constituted authorities, to enlighten
coroners' inquests and courts of justice on subjects strictly medical—such
as involve questions relating to sanity, legitimacy, murder by poisons or
other violent means, and in regard to the various other subjects embraced

in the science of Medical Jurisprudence." But the next sentence insisted that "the public should award them a proper honorarium" if the public expected them actually to perform those duties.[28]

Henry F. Campbell of the Medical College of Georgia became president of the AMA in 1885. Thoroughly disgusted with the way doctors seemed to be suffering in legal situations, Campbell devoted his presidential address to "The Physician as Related to the Tribunals of Law." The speech berated American society for permitting physicians to be commandeered as witnesses, pummelled by lawyers, extorted as experts, and fleeced in malpractice actions. His tone was frankly defensive and elitist; given the situation, no wonder so many of the nation's most able and perceptive physicians were now avoiding the field of medical jurisprudence. But Campbell also recognized that part of the problem lay within the medical profession itself, which seemed to be taking the field less and less seriously. "[I]n the not distant past," he observed, "medical jurisprudence was, in some sort, comprehended in the scope of the regular sections of this association." Yet the traditional study of legal medicine was fast disappearing, both within the AMA and without. "In the organization and subsequent changes of the sections, medical jurisprudence seems at last to have disappeared as a fully recognized platform for our readings and discussions." And while he regretted that deeply, perhaps the time had come to face reality.[29]

To help the AMA address the profession's mounting legal problems, Campbell wanted the delegates to create a separate new section on forensic medicine specifically rather than try to revive the moribund section on medical jurisprudence writ large. This proposal acknowledged openly that medical jurisprudence in the broad sense was no longer a subject that the AMA was prepared to deal with, and the assumption behind the proposal revealed neatly the conceptual inversion that was taking place within the AMA on the subject. Campbell would salvage what he could of the old subject by creating a vehicle the AMA might use to alleviate some of the most pressing medico-legal problems that confronted regular practitioners in the professional marketplace, as distinguished from a vehicle the AMA might use to alleviate some of the most pressing medico-legal problems that confronted the republic. Campbell regarded the problems associated with what he emphatically labeled *"The Doctor in the Courts"* as the worst ones his fellow physicians faced in the United States, and he hoped the new section would take those up first.[30] The subsequent business meeting of the association, however, tabled a motion that would have implemented their president's suggestion, an action that probably indicated lingering uncertainties about the place, the role, and the character of medical jurisprudence within the AMA.[31]

In 1886, delegates to the AMA's annual convention again rejected Campbell's call for a separate section on forensic medicine, but amended the association by-laws to re-create the old section on Medical Jurisprudence writ large. Isaac N. Quimby of Jersey City headed the revived section.[32] Significantly enough, however, Quimby was uninformed about the long history of medical jurisprudence in the United States and did not even realize that the AMA itself had wrestled with the subject since its inception; "medical jurisprudence is but a new comer in the schools," he announced in the first line of his 1887 chairman's address, "and only one year ago received its first recognition as one of the legitimate subdivisions of the working scope of the American Medical Association." As his address made evident, Quimby had accepted the chair in order to complain in a national forum about four of his own pet peeves: the continued high incidence of abortion in America, despite the crusade of the AMA against it; the continued low quality of coroners; the fear that immigrants were shifting the burdens of disease and insanity from Europe to the United States; and the need to prohibit the consumption of alcohol.[33] Though his sectional colleagues agreed to look into the first two problems, the AMA Section on Medical Jurisprudence was plainly in the hands of someone who knew little about the subject, took a narrow view of what it was all about, and would be unlikely to accomplish much.[34]

The Section on Medical Jurisprudence received stronger leadership the following year, when E. Miller Reid assumed the chair.[35] A medical faculty veteran, he taught physiology and diseases of the nervous system at Baltimore University.[36] Reid had a far more profound sense than Quimby of what was really at stake in the AMA's shifting attitudes toward medical jurisprudence, for Reid rightly understood that a serious reconsideration of medical jurisprudence involved not only a wide variety of specific problems at different times and places but also the role and development of the professions in the United States generally. And he rightly identified the fundamental issue from the point of view of those interested in medical jurisprudence: the incentives of American marketplace professionalism.

> There is not at present sufficient incentive to induce the lawyer to investigate the philosophy or latent principles of the law; there is still less to spur him to inquire into that of medicine. Consequently he dips no deeper into the troubled waters of even his special branch of science than is necessary to enable him to fill his coffers. . . . [Similarly,] the busy practitioner of medicine has hitherto imagined he had no time to devote to any division of science which compelled him to go far beyond the pale of symptomatology and therapeutics, and which offered no direct emoluments to compensate him for the time and study that would be diverted from that which he has been inclined to consider the legitimate bounds of his profession.[37]

Given that reality, Reid endorsed a conclusion previously reached as well by the Philadelphia *Medical Register:* "It would best become the dignity of science and truth if legal-medicine were held as a definite and distinct profession, in which the emoluments were sufficient to justify a physician in abandoning all other practice in the interest of this special work."[38] In other words, law and medicine had evolved along tracks that left them no longer able to work together on anything approaching a socially significant scale. Most lawyers cared only for those medical specifics that might aid individual clients in particular cases; most physicians feared and resented court appearances and devoted the vast majority of their legal thoughts and discussions to ways of avoiding malpractice indictments in particular and the witness stand in general. Even if forced into court, physicians could contribute little, since lawyers wanted to use them or break them, not elicit information from them. "No Indian takes greater delight in the agony of his victim," according to Reid, "than the average lawyer takes in the suffering of the medical witness under the treacherous thrust of the cross-examination." Medico-legal discoveries in the United States went "unapplied"; medico-legal laboratories had virtually disappeared from the American scene; and "much useful information" was being "lost to the world."

Reid posed two courses of action. First, he called once again for medical experts "appointed by the State, at adequate salary, to serve" as needed. Surprisingly vague and unspecific, Reid presumably intended this as a ritual ratification of the movement then under way to replace coroners with medical examiners, though he apparently had little sense of how anticlimactic that movement really was. But his comments were brief, and he acknowledged, in a laconic understatement, that "this point has been urged before." More intriguing and revealing was the second proposition: medical jurisprudence in some form should be taught to ordinary citizens through the public schools. If the field had a future, it lay there.

A solid knowledge of medical jurisprudence imparted in the public schools would "do much to prevent crime," especially abortion. By teaching medical jurisprudence to boys and girls, "its doctrines would be carried home by them, and thus kept fresh in the minds of the people" as well. Moreover, "in teaching Medical Jurisprudence in our schools we will be instructing our future legislators in that branch of science and thereby preparing them better to understand the needs of the people, and to frame laws to meet them." Indeed, "if a knowledge of forensic medicine were generally diffused among the laity," Reid foresaw laws forthcoming on such matters as mental assault, to parallel the laws against physical assault that already existed; though such laws or others like them could never be passed under the circumstances that prevailed in 1887.

At one level, this suggestion was not as far-fetched as it might at first appear. Reid was calling for something not unlike the "hygiene" courses of the early twentieth century or the "health" classes of our own era. At another level, however, this suggestion demonstrated just how marginal the whole concept of medical jurisprudence had become to the AMA by the late 1880s. The chairman of the Section on Medical Jurisprudence, after all, was openly arguing that he considered the subject essentially dead as a professional field, and he was urging that its social benefits be salvaged by diffusing its lessons among the nation's schoolchildren and trying to build popular support for its chief contributions.

The Section on Medical Jurisprudence survived into the 1890s, but its national sessions confirmed the impression that Reid left. Almost all of the papers reported by the section through the end of the decade fell into either of two categories. The first group consisted of those that agonized over and complained about the hopeless and helpless situation of the physician as expert witness; the second explored ways to avoid becoming vulnerable to lawsuits.[39] Both types of papers epitomized the inverted and defensive concept of medical jurisprudence Campbell had propounded in his presidential address of 1885. The same concerns prevailed at the local and regional meetings of the AMA's constituent societies as well, even those specifically concerned with medico-legal issues. In March 1888 the Chicago Medico-Legal Society, for example, seriously discussed whether and how to edit their published proceedings, since they feared their internal disagreements and debates would become fodder for malpractice attorneys. *JAMA* considered the discussion worthy of report.[40]

Organized at mid-century to rally regulars, drive out irregulars, upgrade medical schools, and establish a secure place in American society for physicians, the AMA had essentially decided by default as it entered the twentieth century that medical jurisprudence of the sort Beck and his contemporaries once envisioned could no longer advance those agendas. Expert witnesses as often as not made professional knowledge look shaky rather than strong; time spent investigating legal problems tended to go uncompensated; the insanity issue had evoked a popular backlash rather than continued public support; and suits against shabby medical treatments, which might have helped drive quacks from the field, had instead ignited a continuing, even growing, firestorm of malpractice indictments against the regulars themselves. Whereas the leaders of the medical profession early in the century considered cooperation with the legal profession an important part of their mutual professional future, leaders of the medical profession later in the century concluded that medical jurisprudence did not, either metaphorically or practically, pay.

While there is no question that they continued to influence social legislation, especially as silent partners in the process of criminal code revision, and they continued to work for laws that helped advance the medical profession separately, leaders of the AMA by 1890 otherwise wanted as little to do with lawyers and legal processes as they could. Once viewed optimistically as an exciting way for physicians to serve society, medical jurisprudence had become a nearly extinct field within the AMA, pursued by a dwindling handful of medical professionals whose main goal was to protect their fellow physicians rather than the public. In this respect, however, the AMA merely reflected at the national level the activities of its rank-and-file members after mid-century as well as corresponding developments within the nation's medical schools, those institutions to which the AMA had paid such close attention since its founding.

CHAPTER SEVENTEEN

Medical Jurisprudence as a Dying Field in American Professional Schools

Unmistakable trends within American professional schools after 1860 registered the declining fortunes of medical jurisprudence as a professional field in the United States during the second half of the nineteenth century. Influential doctors had once believed that medical jurisprudence would become a central concern of American physicians, that physicians and lawyers would work closely together in the public interest, and that medical jurisprudence, the umbrella under which those developments would take place, was destined to become an increasingly prominent field. Many of the best of those early doctors taught the field themselves at some point in their careers, conducted research related to its various aspects, and insisted that formal training in the subject was essential to the molding of future doctors. Students reciprocated the conviction of their mentors and subscribed to the nation's courses in medical jurisprudence with enthusiasm and in substantial numbers. Extra-curricular lectures for physicians and attorneys already practicing in the community found paying auditors.

Following the decline of the field after mid-century, however, disillusionment and self-interest drove the subject of medical jurisprudence inexorably toward the margins of American professional training, especially in medical schools. By 1900, public-spirited medical jurisprudence of the sort Beck envisioned, cross-professional and broadly conceived, had all but disappeared; even its narrow and more practically applied subspecialties hung perilously on the far edges of medical school curricula and in a few law schools, usually taught by a changing cast of part-time instructors. The process both ratified and reinforced the fact that medical jurisprudence had ceased to be a central field in the United States.

From the end of the Civil War to the end of the nineteenth century, physicians commented often on the decline of medical jurisprudence in American professsional education. Stanford Chaillé's report to the American Medical Association on the status of medical jurisprudence at the time of the nation's centennial laid heavy stress on the fact that the number of

237

professorships of medical jurisprudence, courses in medical jurisprudence, and students of medical jurisprudence had all reached distressingly low levels. Drawing on data about forty-six leading American medical schools (which together were annually graduating more than 90 percent of the nation's M.D.s), Chaillé discovered that only twenty-five of them taught the subject at all. In most of those twenty-five, medical jurisprudence was " 'tacked on as a caudal appendage'" to some other course, and in five of them students were "taught to become *medical* experts by *lawyers.*" Nowhere was medical jurisprudence required for a degree. Chaillé explained those educational developments, as he had the fate of the entire field, in straightforward market terms:

> . . . the States through the[ir] citizens have failed to provide honorable and profitable employment for medico-legal experts, and therefore, the profession has not furnished them; and however enlightened the colleges, however praiseworthy their efforts, they will continue to contend in vain against the obstinate "demand and supply law" of political economy. . . . the colleges, dependent on the student and not on the State for their existence, will be forced by these practical students to realize continually the force of the homely adage, "you may take a horse to water, but you cannot force him to drink."[1]

While an occasional critic took the medical schools themselves to task for spending ever more money on extravagant buildings and "beautiful, delicate, wonderful" apparatus that was "too costly for use," while they spent less and less on the socially crucial subject of medical jurisprudence, most prominent observers agreed with Chaillé's analysis.[2] The president of the Ohio State Medical Society, for example, speaking for a special committee he headed himself in 1877, explained the decline of courses in medical jurisprudence in precisely the same market terms that Chaillé had used. "Supply follows demand," he stated in behalf of Ohio's regulars. "It is the duty of the State to furnish a demand for competent experts. This has not been done, and hence the reason why medical jurisprudence has been so much neglected in our medical schools."[3] From the Michigan State Medical Society came a similar opinion in 1879. There a committee investigating "Our Relations to Jurisprudence" rehearsed Chaillé's depressing numbers and accounted for them essentially as he had done: medical jurisprudence was a difficult subject in the first place "and the remuneration of experts is so small as to offer students little inducement."[4]

The decline that alarmed Chaillé and so many others during the last third of the nineteenth century was neatly illustrated by events at the University of Pennsylvania. That was, after all, the school where Revolutionary veteran Benjamin Rush made his plea for the importance of medical jurisprudence in the new republic, where Thomas Cooper and Charles Caldwell took up the field before carrying it south and west, where R.E. Griffith produced American editions of the most important English texts on the subject during the 1830s and 1840s, and where many of the editorial principals in the *American Journal of the Medical Sciences* had proselytized for medical jurisprudence and promulgated its exciting developments through mid-century. More significant still, the University of Pennsylvania had in its chair of medical jurisprudence in 1865 the nation's most famous expert in the subject, John James Reese. Following the Schoeppe and Wharton trials, where he emerged both times as the victorious professional lion, virtually every doctor and lawyer in the country would have recognized the name of J.J. Reese, and so would a substantial portion of the general public. Reese regularly added to his scholarly reputation with significant and widely read publications on important aspects of the field, especially those involving advances in toxicology.[5] In short, there would be every reason to suppose that medical jurisprudence would continue to thrive at the University of Pennsylvania after the Civil War, if it thrived anywhere.

On the surface, medical jurisprudence did seem to remain strong and sustained at the University of Pennsylvania after the Civil War. The medical department catalogues for the next twenty-five years proudly and continuously listed Professor Reese in a capacity that would now be styled clinical professor, and they advertised his course in medical jurisprudence annually without a break through 1890.[6] But beneath the surface the course was in trouble, primarily because few students were taking Reese's classes. Teaching income was still directly related to the number of students who purchased admission to particular courses separately, which prompted Reese to grow restive and frustrated. Offering classes for a small number of students was economically dysfunctional and personally embarrassing for a professional of Reese's steadily growing national fame.[7]

In the spring term of 1874 the University of Pennsylvania board of trustees proposed a possible solution. While continuing him in his medical department professorship, the trustees simultaneously appointed Reese to a chair in the university's law department as well.[8] Separate departments of law and separate law schools were emerging in universities in this era much as separate medical departments and separate medical schools had proliferated a generation earlier.[9] By drawing from both student populations, the trustees hoped Reese could bolster his enrollments; and by adding Reese's name to the law faculty, they hoped to give a boost to recruiting efforts in that rather vulnerable department. Reese himself was encouraged to hope that direct access to law students might allow him to establish a new professional base for the subject medical students seemed to abandoning.

From Reese's point of view, however, the results proved quickly disappointing. By the end of the 1874–75 academic year, Reese had so few students from the law school that he submitted a letter of resignation in which he explained the situation as he saw it and implicitly asked for support. "Although the chair of 'Medical Jurisprudence' is announced as *one* of the five chairs in the Faculty of Law," Reese protested to the trustees, "it is afterwards stated that attendance upon the Lectures of this Chair is not obligatory upon the students, and that an examination on the branch is not required for their graduation. The consequence," he continued, "is what might naturally be expected: -the students will *not* attend lectures that are not regarded as necessary to their graduation, and the Chair of 'Medical Jurisprudence' is virtually ignored."[10] In short, the field of medical jurisprudence was not going to be saved, even at the institution with the field's best-known star, by any voluntary outpouring of interest on the part of law students. Unless coerced, the latter were not about to embrace a traditionally medical subject that the medical students themselves no longer found attractive enough to study.

At their July 1875 session the trustees refused to accept Reese's resignation from the law faculty and cajoled him into staying by referring his problems to the university's committee on the law department.[11] But the situation failed to improve during the 1875–76 academic year, and Reese submitted yet another letter of resignation, probably to force a formal response from the committee. "My experience of my failure to make this department of science *practically* available to the Law Students of the University, under the present arrangements," he wrote curtly, "convinces me of the propriety of relieving both the Trustees and myself of the embarrassment of my present anomalous position."[12]

Again, however, the trustees refused to accept his resignation from the law faculty.[13] They still wanted Reese's famous name on both faculties for recruiting purposes whether he had many students or not. Indeed, in their private report to the trustees the members of the law committee were straightforward about their desire to keep using Reese's academic celebrity to maximum advantage. "The object of attaching him to the faculty of Law was that the students of Law or those proposing to matriculate might understand that they would have the privilege of taking his ticket and attending his courses of lectures delivered before his class in the [medical school]." But the law committee felt "it would not be advisable . . . to make attendance upon his course essential to a degree" in law. American legal scholars had never considered medical jurisprudence part of the core of their enterprise, and those legal scholars who were shaping the new law school curricula, and hence trying to shape the future of their profession, showed no inclination to appropriate the field now, even if it was available for the taking. If anything, law faculties were narrowing their focus after the Civil War and teaching the law in an ever more technical fashion.[14] The law committee did believe, no doubt sincerely, that it was "certainly to be lamented that so few of the Law students have thus have [sic] availed themselves of the benifit [sic] of his lectures, but it is to be hoped that this want of interest in a subject so interesting and important will not long endure." Still, the trustees would go no further than a formal resolution that all other law faculty "be instructed to urge upon their classes the importance of attending [Reese's] course."[15]

Medical jurisprudence limped along at the University of Pennsylvania for another eleven years in this anomalous fashion: the nation's most famous practitioner actually teaching a small number of medical students in the medical school, while maintaining a largely symbolic professorship in the

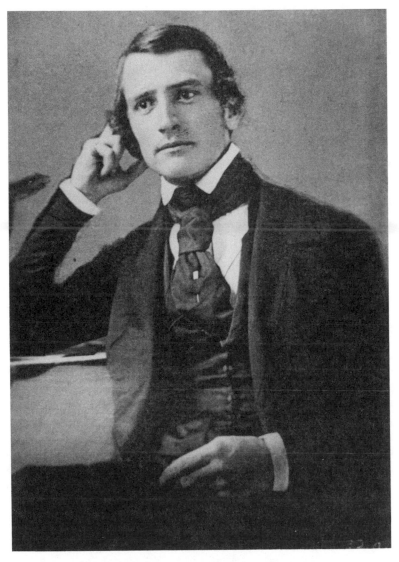

John J. Reese, the forensic toxicologist who gained national attention in the Schoeppe and Wharton trials and taught medical jurisprudence at the University of Pennsylvania. *(From the Sturgis Collection, College of Physicians of Philadelphia)*

law school, teaching few or no law students. Then in 1887 the University of Pennsylvania reorganized its law school. Student fees would henceforth be collected centrally by the administration and the faculty would be paid salaries regardless of class size. By no coincidence, the trustees that same year suddenly accepted Reese's long-standing resignation as a law professor.[16] Since Reese taught essentially no law students, the reorganized law school did not want to negotiate a salary for him, eloquent testimony indeed to the marginal attraction of Reese's field in the calculus of those who defined what lawyers should be required to know. Put differently, as long as Reese was free advertising for the law school, the lawyers had virtually forced him to remain at least on paper a chaired professor of law, thereby padding their catalogue; as soon as the law school would have to pay Reese a salary, however, both the professorship and the course on medical jurisprudence were promptly jettisoned.[17]

Although Reese continued to offer medical jurisprudence in the medical school, as he had been doing all along, through the 1890–91 academic year, he finally resigned his medical professorship as well before the beginning of the 1891–92 academic year.[18] He was then seventy-four years old and his health was failing. He would die the following year. Germane to the present discussion, however, was the fact that the University of Pennsylvania did not replace him. Medical jurisprudence was not offered again until 1893, when the dean of the medical school advertised a willingness to address the subject. By 1900, lectures in medical jurisprudence were listed as part of a pastiche of subjects presented after the fact, as it were, to fourth-year students whose real professional training was essentially complete.[19] But serious instruction in medical jurisprudence had essentially ceased at the University of Pennsylvania with the resignation of John James Reese in 1890, if not before.[20] Even had it survived, Reese's version of medical jurisprudence in the final decades of the nineteenth century had already become much more narrowly forensic in conception than the civic-minded approach advocated in the early decades of the century by his predecessor, Benjamin Rush.

Elsewhere around the nation's professional schools, medical jurisprudence often declined even more rapidly and more obviously than it did at the University of Pennsylvania. Across town at Jefferson Medical College, the subject disappeared during the 1890s.[21] Columbia abolished Ordronaux's chair when he retired in 1897.[22] Ira Harris, a former United States senator, had tried to revive medical jurisprudence at Albany Medical College after the Civil War, but the subject became a part-time course in the hands of part-time instructors when Albany went to a graded curriculum in 1890. When Albany reorganized into departments in 1914, medical jurisprudence vanished completely; the only faint echo of Beck's once towering presence was a promise by the new department of pathology to teach "certain phases of legal medicine."[23] In a similar fashion, the University of Missouri Medical School went to a laboratory-intensive four-year curriculum in 1899, which certainly positioned it to face the twentieth century near the forefront of professional training; but in the process, medical jurisprudence disappeared.[24]

At Yale, where medical jurisprudence had been a central concern of the faculty through mid-century, no one bothered to teach the subject during or immediately after the Civil War. Prospective doctors wanted as little interaction with legal processes as possible, and they were voting those sentiments with their feet. In 1868 the Connecticut Medical Society, responding to resolutions passed by the AMA in 1867, pressed the state's medical colleges to require three years of study for an M.D. degree, and in the second year of the recommended sequence was a course on "medical jurisprudence and medical ethics."[25] The Yale faculty demurred; forty years earlier they had been badly burned when they stiffened their degree requirements and other schools failed to follow suit. Yale did announce a tentative curricular reform for 1869, and the faculty reintroduced medical jurisprudence texts to their published list of student readings (Taylor was required; the Becks' *Elements* and Casper's *Forensic Medicine* were both recommended). But no new faculty members were retained to offer work in the field and no separate course on medical jurisprudence was actually scheduled by any of the existing faculty.[26]

A decade later, the Yale catalogue of 1880–81 revealed the way medical jurisprudence was being handled: "Several of the professors will give lectures on medical jurisprudence as it is related to their respective departments of instruction." In other words, some professors might allude to legal problems in passing, but the field of medical jurisprudence itself was not taught separately as an integrated way of examining the relationships between medicine and law. Moreover, medical jurisprudence was not listed among the subjects upon which students would be examined.[27] Only in 1885, with the AMA under President Campbell making its last serious effort to promote medical jurisprudence nation-wide, did Yale appoint William H. Brewer to lecture separately on the subject. Brewer was the sole Ph.D. on a faculty with twenty M.D.s, and the students were not examined on his course work.[28]

By 1890 Brewer was teaching public health, and a long-term part-time instructor from the Hartford Retreat, a private asylum, was offering lectures on insanity. Between them they uneasily shared what was left of medical jurisprudence. The catalogue told prospective students that "instruction in this subject is given by lectures and demonstrations," but no classes on medical jurisprudence appeared in the annual schedules. Moreover, in 1890 the faculty demoted medical jurisprudence to a subsection of pathology, as distinguished from being listed as a separate subject worthy of notice by itself.[29] By 1895 students would still be exposed to "reports of cases coming before the medical examiner and the coroner of New Haven County," and they would review "cases occurring in the courts," but they would have no independent work in the field.[30] In the final year of the nineteenth century, medical jurisprudence disappeared completely from the catalogue of the Yale Medical School, even as a subsection of pathology. Henceforth it would be dealt with under general medicine "from the standpoint of the medical practitioner," a phrase which inadvertently revealed the larger shift in medical perspective that had taken place: interaction with the nation's legal processes, once viewed as a civic opportunity, was now something the profession needed to be forewarned about.[31]

At Harvard Medical School, where Channing had been appointed pro-

fessor of obstetrics and medical jurisprudence in 1815, interest in legal medicine had also languished after the Civil War. In 1877, after the legislature
created medical examiners, Harvard separated medical jurisprudence from
obstetrics and organized a new offering in forensic medicine. F. W. Draper,
one of the principal leaders behind the medical examiner movement and
president of the Massachusetts Medico-Legal Society, the examiners' professional organization, was named an instructor to teach the new offering.
Draper's course, optional for the general medical students, was designed
primarily to train future examiners. Although Draper was promoted to assistant professor in 1884 and to professor in 1889, when he retired in 1903
"the vacancy was not filled."[32]

In 1907 Harvard finally asked George Burgess Magrath, medical examiner for the Northern District of Suffolk County, to serve as instructor
in legal medicine for those students who might be interested in becoming
examiners themselves. Though he served nominally in that capacity for the
next quarter-century, "Magrath's connection with the School was not strong
during most of his years, . . . and the course he taught was voluntary." In
1932 a private donor endowed a chair in legal medicine at Harvard Medical
School. Though some members of the medical faculty saw this as an opportunity to reconsider "the broad aspects of the subject," including such
questions as the relationship between health and crime, the donor insisted
upon emphasizing "the medicolegal investigation of death." The faculty acquiesced, and Harvard's professors of legal medicine continued to teach a
narrow version of forensic pathology well into the 1960s. As a special *ad
hoc* committee of the faculty openly recognized with real regret in 1968,
medical jurisprudence of the old sort had been moribund at Harvard Medical School for nearly a century.[33]

Additional examples abound. Starling Medical College, the Columbus,
Ohio, school where Judge Thurman had assessed the status of the medical
expert witness in 1857 and where Theodore G. Wormley, Reese's chief ally
in the witness stand during the Schoeppe trial, taught medical chemistry
and toxicology, abandoned medical jurisprudence after the Civil War first
to a relative of the college's founder, then to a parade of local judges. By
the end of the first decade of the twentieth century, Starling dropped the
course altogether.[34] The Medical College of Ohio in Cincinnati, which had
featured the subject during the 1850s, offered nothing in medical jurisprudence from the Civil War through 1885. Local judges lectured occasionally
thereafter until 1896, when the Medical College of Ohio merged with a
former rival to create the University of Cincinnati Medical School. In the
new institution medical jurisprudence was initially allotted one lecture per
week for one-third of a term in the fourth year of an otherwise greatly
expanded program, before being submerged, significantly enough, in "medical economics" in 1907.[35] A long line of local lawyers and judges also offered medical jurisprudence at Western Homoeopathic Medical College in
Cleveland in the decades following the Civil War, but their emphasis was
on how homoeopaths should handle legal challenges.[36] By the end of the

century Western's course on medical jurisprudence had been pushed back to the fourth year of a new four-year curriculum, where it was addressed by a Cleveland judge who took the students on field trips to his probate court and to the morgue.[37] Clearly, the subject lost its centrality at Western Homoeopathic as surely as it did in the regular medical colleges.

In the same years that president Henry F. Campbell tried unsuccessfully to revive the AMA's interest in medico-legal issues, his own school back home in Augusta, Georgia, was reflecting almost perfectly the national patterns he decried. The Medical College of Georgia had been founded in 1829 by the venerable Lewis Ford, who had a powerful personal interest in medical jurisprudence and taught the subject himself for half a century. But medical jurisprudence fell precipitously at MCG following Ford's retirement in 1881. The son of an influential faculty member was initially given the course to carry forward, but he failed to do much with it. He was followed in rapid succession by the son of another faculty member, then by the nephew of a third, neither of whom proved effectual. The field that seemed to obsess Campbell at the national level was moribund at his own college by 1890. The institutional biographer of MCG characterized the 1880s as an era when the school placed a heavy "emphasis on profit." The lesson was clear: medical jurisprudence no longer paid, either in cash or in professional advancement.[38]

The Johns Hopkins Medical School at Baltimore, self-consciously established as a model for medical education in the twentieth century and hailed in 1910 in the famous Flexner Report as the sort of medical school to which all the others should aspire, offered a final confirmation of the overall pattern. Hopkins Medical School was planned and developed from 1867, when its founding trust was set up, through 1893, when the first class of regular medical students began full-time study; or in other words, exactly during the era when medical jurisprudence began to fall from grace. And the Hopkins story reflects both the concern of medical leaders about the disappearance of medical jurisprudence and the ultimate power of the national trends.[39]

John Shaw Billings, one of the country's leading medical administrators, served as chief consultant to the board of trustees that built the Hopkins Medical School. A sanitarian and a U.S. Surgeon General, Billings was personally and professionally committed to the importance of medical jurisprudence. In a series of lectures that began in the fall of 1877, Billings outlined his vision of medical education at Hopkins. In addition to its most famous aspects, including a strong commitment to scientific research and hospital training, that vision included specific endorsement of "the study of 'state medicine' with reference to registration of physicians, statistics, public hygiene, sewerage, ventilation of public buildings and schools; for the study of medical jurisprudence, with special reference to expert testimony in courts of law on insanity and other subjects, and a special course for the education of medical officers of the army and navy."[40]

While research on some of those and related subjects went on at Hopkins, the medical school itself actually opened without serious instruction in medical jurisprudence. Physicians who regretted the decline of medical jurisprudence were disappointed that "an institution so richly endowed and officered by such distinguished gentlemen" had failed to do "justice to medico-legal science. . . . Johns Hopkins University has lost a great opportunity."[41] William Welch, one of those distinguished gentlemen and a guiding director of the Hopkins experiment, was in fact an unusually public-spirited physician who maintained a lively interest in problems that once fell under the umbrella of medical jurisprudence; but the Hopkins medical students he and his colleagues taught were rigorously and almost exclusively trained in the scientific care of individual patients, while Welch pressed another twenty years for a separate and distinct school of hygiene and public health. He finally succeeded in establishing such a school after World War I, but its very existence as a separate institution paradoxically institutionalized the nearly complete excision by then of medical jurisprudential concerns from the regular training of mainstream physicians.[42] As an almost comic after-thought, the medical school itself eventually brought Judge Eugene O'Dunne, "one of the more colorful members of the Supreme Bench of Baltimore City," to lecture the fourth-year students on medical jurisprudence four to six times a year from 1926 to 1946. O'Dunne was succeeded by Judge Emory H. Niles of the same bench, who continued the series until his own retirement in 1968.[43] Between them they constituted medical jurisprudence through the first two-thirds of the twentieth century at America's model medical school.

While the trends were unmistakable and easy to document in school after school throughout the United States,[44] exactly what to make of them is rather more difficult and raises a number of subtle problems. First, even though courses in medical jurisprudence disappeared, many of the specific skills and pieces of information once taught in those courses were still being offered elsewhere in the curriculum or in other ways. There is little doubt, to take an obvious example, that a larger percentage of American medical students was at least theoretically able to perform effective chemical analyses in 1895 than had been the case in 1835; if called upon to do so, these students could presumably put those skills to civic and forensic purposes. And many of the component parts of what once constituted medical jurisprudence were being covered by the end of the century in courses that did not formerly exist as separate units of inquiry: insanity, in classes now labeled neurology or psychiatry, for example; or a smattering of public health, in classes now labeled hygiene or sanitary science. A number of medical schools were offering separate electives on the medical aspects of life insurance, thereby suggesting that at least one part of nineteenth-century medical jurisprudence had proved eminently practical and profitable for ordinary practitioners.[45] And during the early years of the twentieth century a handful of schools even experimented briefly with designated professorships and formal classes in "state medicine."

Second, many of the problems that Beck's generation hoped to solve had, in fact, been solved and no longer required continued professional attention. Improved microscopy, for example, led to advances in blood typing and the analysis of wounds. Physiologists finally understood the basic mechanisms of human conception by the end of the nineteenth century, and the length of normal gestation no longer remained a subject of serious dispute. The bacteriological revolution, which was also finally taking hold in the United States by the end of the nineteenth century, rendered straightforward many determinations of death that might once have been debated. Advances in organic chemistry were revolutionizing the subject of toxicology.

In light of the foregoing, it would be tempting to argue that the disappearance of medical jurisprudence from American medical schools might be easily, even positively, explained as a consequence of the combined effects of two well-known processes: specialization, which divided the component parts of a no longer manageable whole into separate units capable of more intense examination; and scientific progress, which rendered moot many of the questions that puzzled previous investigators. Without doubt, both factors played a role in the process outlined in this chapter, and there is no reason to gainsay or minimize their roles. But much more was involved, for the disappearance of medical jurisprudence from American professional schools did not occur in a vacuum.

The larger context in which these professional school changes took place must be borne in mind. That context, as previous chapters have made clear, included at minimum a growing alienation between doctors and lawyers (which had been evident from mid-century onward), a crisis of the medical expert witness (which had peaked in the 1870s), futile efforts by the AMA to revive medical jurisprudence (which had produced a jeremiad to the subject in 1876 and finally ceased altogether in the 1880s), the structural demotion of professional medical examiners (which had devalued and subordinated traditional jurisprudential skills and activities), and the insignificance of medico-legal societies (which indicated a lack of professional interest and commitment). While specialization and progress played a role, the demise of medical jurisprudence ultimately mirrored profound shifts in the fundamental ethos of American professionals.

The republican, holistic, civic-minded, and intellectually integrated professional ideals of the early national period had disappeared in the face of social and professional realities by the end of the nineteenth century. Doctors and lawyers constituted two sharply differentiated professional categories. Both had developed separate schools of training and fixed mechanisms of professional access; few professionals any longer passed back and forth between the demarcated spheres of the two; no third group arose to bridge the chasm between them. Aspiring physicians were no longer exposed in their course work even to the possibility of practicing in a community of interactive professionals, much less were they trained to be able to do so. The vast majority of American doctors ministered almost exclusively to individual paying patients and seldom to the public as a whole.

The public as a whole, after all, and with good reason, had proved quite profoundly skeptical of officially sanctioned professionals and had failed since the great watershed era of the 1830s to afford them the support of the state.

The professionals themselves responded accordingly and largely abandoned their integrative ideals after mid-century. Public interaction with the law became a nightmare for most physicians during that period, rather than a source of professional elevation and pride. Medical jurisprudence, once a central subject both in the actual training and in the intellectual socialization of American physicians, was dead or dying in every medical school in the United States by 1900. As the contemporary analyst Thomas Hall Shastid correctly observed in a widely read essay first published in 1912, the teaching of medical jurisprudence in American medical schools "progressed in a retrograde direction" during the second half of the nineteenth century.[46] And even where the subject survived in name, it was a different undertaking with different purposes from the courses both offered and envisioned sixty years before.

A final irony stands out. Courses in medical jurisprudence had arisen at a time when American medical schools were extremely sensitive to student demand. Had no students wanted to take those courses, those courses would not have survived even as long as they did. At least implicitly, students anticipated that medico-legal interactions would comprise a significant component of their professional future and they wanted to know about the field.

From mid-century on, however, students saw practicing physicians increasingly battered by medico-legal interactions, most of which seemed to backfire on their profession. Forensic investigations went uncompensated; testimony in court made doctors look unprofessional and gave charlatans a chance to persuade the community they were right; insanity shifted from an area in which physicians were humane heroes to one in which they were imprisoning the innocent and making excuses for the guilty; and so forth. Under such circumstances, students no longer welcomed the notion that medical jurisprudence would play a significant role in their professional lives, and they concentrated their studies elsewhere. Since American medical schools remained quite sensitive to student demand, courses in medical jurisprudence declined in the fashion documented in this chapter. Indeed, something of a reciprocal process was probably under way during the second half of the nineteenth century in American medical schools, which produced a vicious cycle of disaffection: fewer students found the field potentially attractive and fewer first-rate professors were taking it up.

The irony comes at the end of the period discussed in this chapter. As William Rothstein, Kenneth Ludmerer, and others have demonstrated, American medical schools began finally to gain control of their own curricula toward the end of the nineteenth century.[47] Medical schools became gateways through which aspiring physicians had to pass, rather than optional training centers that offered students what they thought they needed or might someday want. By the first decade of the twentieth century, medical schools could actually begin to impose requirements and make them stick. But medical jurisprudence was not one of the requirements they imposed, for the shift that empowered medical schools was rooted firmly in the ethos of marketplace professionalism, controlled and ultimately licensed by separate professional organizations. Doctors would henceforth train to serve the specific medical needs of individual paying patients and stay away from the law, except insofar as they needed to know how to defend themselves against its incursions. To put it differently, the very processes that might have enabled those who shaped the American medical profession at the beginning of the twentieth century to reintroduce the republican, civic, and integrative aspects of medical jurisprudence to the training of future professionals instead sealed the sorry fate of the field. For all intents and purposes medical jurisprudence had ceased to exist.

Afterword

Looking back from the last decade of the twentieth century at the history of medical jurisprudence in the United States during the nineteenth century, several overarching observations come into focus. Together they help link those nineteenth-century developments to our own times. First, medical jurisprudence, though hardly discernible as a field today, figured prominently in early American medical history and in the evolution of the current configuration of the American professions; neither subject can be fully understood in its modern context without taking the history of legal medicine into account. Particularly during the first half of the nineteenth century, physicians interested in the law and in legal processes affected medical education, advanced an ideal of republican professionalization, and stimulated genuinely scientific investigations at a time when most of American medicine remained diffuse, provincial, and archaic in its theories and superficially observational in its inquiries. Medical jurisprudence was also the first field in which an American physician gained international recognition.

Second, even though their ideals proved unworkable, physicians interested in medico-legal issues had a profound impact upon the socio-cultural history of the nation as a whole; what they did in the nineteenth century still directly affects the lives of American citizens in the late twentieth century. Through court testimony, professional writing, and public involvement, they helped shift both popular attitudes and specific legal positions on a number of key subjects. And by the 1820s they had already established what became enduring and characteristic patterns of shaping official policies in an effective, if seldom analyzed, fashion. Much more research needs to be done on the history of state codes, omnibus crime acts, and related subjects in the nineteenth century; on the activities of medical and health committees in state legislatures in the nineteenth and twentieth centuries; and on the decision-making processes of executive and administrative medical agencies in the twentieth-century (the lineal descendants of nineteenth-century code revision and health committees). But the material in this study makes abundantly clear the fact that medico-legal perspectives have played a significant role in the formation of America's basic social rules. Physicians had a great deal of influence over what Americans decided to proscribe as criminal behavior and encourage as civic benefit; in short, they influenced significantly during the nineteenth century the fundamental infrastructures that still shape American social behavior in the late twentieth century.

Third, the shift in national ethos from revolutionary republicanism to liberal democracy, which so many historians have chronicled in so many ways, is no mere academic curiosity. The shift, which seems to have engulfed the national consciousness like a great wave about 1830, had real consequences for the evolution of American society. Prominent among those consequences was the impact it had upon the history of the professions in America, particularly medicine and law, which had to accommodate themselves to the triumph of marketplace professionalism by mid-century. Nascent assumptions about the place and role of the medical profession in the legal processes of the early republic were undercut and redirected after 1830, altering profoundly the collective behavior of what would eventually become one of the most powerful and influential groups in American society. The nation's present medico-legal system is the product of that nineteenth-century accommodation, which involved the subsequent working out of a series of relationships involving the public, the state, and the professions.

Fourth, a long perspective makes clear the fact that the medical profession and the state have continuously maintained a deeply ambiguous relationship over medico-legal matters in the United States. On the one hand, the influence of physicians on public policy has been substantial; on the other, the state has consistently refused to put medico-legal decision-making directly into the hands of the profession. And this eminently nineteenth-century pattern has persisted through the twentieth century, even though the medical profession is now a licensed entity of the state. More than a century of pressing for some modified version of Continental-style medical jurisprudence in the United States finally came to naught by the end of the nineteenth century. Physicians thereafter largely abandoned their collective efforts to persuade the state to create a system of official medico-legal experts, and instead adjusted their professional responses to the circumstances that actually prevailed, and to the ways in which those circumstances had been changing during the nineteenth century.

Fifth, after decades of trying to persuade the state that medico-legal officers would be a great benefit to society, the medical profession, consolidating itself around the concept of individual practice, finally helped engineer the politico-professional compromise that created medical examiners. From the outset, however, medical examiners were viewed as a sort of desultory second-best, essentially powerless functionaries rather than influential professional agents. In the eyes of most physicians, the chief attraction of medical examiners lay in the promise of ending the old system of political coroners impressing medical expertise. This is not meant to disparage modern medical examiners as individual professionals; they continue to perform essential services for American society at extremely modest rates of pay by the standards of the medical profession as a whole. Sometimes they gain moments of fame in sensational situations, and on the prime-time television show "Quincy" during the 1980s, they even enjoyed a heroic image. More often, they serve the public interest in silent and sometimes thankless ways, and they are afforded minimal status in the larger medical profession.

Massachusetts medical examiners, as if to emphasize the foregoing, felt compelled to spend their centennial year, 1977, symbolically enough, organizing yet another "coalition of medical, law-enforcement and legal" groups to press the state legislature for improvement of their status, conditions, and pay. Their efforts and their arguments closely resembled the efforts and the arguments of their predecessors a hundred years before. But the act of 1978 that resulted from their efforts, as they themselves recognized, did almost nothing to improve their circumstances.[1] All across the United States modern medical examiners remain officers for the most part quite different from the proactive medico-legal facilitators of public justice and public well-being once envisioned by medical leaders like Rush, Beck, and Gross. Nor did the spread of medical examiners eliminate by any means all of the problems traditionally associated with political coroners.[2]

Sixth, the role of the expert medical witness, which most Americans now take for granted in a medico-legal context, evolved during the nineteenth century in an awkward series of fits and starts. During the 1830s and 1840s, physicians who were originally committed to republican assumptions about professional service came face to face with the practical problems of adversarial justice and marketplace professionalism in an era when the basic concept of the expert medical witness was still being refined. Those who considered themselves most knowledgeable and potentially most helpful found themselves without special standing in courts and without special compensation, and they made no headway in adapting aspects of the French system of court-appointed medical investigators to American circumstances. The nineteenth-century evolution of the expert witness also made plain some of the inherent ambiguities in the fundamental concept of expertise itself, forced physicians to face the reasons why the public did not trust them to administer justice, and underlined boldly the often distressing and sometimes ironical interrelationships in the United States between expertise, on the one hand, and power (often in the form of cash), on the other.

Following a prolonged period of frustration and agitation, physicians after the Civil War eventually reached a modus vivendi with the professional, political, and legal realities they actually faced as witnesses in American courtrooms. With medical examiners taking much of the burden of uncompensated public testimony off the vast majority of physicians, would-be medical witnesses in private actions could weigh for themselves the rising financial benefits of testifying as an expert, on the one hand, against the diminishing professional risks of doing public battle, on the other hand, while most physicians steadily and successfully consolidated their collective position in American society in other ways.[3] Once a license, as distinguished from a personal reputation, all but guaranteed a successful professional practice for most physicians in the twentieth century, the process of offering expert testimony began to look considerably less forbidding than it had in the nineteenth century.

By 1984, even the editor of the *Journal of the American Medical Association* acknowledged forthrightly that the AMA's official policy, that "the physician should not allow himself [sic] to become an advocate or a partisan" in legal cases, had become a farce. Commenting on the "burgeoning medical expert consultant and witness business," George Lundberg correctly and courageously observed that the "money available for such consultation, and possible subsequent appearance as a witness, is often 'whatever the market will bear.' And if the client is a large industry or insurance company in civil litigation or a wealthy defendant in criminal action, the market may bear very great fees indeed."[4] In short, many of the most unsettling aspects of nineteenth-century advocacy persisted, while the checks and balances that might formerly have restrained the participants, however imperfectly, all but disappeared. Indeed, would-be medical experts now advertise vigorously in legal journals, thereby quite openly selling medico-legal expertise to the highest bidder. That system, which Americans are having a hard time dealing with in the late twentieth century, is one of the most expensive and legally awkward legacies of nineteenth-century medical jurisprudence.

Seventh, the modern problems associated with the insanity defense, which hardly existed in a significant sense when the republic was established during the 1780s, had assumed by the 1880s the basic outlines they still present to American society in the 1990s. Early in the nineteenth century physicians interested in medical jurisprudence had found in mental aberration a subject that allowed them to enhance their civic and humanistic roles in American society and to augment their legal authority. By the 1880s, however, insanity had become a medico-legal nightmare, and it has largely remained one since. When John Hinckley, Jr., stood trial for the shooting of President Ronald Reagan in 1982, he was found not guilty by reason of insanity and remanded to a mental hospital, where theoretically he might have been declared well the next day and released. The verdict evoked furor throughout the nation as the Attorney General of the United States, the Secretary of the Treasury, and several key members of Congress called for changes in the law of insanity. The *New York Times* and many other papers urged the separate state legislatures to experiment with new verdicts and new rules.[5]

The AMA Committee on Medicolegal Problems recognized that the insanity plea was producing "public cynicism" and discrediting the profession. Following the Hinckley uproar, the committee drafted a special report on the subject that concluded with a series of recommendations, the first of which declared bluntly that "the special defense of insanity should be abolished. . . ."[6] The AMA's House of Delegates debated the report in terms that might have been lifted almost verbatim from discussions of the New York Medico-Legal Society a hundred years before. Despite pleas for moderation from the presidents of the American Bar Association and the American Psychiatric Association, the AMA's House of Delegates voted in 1983 to accept their committee's report, thereby officially disassociating mainstream physicians from the implications of what their predecessors had brought about.[7]

In 1988 the highly respected journal *Science* published a key article, later more widely disseminated and discussed by the electronic media and the popular press, that may bring the debate over legal insanity full circle. On strong evidence, the article demonstrated that "professionals often fail to reach reliable or valid conclusions and that the accuracy of their judgments does not necessarily surpass that of laypersons" in matters related to insanity.[8] The logic of the situation would return the jurisprudence of insanity, at least in a rough sense, to the circumstances Rush and Beck confronted at the outset of the nineteenth century. Whether modern theorists of medical jurisprudence would, like them, consider that an opportunity, however, remains an open question.

Eighth, though the subject of malpractice now dominates most discussions of medical jurisprudence, medical malpractice hardly existed in American law through the first quarter of the nineteenth century. Then, quite suddenly, in the second quarter it assumed essentially its present form, and has continued to grow as a professional concern ever since. Intraprofessional and interprofessional efforts for the next century and a quarter failed to check its most counter-productive aspects.[9] By the mid-1970s, as jury awards in malpractice cases rose dramatically, both the public and professional press expressed grave concern about what was characterized as a nationwide malpractice crisis.[10] Physicians began to abandon the most vulnerable specialties, to practice defensive medicine, and to reconsider their so-called "good Samaritan" obligations to help strangers. Insurance companies claimed to be caught in the middle; the *New York Times* accused lawyers of "legalized larceny"; and several state legislatures agonized without much result over ways to balance public protection, professional regulation, medical quality, ordinary justice, and fiscal reality.[11] Though Americans have continued to debate medical malpractice fervently ever since, they have seldom viewed it as the product of specific nineteenth-century historical circumstances or placed it in the larger context of evolving relations between American physicians and the nation's legal processes; one aspect, albeit a highly visible aspect, of the history of medical jurisprudence in the United States.

Ninth, some of the reasonably standard assumptions about the processes of professionalization in the United States need to be reassessed in light of the history of medical jurisprudence. Most theories of professionalization have been derived implicitly or explicitly from the study of successful professional groups; analysts have tried to generalize about how those groups achieved professional status. Yet the subject of medical jurisprudence offers a challenging counter-example. Medical jurisprudence, after all, fulfilled most of the customary criteria for professional advancement: an educational base, a literature, a group of influential and unusually able champions, and by the 1860s, formal professional societies. Moreover, medical jurisprudence already functioned as a long-established and reasonably independent field in Europe. Yet, despite every reason to assume in theory that a new profession might arise, none did. Indeed, the specialty of medical jurisprudence that already existed in the first half of the nineteenth century steadily withered during the second half of the nineteenth century and has all but disappeared in the twentieth century.

The foregoing helps underscore a tenth observation that emerges from the overall history of medical jurisprudence in the nineteenth century: there is great analytical value and much insight to be gained from recognizing the deceptively elemental fact that professions do not exist in a vacuum. American physicians certainly had their own agendas and took independent action at many points in American history, not just in the area of medical jurisprudence but in many other areas as well; and the internal history of the medical profession as an independent entity certainly needs continued scrutiny. But the medical profession, like all other professions, also influenced the larger society in which it developed and was, in turn, influenced by. Without some historical knowledge of the way marketplace professionalism offered medico-legalists counter-incentives rather than inducements after the middle decades of the nineteenth century, for example, it would be difficult to understand why medical jurisprudence failed to continue to flourish within the American medical profession. Without some appreciation of the bedrock anti-power bias and altogether-merited skepticism of the American public toward medical experts during the nineteenth century, it would be difficult to understand why twentieth-century Americans inherited a gulf between medicine and law with no profession to bridge it. Especially in the United States, where the professions have played such significant historical roles in the absence of legally privileged classes, those influences and interrelationships are crucial not only to the history of the professions themselves but more importantly to an understanding of larger American history itself.

As the twentieth century draws to a close and Americans consider which aspects of their society seem to have developed satisfactorily and which are in need of serious restructuring in the century ahead, few Americans seem much enamored of the way the medical profession currently interacts with the nation's legal processes. The role of physicians in the making of public policy continues to be at once disquietingly powerful and strangely unsystematic. Physicians serving as expert witnesses in court all too often battle one another to expensive stalemates; costly to the parties involved, to the time and trouble of the courts, and to the cause of justice. Exactly what those stalemates achieve is frequently unclear. Almost everyone, especially physicians themselves, will readily express some degree of frustration with the way actions for medical malpractice now operate. The social costs associated with that nineteenth-century system have become enormous in the late twentieth century. And however they might behave personally, as individual citizens, when modern physicians act collectively, as a professional group, they seem all too often to lack what might be called a civic sensitivity.

As this book has tried to demonstrate, those current disaffections are for the most part products of the nineteenth-century history of medical jurisprudence: the legacy of professional developments that took place in an era when the essential socio-professional outlines of American life were being shaped. Those developments and their consequences were not accidents, but responses in context to specific historical situations, and anyone who understands those situations will not be surprised by the circumstances that now confront the country. This book has attempted to tell the story of those developments and to explain who was involved, when the key developments took place, why public policies and professional responses evolved as they did, and how shifting circumstances affected interactions between the medical profession, on the one hand, and the legal processes of the republic, on the other. In doing so, it has attempted to provide background, context, perspective, and understanding for future discussion. The time may be at hand either to reaffirm those nineteenth-century developments and consider how to continue paying for them, literally and metaphorically, or to adjust them in the context of twenty-first-century circumstances.

Abbreviations
Used in Notes

AJMPS   *American Journal of the Medical and Physical Sciences*

AJMS   *American Journal of the Medical Sciences*

ALJ   *Albany Law Journal*

BHM   *Bulletin of the History of Medicine*

BMSJ   *Boston Medical and Surgical Journal*

DAB   *Dictionary of American Biography*, Allen Johnson and Dumas Malone, eds. (New York, 1930)

DAMB   *Dictionary of American Medical Biography*, Martin Kaufman et al., eds. (Westport, Conn., 1984)

DNB   *Dictionary of National Biography*, Leslie Stephen and Sidney Lee, eds. (London, 1917)

JAMA   *Journal of the American Medical Association*

JHU   Johns Hopkins University

JWFP   John W. Francis Papers, Manuscripts Division, New York State Library, Albany

LC   Library of Congress, Washington, D.C.

NCAB   *National Cyclopaedia of American Biography* (New York, 1898–1984)

NLM   National Library of Medicine, Bethesda, Maryland

NYAM   New York Academy of Medicine, New York, New York

NYMPJ   *New-York Medical and Physical Journal*

NYPL   New York Public Library, New York, New York

PJMPS   *Philadelphia Journal of the Medical and Physical Sciences*

TAMA   *Transactions of the American Medical Association*

TC   Toner Collection, Rare Books Room, Library of Congress, Washington, D.C.

TMMLS   *Transactions of the Massachusetts Medico-Legal Society*

UP   University of Pennsylvania

Notes

CHAPTER ONE

1. For a brief overview of the old British system, see A. Keith Mant, "Milestones in the Development of the British Medicolegal System," *Medicine, Science, and the Law,* 17, no. 3 (1977): 155–63, which also contains a useful list of references on the subject. Many historians of American medicine have commented upon the provincial and uneducated qualities of colonial physicians. One of the best summary statements of this sort is Whitfield J. Bell, Jr., "Medical Practice in Colonial America," *BIIM* 31 (1957): 442–53.

2. The best short overview of early Continental developments is Erwin H. Ackerknecht, "Early History of Legal Medicine," *CIBA Symposia* 2, no. 7 (Winter 1950–51): 1286–89. For the early spread of "medicalized law" from Italy westward around the Mediterranean to Spain, I am indebted to Michael McVaugh, "Medical Testimony in Medieval Trials," seminar presentation, Institute for the History of Medicine, April 18, 1991, JHU.

3. Duncan's papers are full of orders for books and correspondence of various sorts with German medical centers. See Letters and Papers of Andrew Duncan, Junior, M.D., Special Collections, University of Edinburgh Library.

4. Alvin R. Riggs, "The Colonial American Medical Student at Edinburgh," *University of Edinburgh Journal* 20 (1961): 141–50.

5. See "Observations on Medical Jurisprudence delivered in Lectures in the University of Edinburgh, by Andrew Duncan [Sr.], M.D. & P. Taken by David Pollock," 2 vols. (1797–98); and "Notes on Medical Jurisprudence by Andrew Duncan [Senior], M.D., Edinburgh, 1800, taken from lectures by J. Lee." The quotation is from Pollock, 1: 106. Both sets of student notes are in Special Collections, University of Edinburgh Library

6. Henry Harvey Littlejohn, "Department of Forensic Medicine, University of Edinburgh," *Methods and Problems of Medical Education* (9th series, New York, 1928), 187–91; Theodric Romeyn Beck and John B. Beck, *Elements of Medical Jurisprudence* (11th ed., Philadelphia, 1860), vol. 1: xx-xxi. The lives and careers of both Duncans are sketched in *DNB* 6: 161–63.

7. *Philadelphia Medical Museum,* 5 (1808) [74–82].

8. *DNB* 6: 829.

9. The word "police" was used in this fashion on both sides of the Atlantic at the end of the eighteenth century and through the first decades of the nineteenth century. When Thomas Jefferson established a legal professorship at William and Mary in 1779, he had styled its first incumbent, George Wythe, Professor of Law and Police. By "police" he meant, roughly, public administration.

10. Elijah Griffiths, M.D., "An Essay on the Means necessary to be employed for correcting and rendering wholesome the Atmosphere of Large Cities," *Philadelphia Medical Museum* 5 (1808): 49–54; the announcement about lectures in New York, *ibid.*, 152.

11. *William Hunter and the Eighteenth-Century Medical World*, W. F. Bynum and Roy Porter, eds. (Cambridge, UK, 1985); C. H. Brock, ed., *William Hunter, 1718–1783: A Memoir by Samuel Foart Simmons and John Hunter* (Glasgow, 1983), 62–63.

12. Rush is certainly the best-known physician of the Revolutionary period and his career is well documented in several books, including Nathan G. Goodman, *Benjamin Rush, Physician and Citizen, 1746–1813* (Philadelphia, 1934); and David Freeman Hawke, *Benjamin Rush: Revolutionary Gadfly* (Indianapolis, 1971).

13. Benjamin Rush to James Rush, June 8, 1810, in *Letters of Benjamin Rush*, L.H. Butterfield, ed., vol. 2 (Princeton, N.J., 1951), 1051.

14. Benjamin Rush to James Rush, Oct. 4, 1810, *ibid.*, 1069.

15. These sentiments were remembered by Robert Eglesfeld Griffith and quoted by him in, "On Medical Jurisprudence," *PJMPS* 10 (1825): 46.

16. Rush, "Introductory Lecture," in Benjamin Rush, *Sixteen Introductory Lectures, to Courses of Lectures upon the Institutes and Practice of Medicine, with a Syllabus of the Latter* (Philadelphia, 1811), 363–95.

17. Griffith, "On Medical Jurisprudence," 46.

18. Benjamin Rush to Thomas Jefferson, Jan. 2, 1811, in Butterfield, ed., *Letters*, 1074.

19. William G. Rothstein, *American Medical Schools and the Practice of Medicine: A History* (New York, 1987), 56–61.

20. Charles Caldwell, *Autobiography of Charles Caldwell, M.D.* (originally published 1855; rpt. with new introduction by Lloyd G. Stevenson, New York, 1968), 330–31.

21. See, for example, Charles Caldwell, *Outlines of a Course of Lectures on the Institutes of Medicine* (Lexington, Ky., 1823), 3, 188.

22. Dumas Malone, *The Public Life of Thomas Cooper, 1783–1839* (Columbia, S.C., 1961).

23. Thomas Cooper, *Tracts on Medical Jurisprudence* (Philadelphia, 1819).

24. *Ibid.*, esp. 87–109, 418–30.

25. There is a convenient summary of Cooper's career in *DAB* 6: 414–16, which was done by Malone; and another in *Who Was Who in America: Historical Volume* (Chicago, 1963), 121.

26. Cooper, *Tracts*, 449.

27. Cooper had previously presented some of his toxicological research to the American Philosophical Society. See *ibid.*, 49, 52, 431–45.

28. *Ibid.*, 455, and Malone, *Thomas Cooper*, 311–47. Samuel Haber, *The Quest for Authority and Honor in the American Professions, 1750–1900* (Chicago, 1991), 3–87, lays heavy stess upon this point. Though Haber's *Quest* appeared too late to be integrated into this study, his analyses of professional ideology and the analyses offered in this book, while clearly different, nonetheless mesh well at several points.

29. Cooper, *Tracts*, 89, 96, 97, 100, 109, 224–26, 243–47; quotes: 96, 243.

30. James Thacher, *American Medical Biography: Or Memoirs of Eminent Physicians Who Have Flourished in America*, vol. 2 (Boston, 1828; rpt. New York, 1967), 104–6; and T[homas] H[all] S[hastid], "James S. Stringham," in Howard A. Kelly, ed., *A Cyclopedia of American Medical Biography*, vol. 2 (Philadelphia, 1912), 423. The latter contains some inaccuracies. An announcement of Stringham's appointment as professor of chemistry at Columbia appears in *Medical Repository* [New York] 6 (1803): 236.

31. John W. Francis to James Thacher (n.d., but *c.* mid-1820s), rpt. in part in Thacher, *Medical Biography*, 105–6.

32. *Ibid.*, 105.

33. See, for example, the Columbia announcement in *Philadelphia Medical Museum* 5 (1808) [152].

34. On these battles over medical education in New York City see Joseph F. Kett, *The Formation of the American Medical Profession: The Role of Institutions, 1780–1860* (New Haven, 1968), esp. 35–40; and David Hosack to James S. Stringham, May 4, 1811, printed as "Observations on the Establishment of the College of Physicians and Surgeons in the City of New York and the late Proceedings of the Regents of the University, Relative to That Institution," in Rare Book Room, NYAM.

35. On Samuel Latham Mitchill, see *DAMB* 2: 531.

36. Erwin Ackerknecht, *Medicine at the Paris Hospital, 1794–1848* (Baltimore, 1967).

37. The best surviving student notebook is that of George B. McKnight, in TC. McKnight took Stringham's course twice, a practice then common in medical schools, once in 1814–15 and again in 1815–16. Thus his notes are a thorough record: the basic course as given the first time through and corrections as necessary the second. Stringham's syllabus was published in the *American Medical and Philosophical Register* 4 (1814): 614–15.

38. *Ibid.*

39. Stringham's contributions to the prominent *Medical Repository*, which was run by colleagues in New York City, were typical. In 6 (1803): 325–26, Stringham published under the title "Violent Effects of Oxygenated Muriate of Mercury" what amounted to an exposé of a false method of curing gonorrhea. In 8 (1805): 38–42, he published a perfunctorily descriptive account of a case involving an enlarged head. While both of these subjects were sometimes dealt with in medical jurisprudence, under the headings of poisons and birth defects respectively, these essays can hardly be considered the rich fruits of a professorship in the subject.

40. Thacher, *Medical Biography*, 105; Shastid, "Stringham," 423; Theodric Romeyn Beck, *Elements of Medical Jurisprudence* (1st ed., Albany, 1823), xxxi.

CHAPTER TWO

1. On the founding of the college at Fairfield see William Frederick Norwood, *Medical Education in the United States Before the Civil War* (Philadelphia, 1944), 150.

2. Most of the biographical material that follows has been drawn from Frank H. Hamilton, *Eulogy on the Life and Character of Theodric Romeyn Beck* (Albany, 1856), 87 pps. This pamphlet, published by order of the New York State Senate, remains the standard chronicle of Beck's life, though it is not, of course, a scholarly study. Hamilton was a student, friend, and successor to Beck at the Albany Medical College, and did not consult Beck's private papers in preparing his oration. Where

Hamilton's material is supplemented with information drawn from other sources, the other sources will be noted separately. There is a crying need for a scholarly biography of T.R. Beck, or perhaps a group study of Beck and his brothers, all of whom also went on to become influential professionals in the period when the American professions were just beginning to take their modern forms.

3. For supporting statements about the family tradition of education, see Catherine E. Van Cortlandt (Beck's daughter), "Theodric Romeyn Beck," in Albany Medical Society, *Annals, 1806–1851* (Albany, 1864), 258; and Van Cortlandt, "Lewis C. Beck," (a biographical pamphlet in TC) 12.

4. Theodric Romeyn Beck, *Elements of Medical Jurisprudence* (1st ed., Albany 1823), xxxi.

5. Van Cortlandt, "Theodric Romeyn Beck," 268.

6. Theodric Romeyn Beck, *An Inaugural Dissertation on Insanity* (New York, 1811); quotes: 27–28. This dissertation has also been reprinted in Gerald N. Grob, advisory ed., *The Beginnings of American Psychiatric Thought and Practice: Five Accounts, 1811–1830* (New York, 1973).

7. The most valuable source of information on Beck's early years in Albany is a series of letters he wrote to John W. Francis, who remained in New York City after the two graduated from the College of Physicians and Surgeons. Francis saved these letters and they are in Folder 8, JWFP. The quote here is from TRB to JWF, n.d., but almost certainly, on the basis of internal evidence, sometime in the spring of 1812.

8. TRB to JWF, Oct. 22, 1811, JWFP.

9. On Beck's intense nationalism see Van Cortlandt, "Theodric Romeyn Beck," 269.

10. TRB to JWF, Oct. 1812, JWFP

11. TRB to JWF, Feb. 10, 1813, JWFP.

12. TRB to JWF, Oct. 29, 1813. On Zacchia's great work, see Jaroslav Nemec, *Highlights in Medicolegal Relations* (Washington, D.C., 1976), 44.

13. TRB to JWF, May 19 and Oct. 29, 1813, JWFP.

14. TRB to JWF, May 19, 1813, JWFP.

15. TRB to JWF, Feb. 15, 1815, JWFP.

16. William G. Rothstein, *American Medical Schools and the Practice of Medicine: A History* (New York, 1987) and Kenneth M. Ludmerer, *Learning to Heal: The Development of American Medical Education* (New York, 1985) are the two most important recent surveys of the subject. Though they approach the subject from different perspectives, both support the generalizations advanced in this paragraph.

17. The allusion to Romeyn's lectures is contained in Stephen W. Williams, *A Catechism of Medical Jurisprudence; Being Principally a Compendium of the Opinions of the Best Writers Upon the Subject . . . Designed for Physicians, Attorneys, Coroners and Jurymen* (Northampton, Mass., 1835), 30–31, who misspells the name Romayne.

18. Quoted in Hamilton, *Eulogy*, 13.

19. TRB to JWF, n.d., but late 1815 or early 1816, JWFP.

20. The quotes are from TRB to JWF, Feb. 15, 1815, JWFP.

21. TRB to JWF, n.d., but late 1815 or early 1816, JWFP.

22. TRB to JWF, n.d., but probably 1813, JWFP.

23. TRB to JWF, n.d., but late 1815 or early 1816, JWFP.

24. Nathan Reingold, ed., *The Papers of Joseph Henry*, vol. 1 (Washington, D.C., 1972), xxi-xxii, 107, 114; and Reingold, ed., *Science in Nineteenth-Century America: A Documentary History* (London, 1966), 63–64, 71.

25. Beck's connections with such local organizations as the Society for the Promotion of Agriculture, Arts and Manufactures; the Society for the Promotion of Useful Arts; the Albany Lyceum of Natural History; and the Albany Institute are evident in two excellent studies: Michele A. L. Aldrich, "New York Natural History Survey, 1836–1845" (Ph.D. dissertation, University of Texas, 1974); and James M. Hobbins, "Shaping a Provincial Learned Society: The Early History of the Albany Institute," in Alexandra Oleson and Sanborn Brown, eds., *The Pursuit of Knowledge in the Early American Republic: American Scientific and Learned Societies from Colonial Times to the Civil War* (Baltimore, 1976), 117–50. Beck's correspondence also makes clear that he was attempting during this period to use some of his considerable influence in the capital city to push for passage of bills that would aid the state's medical community. See, for example, E. T. Foote to TRB, Feb. 23, 1820, and Stephen Van Rensselaer to TRB, Dec. 16, 1821, both in the Beck Manuscripts, NYPL.

26. TRB to JWF, n.d., but probably 1818, JWFP.

27. Beck Manuscripts, NYPL.

28. New York State, Assembly, *Journal . . . Session of 1818* (Albany, 1818), 25.

29. Beck, *Elements* (1st. ed.), 41–42.

30. *Ibid.*, 86–99; quote: 99.

31. John B. Beck became one of New York City's best known and most influential physicians. For a nearly contemporary vignette of his life and career written by a colleague on the faculty of the College of Physicians and Surgeons, see C[handler] R. Gilman, *Sketch of the Life and Character of John Brodhead Beck, M.D., Late Professor of Materia Medica and Medical Jurisprudence in the College of Physicians and Surgeons, New-York* (New York, 1851), in the bound pamphlet collection, Rare Book Room, NYAM; and Samuel D. Gross, ed., *Lives of Eminent American Physicians and Surgeons of the Nineteenth Century* (Philadelphia, 1861), 605–13.

32. For a discussion of the way in which John Beck's work helped influence American abortion policy, see James C. Mohr, *Abortion in America: The Origins and Evolution of National Policy, 1800–1900* (New York, 1978), 35 and *passim*.

33. John Beck was considered an outstanding teacher, whose personal popularity helped carry the College of Physicians and Surgeons through its great political battles of the late 1820s. Gilman, *John Beck*, 6–7. The Rare Book Room of the NYAM holds two student notebooks from John Beck's classes in medical jurisprudence: [John Clarkson Jay] "Medical Jurisprudence by Dr. [John B.] Beck" (Nov. 27, 1829 and thereafter); and [Benjamin S. Downing] "Lectures on the Materia Medica and Medical Jurisprudence Delivered at the College of Physicians and Surgeons at the University of the State of New-York by John B. Beck, M. D., Professor &," Vol. 2 (n.d.).

34. Theodric Romeyn Beck and John B. Beck, *Elements of Medical Jurisprudence* (5th ed., Albany, 1835). In this version of the book, Chapter Eight, "Infanticide," had already grown to 177 pages; it would eventually get longer. In truth, however, the gesture of making John a co-author appears to be more the affectionate response of an older brother than a reflection of shared duties. There is no evidence that John had a real hand in anything except the infanticide chapter. Because John was such a prominent medical professor in the nation's leading city, his name on the book might also have helped sales and marketing.

35. Natalie Z. Davis, *The Return of Martin Guerre* (Cambridge, Mass., 1983). The story was also made into a commercially successful film with the same title.

36. Beck, *Elements* (1st ed.), 335.

37. Burcard. Dav. Mauchartus, *De Inspectione et Sectione Legali* (Tübingen, 1736); Jno. Ern. Hebenstreit, *Anthropologia Forensis* (Leipsic, 1751); Gottleib Ludwig, *Institutiones Medicinae Forensis Praelectionibus Academicis accommodatae* (Leipsic, 1765); and Joan. Christ. Traugott Schlegel, *Collectio Opusculorum Selectorum ad Medicinam forensem spectantium* (Leipsic, 1785–91) were all cited by Beck in the *Elements*.

38. Beck, *Elements* (1st ed.), vol. 2, 10; italics in original.

39. *Ibid.*

40. *Ibid.*, 20.

41. *Ibid.*, 122.

42. On the pervasive influence of French science in Beck's own Hudson Valley, see Aldrich, "New York Natural History Survey," 21, 29, 47–55, 101–2, 104–13. On Orfila, see Hoefer, ed., *Nouvelle Biographie Général*, vol. 37 (Paris, 1863), cols. 779–83. For more on Orfila and the influence of the French, see Chapter Four.

43. Orfila, *Traité des poisons tires des règnes minéral, végétal et animal, ou toxicologie générale* (Paris, 1813–15).

44. J. G. Nancrede, *A General System of Toxicology* (Philadelphia, 1817); R. H. Black, *Directions for the Treatment of Persons Who Have Taken Poison and Those in a State of Apparent Death* (Baltimore, 1819). A third translation appeared in 1826: J.G. Stevens, *Poisons* (Boston, 1826). These translations are cited in S.K. Niyogi, "Historic Development of Forensic Toxicology in America up to 1978," *American Journal of Forensic Medicine and Pathology* 1 (1980): 249–64.

45. Orfila, *Élemens de chimie appliquée a la médecine et aux arts* (Paris, 1817).

46. Beck, *Elements* (1st ed.), vol. 2: 216–17. The debate hinged not upon Cooper's results but upon whether his test was reliable for arsenic specifically or for a larger class of substances with similar properties.

47. *PJMPS* 8 (1824): 152–57.

48. R.E. Griffith, "On Medical Jurisprudence," *ibid.* (1825): 46.

49. *NYMPJ* 3 (1824): 95–112.

50. This statement is based upon a survey of the collection of early medical school catalogues in the NLM and in the Sterling Library at Yale University. Catalogues generally listed required texts along with course descriptions.

51. This observation is based upon several years of reading nineteenth-century medico-legally related court cases. While that reading does not constitute anything like a systematic sample, the impression is unmistakable that the *Elements* assumed a paramount position in American courtrooms almost from the date of its publication, and held that place until after the Civil War. In many courts it was still being cited as a leading authority into the 1890s.

52. James Kent to TRB, Sept. 29, 1823, Beck Papers, NYPL.

53. This is not to suggest that the *Edinburgh Medical and Surgical Journal* was a journal exclusively of medical jurisprudence, for it certainly was not. But of the British journals that paid attention to medical jurisprudence, the *EMSJ* was the most important.

54. *Edinburgh Medical and Surgical Journal*, July 1824.

55. Andrew Duncan, Jr., to TRB, July 22, 1822, Beck Papers, NYPL. This letter is almost certainly misdated. The year should be 1824; Duncan probably repeated the 22 of the date.

56. George Edward Male, *Epitome of Juridical or Forensic Medicine for the Use of Medical Men, Coroners, and Barristers* (London, 1816) and *Elements of Juridical or Forensic Medicine: For the Use of Medical Men, Coroners, and Barristers* (London, 1818). Male had submitted his dissertation at Edinburgh in 1802.

57. Reprinted in Beck, *Elements* (2nd ed., London, 1825), xvii.

58. Rutter, M.D., to TRB, Dec. 13, 1825, Beck Papers, NYPL.

59. Thomas Weatherill, M.D., to TRB, Feb. 17, 1826, Beck Papers, NYPL.

60. See "Preface" to Alfred S. Taylor, *Treatise on Medical Jurisprudence* (American ed., Philadelphia, 1873); rpt. in *ALJ* 10 (1874): 62–63.

61. Beck, *Elements* (3rd ed., London, 1829).

62. Theodor Romeyn Beck, Professor an dem Collegium des Westlichen Districts des Staates New York. *Elemente der gerichtlichen Medicin. Nach der zweiten von Dr. Dunlop, Mitgliede des Konigl. Collegiums der Wondarzte zu London, mit noten and zusartren versehenen Ausgabe aus dem Englischen ubersetzt* (Weimar, 1827), 2 vols.; see also the congratulatory announcement of the translation in *NYMPJ* n.s. 1 (April 1829): 215.

63. Theodric Romeyn Beck and John B. Beck, *Elements of Medical Jurisprudence* (5th ed., Albany, 1835).

64. Beck and Beck, *Elements* (7th ed., London, 1842). The inscription was partly an acknowledgment of Christison's substantial contributions to forensic toxicology, which the Becks had incorporated into their book, and partly a not-so-subtle merchandising tactic. For this edition, the Becks contracted directly with a consortium of book distributors in London and Edinburgh to sell the book in Great Britain, thereby becoming principals in the marketing process. They probably thought the inscription would help in that process.

65. Beck and Beck, *Elements* (10th ed., Albany, 1850).

66. On the Becks' deaths, see Van Cortlandt, "Theodric Romeyn Beck," 266–68; and Hamilton, "Eulogy," 58–59. Both brothers, appropriately enough, had autopsies performed on their remains.

67. Beck and Beck, *Elements* (11th ed., Philadelphia, 1860).

68. Beck and Beck, *Elements* (12th ed., Philadelphia, 1863).

CHAPTER THREE

1. Charles Caldwell, *Autobiography of Charles Caldwell, M.D.* (originally published 1855; reprint with new introduction by Lloyd Stevenson, New York, 1968), 330–31.

2. Charles Caldwell, *Outline of a Course of Lectures on the Institutes of Medicine*, (Lexington, Ky., 1823), 3, 188.

3. Dumas Malone, *The Public Life of Thomas Cooper, 1783–1839* (Columbia, S.C., 1960), 251–253.

4. *Statutes at Large of South Carolina* (5 vols., Columbia, 1836–39).

5. George B. McKnight, "Notes of Lectures on Legal Medicine," entry for Dec. 2, 1815, TC.

6. *DAMB* 2: 549; and Chester R. Burns, "Medical Ethics and Jurisprudence," in Ronald L. Numbers, ed., *The Education of American Physicians: Historical Essays* (Berkeley, 1980), 274.

7. *DAMB* 1: 129; Henry K. Beecher and Mark D. Altschule, *Medicine at Harvard: The First Three Hundred Years* (Hanover, N.H., 1977), 53–54; Burns, "Medical Ethics and Jurisprudence," 274; Amalie M. Kass, "Establishing a Career in Obstetrics: The Case Book of Walter Channing," paper presented at the annual convention of the American Association for the History of Medicine, Cleveland, May 1991.

8. William Frederick Norwood, *Medical Education in the United States Before the Civil War* (Philadelphia, 1944), 211–13. The student notebooks are in the manuscript collection, NLM. Direct quotations from them will be cited separately.

9. Eaton was a solid scholar who would eventually establish a strong scientific reputation. Like the Beck brothers, Eaton was close to DeWitt Clinton and to the Van Rensselaer family. He joined the faculty at Rensselaer Polytechnic Institute in the mid-1820s and remained there until his death in 1842. Eaton wrote manuals on botany and conducted for the State of New York a geologic survey of the route of the Erie Canal. For more on Eaton see *NCAB* 5: 312–13; and *DAB* 3: 605–6.

10. Notebook from the September term of 1822, "Medical Jurisprudence" as taught by John P. Batchelder, in Berkshire Collection, NLM. On Batchelder himself, see *NCAB* 9: 351.

11. *DAMB* 2: 809; *NCAB* 1: 182–83. Williams was active in his local medical society, a publisher of articles, and apparently anxious to gain an academic appointment. He would eventually become a pioneer in medical biography and medical history.

12. Stephen W. Williams, *A Catechism of Medical Jurisprudence; Being Principally a Compendium of the Opinions of the Best Writers Upon the Subject . . . Designed for Physicians, Attorneys, Coroners and Jurymen* (Northampton, Mass., 1835), 5.

13. *Ibid.*, 3–6.

14. Notes from Williams's first term have not surfaced, but a complete set taken from his second time through the course, which was in the autumn of 1824, are in the NLM collection noted earlier.

15. For a critical review of Williams's published work on medical jurisprudence see R.E.G[riffith], review of *A Catechism of Medical Jurisprudence*, in *AJMS* 16 (1835): 159–62.

16. "Lectures on Medical Jurisprudence" by Stephen W. Williams, M.D., October term, 1824, NLM collection.

17. Joseph Kett, *The Formation of the American Medical Profession: The Role of Institutions, 1780–1860* (New Haven, 1968), 85–88, documents the ways in which these posts figured in the medical school rivalries of the period.

18. *DAB* 8: 99–100; *A Catalogue of the Officers and Students of the Cincinnati College in its Medical, Law and Academical Departments, for 1836–7* (Cincinnati, 1836), NLM. Samuel Gross was professor of anatomy and physiology at Cincinnati at this same time, and he reported that Rogers was an excellent lecturer.

19. *DAMB* 1: 219; Robley Dunglison, *Syllabus of the Lectures on Medical Jurisprudence and on the Treatment of Poisoning & Suspended Animation, delivered in the University of Virginia* (printed by Clement P. M'Kennic for the University of Virginia, n.p., 1827); Norwood, *Medical Education*, 89.

20. R.E.Griffith, "On Medical Jurisprudence," *PJMPS* 10 (1825): 36–46; Norwood, *Medical Education*, 231–32.

21. *University of Maryland Medical School Catalogue* (1840–41 through 1846–47).

22. On Ford personally, see *DAMB* 1: 259–60. On Ford's activities at the Medical College of Georgia, see Phinizy Spalding, *The History of the Medical College of Georgia* (Athens, Ga., 1987), 14–17, 28, 32.

23. Norwood, *Medical Education*, 396.

24. Chester R. Burns, "Medical Ethics and Jurisprudence," in Ronald L. Numbers, ed., *The Education of American Physicians: Historical Essays* (Berkeley, 1980), 277–278.

25. *Ibid.*, 277, identifies some of the lawyers who taught medical jurisprudence in American medical schools during the first half of the nineteenth century.

26. On Armsby, see *DAMB* 1: 18; on March, *ibid.* 2: 495.

27. *A Catalogue of Students Attending Docts. March & Armsby's Lectures on Anatomy, Physiology and Surgery, in Albany, Jan., 1836* (Albany, 1836) in the Surgeon General's collection, NLM.

28. *Historical Sketch of the Albany Medical College* (Albany, 1876) [revised and separately published version of a piece with the same title that appeared in 1867 in *Munsell's Historical Collections of Albany*], Surgeon General's Collection, NLM.

29. See the sketch in *Union College Magazine* 11, no. 2 (March, 1873): 148–60, in Surgeon General's Collection, NLM. The first board included Daniel D. Barnard (later U.S. Minister to Berlin), Ira Harris (later U.S. Senator), John Pruyn (a leading legislative leader and later Minister to Japan), Bradford R. Wood (later Minister to Denmark), plus members of the Ten Eyck, Groesbeck, and Van Rensselaer families. The appropriations were granted in 1841.

30. *Catalogue and Circular of the Albany Medical College* (Albany, 1839), in Surgeon General's Collection, NLM.

31. As was so often the case during this era, the founding of the Albany Medical College was inextricably bound up with professional politics. In this case the founders were willing to be accommodating to Albany's Thomsonian practitioners and Beck probably boycotted the college for this reason; Beck was a fierce defender of "regular" medicine against competing theories and sects, such as the Thomsonians. For more on these battles, see the standard histories of medical education already cited and the *AJMS* 24 (1839): 523, 528; and 25 (1839–40): 258–59. The Albany Medical College later issued a statement that allowed regulars in the area to support it.

32. See the Albany Medical College *Catalogue* for 1839, 1840, 1842, 1847, 1850, 1853, 1859, and 1889. The catalogues list professors, required books, and course fees. The last catalogue of 1889 contains a useful "Historical List of Faculty, 1839–1889."

33. Robley Dunglison, *Syllabus of the Lectures on Medical Jurisprudence and on the Treatment of Poisoning & Suspended Animation, delivered in the University of Virginia* (Charlottesville, 1827). Dunglison's *Syllabus* was not a mere outline, as the title might suggest, but a substantial volume of over 140 pages.

34. The Smith book was John Gordon Smith, *The Principles of Forensic Medicine, Systematically Arranged, and Applied to British Practice* (2nd ed., London, 1824).

35. Dunglison, *Syllabus*, 22.

36. *Ibid.*, 142.

37. Henry Howard, *A Synopsis of Medical Jurisprudence, from the Latest and Best Authorities, Forming the Basis of Lectures on the Science . . . in the University of Virginia* (Charlottesville, 1851); material on insurance, 86–87.

38. Williams, *Catechism*.

39. See the review in *AJMS* 16 (1835): 159–62. Griffith was extremely critical of the Williams book.

40. The Yale Americana Collection contains a copy of the 1840 imprint; I have seen no other reference to it. The better known version, discussed in this section, is Amos Dean, *Principles of Medical Jurisprudence: Designed for the Professions of Law and Medicine* (Albany and New York, 1850).

41. Dean, *Principles*, vi.

42. The original book was Michael Ryan, *A Manual of Medical Jurisprudence, compiled from the best medical and legal Works, comprising an account, 1st, Of the Ethics of the Medical Profession; 2d, The Charters and Statutes relating to the Faculty; 3d, All Medico-legal Questions, with the latest decisions: being an Analysis of a course of Lectures on Forensic*

Medicine, annually delivered in London (London, 1831), 309 pps.. Griffith's review appeared in *PJMPS* 9 (1831–32): 146–49, and boosted medical jurisprudence generally as well as the Ryan book specifically. The American edition was Philadelphia, 1832, noticed in *ibid.* 10 (1832): 271.

43. See, for example, R.E. Griffith's review in *AJMS* 15 (1834–35): 468–70. Chitty approached the subject from the legal side.

44. Reviews of these books appeared in *AJMS* n.s. 3 (1842): 187–89; n.s. 9 (1845): 431–35; n.s. 10 (1845): 524. In reviewing the American edition of Trail, the *BMJS* 24, no. 26 (Aug. 4, 1841): 430, could not resist a patriotic plug for the *Elements*. The editor found "nothing particularly novel or striking in [Trail], to give it claims to precedence, or even abiding place, by the side of our countrymen, the Drs. Beck."

45. Francis Wharton and Moreton Stillé, *A Treatise on Medical Jurisprudence* (Philadelphia, 1855).

46. On Wharton see Janet A. Tighe, "Francis Wharton and the Nineteenth-Century Insanity Defense: The Origins of a Reform Tradition," *American Journal of Legal History* 27, no. 3 (July 1983): 223–53.

47. See Thomas Hall Shastid, *A History of Medical Jurisprudence in America* (bound pamphlet in NYAM Library, 1912), lxxix; reprint from Howard A. Kelly, *A Cyclopedia of American Medical Biography*, Vol. 1 (Philadelphia, 1912), lxxv–lxxxv; a glowing review by E[dward] H[artshorne], himself a prominent writer and editor on medical jurisprudential subjects, in *AJMS* n.s. 31 (1856): 169–73; and the enthusiastic review of the book in *Medical Examiner of Philadelphia* (1855): 728–43.

48. E[dward] H[artshorne], review of Wharton and Stillé in *AJMS* n.s. 31 (1856): 170.

49. The fifth edition appeared in 1905.

50. Patricia German, "Medical Textbooks in American Medical Schools, 1860–1900" (M.A. thesis, Department of History, University of Maryland Baltimore County, 1991).

51. These dates are, of course, arbitrary and suggestive, not definitive. This entire discussion is based upon wide reading in the history of the professions generally as distinguished from a single source or set of sources, but essential to the present context are Burton J. Bledstein, *The Culture of Professionalism: The Middle Class and the Development of Higher Education in America* (New York, 1976); Thomas Bender, *Community and Social Change in America* (New Brunswick, 1978), and Bender, "Science and the Culture of American Communities," *History of Education Quarterly* (Spring 1976): 63–77; Thomas Haskell, *The Emergence of Professional Social Science: The American Social Science Association and the Nineteenth-Century Crisis of Authority* (1977); and Haskell, ed., *The Authority of Experts: Studies in History and Theory* (Bloomington, 1984).

52. On these subjects generally, the books to start with would include Norwood, *Medical Education*; William G. Rothstein, *American Physicians in the Nineteenth Century: From Sects to Science* (Baltimore, 1972); and *American Medical Schools and the Practice of Medicine: A History* (New York, 1987); Kenneth M. Ludmerer *Learning to Heal: The Development of American Medical Education* (New York, 1985); Numbers, ed., *Education of American Physicians*; and Paul Starr, *The Social Transformation of American Medicine: The Rise of a Sovereign Profession and the Making of a Vast Industry* (New York, 1982).

53. While most historians of American medical education would agree with the basic argument advanced here, the most forceful discussion of nineteenth-century

medical schools as demand-driven institutions (in a fundamentally positive sense) is in Rothstein, *Medical Schools*.

54. Dean, *Principles*, v.

55. "Rush Medical College and the National Medical Association," *BMSJ* 38 (March 1, 1848): 107.

56. Norwood, *Medical Education*, 397, observed: "Medical jurisprudence was added to most any chair, but was more often combined with chemistry or obstetrics and diseases of women and children because of the legal aspects of practice in such a field." Ultimately, however, Norwood considered the combinations "curious" and the result of unique circumstances rather than rational planning. The link to chemistry and materia medica, however, seems clear: those were the areas where the most interesting medico-legal work was being done during the first half of the nineteenth century. The link to obstetrics has traditionally been explained as a function of the importance of procreative matters in aristocratic societies. According to the historians of Harvard Medical School, the link to obstetrics and diseases of women was also a result of early French theories about psychiatry. Those theories postulated a relationship between the female reproductive processes and psychotic behavior. The frankly sexual understanding of evil in the early republic may also have played a role. See Beecher and Altschule, *Medicine at Harvard*, 53–54. Whatever its origins, the link to obstetrics remained common through the first half of the century. See, for example, T.D. Mitchell, "Lecture on Medical Jurisprudence," *Western Lancet* 5 (1846): 275–86. For Hall's chair see University of Maryland catalogue for 1840–41; for Rogers's see the Cincinnati catalogue for 1836–37; for Leonard's chair at Washington see *BMSJ* 35 (1846): 166; for Smith's chair at Willoughby, *ibid.* (Oct. 20, 1847): 247; for Bullit's chair at St. Louis, *ibid.* 39 (1848): 346; for Dalton's chair at Buffalo, *ibid.* 366.

57. Kett, *American Medical Profession*, 86–87.

58. Samuel D. Gross, *Autobiography of Samuel D. Gross, M.D.* (Philadelphia, 1893), vol. 1: 37.

59. Stephen J. Kunitz, "The Historical Roots and Ideological Functions of Disease Concepts in Three Primary Care Specialties," *BHM* 57 (Fall 1983): 412–32, argues that different medical specialties tend to attract self-selected subsets of physicians at least in part for ideological and socio-political reasons rather than strictly for scientific reasons or reasons of inherent interest. Specifically, he believes that "the degree to which a field is seen as a vehicle for social change" will determine "the liberalism or conservatism of its recruits" in the modern era (p. 412). Though it is not possible to apply Kunitz's methods directly to the historical record, it seems safe to assume that similar forces acted upon physicians in the past. If so, the suggestion here is that medical jurisprudence seemed to be attracting a disproportionate share of those members of the profession most attuned to civic service, public responsibility, and upgraded professionalism.

CHAPTER FOUR

1. See *NYMPJ* 1, no. 1 (1822) for editorial announcements and *ibid.* n.s. 1 (1829): vii–xiv, for a discussion of the transition to new management. The journal ceased publication after 1830.

2. T.R. Beck, "A Sketch of the Legislative provision of the Colony and State of New-York, respecting the Practice of Physic and Surgery," *NYMPJ* 1 (1822): 139–51.

3. *Ibid.*, 441–63.

4. *Ibid.*, 513–14, 515.

5. T.R. Beck, "Contributions in Medical Jurisprudence, No. I: Of Insurance Upon Lives," *NYMPJ* 5 (1826): 26–43; quote, 28.

6. T.R. Beck, "Contributions in Medical Jurisprudence and Police, No. II: Results taken or deduced from the Census of the State of New-York for the Year 1825, as communicated by the Secretary of State to the Legislature, Feb. 4, 1826," *ibid.*, 205–8.

7. T.R. Beck, "Contribution in Medical Jurisprudence and Police, No. III: Trials for Murder," *ibid.*, 427–41; quote: 441; parentheses in original.

8. A Correspondent [T.R. Beck], "Contributions in Medical Jurisprudence and Police, No. IV: Duration of Human Pregnancy," *ibid.* 6 (1827): 224–42.

9. T.R. Beck, "Contributions in Medical Jurisprudence and Police, No. V," *ibid.* 7 (1828): 492–518.

10. The piece on medical evidence is T.R. Beck, "Annual Address delivered before the Medical Society of the State of New-York, Feb. 6, 1828," *ibid.*, 9–34; the piece on asylums is "An Account of some of the Lunatic Asylums in the United States," *ibid.*, 186–206; and "Supplement to the Account of some of the Lunatic Asylums of the United States," *ibid.*, 251–54.

11. Alexander H. Stevens to T.R. Beck, in *ibid.* 5 (1826): 314; Charles A. Lee, "Case of Poisoning by Laudanum, in which the Stomach Pump was successfully used," *ibid.* 7 (1828): 518–20.

12. *Ibid.* 1 (1822): 237–39; *ibid.* 6 (1827): 142–43; *ibid.* n.s. 2 (1830): 449–52.

13. Lewis Caleb Beck, born in 1798, studied medicine, law, geology, and mineralogy; served variously as professor of botany, natural history, and chemistry at several colleges; participated in the geologic surveys of Missouri and New York; and published more than 100 articles, essays, and books. He died in 1853. For brief biographical sketches of his life, see Samuel D. Gross, *Lives of Eminent American Physicians and Surgeons of the Nineteenth Century* (Philadelphia, 1861), 679–96; and Catharine E. Van Cortlandt, "Lewis C. Beck," a pamphlet in TC. For a discussion of his place in the scientific world of Jacksonian New York, see Michele A. L. Aldrich, "New York Natural History Survey, 1836–1845" (Ph.D. dissertation, University of Texas, 1974), esp. 99–103, 139–40, 160, 181, 240, 279–81, 336.

14. Lewis C. Beck, "On the Nature of the Compounds, usually denominated Chlorides of Soda, Lime, &c., with Remarks on Their Uses as Disinfecting Agents," *NYMPJ* 7 (1828): 47–65; quotes: 63, 64. For the French background upon which Lewis Beck drew, see Alain Corbin, *The Foul and the Fragrant: Odor and the French Social Imagination* (Cambridge, Mass., 1986), 121–22. Corbin suggests that the "chloride revolution" made post-mortems and dissections more tolerable procedures, hence more common, in France as well as in the United States. Orfila had been the first to try the chlorides in post-mortem examinations.

15. "Toxicological Tables, in which are Exhibited at one view the Symptoms, Treatment, and Modes of Detecting the Various Poisons, Mineral, Vegetable, and Animal; According to the Latest Experiments and Observations, by a Member of the Royal College of Surgeons in London," *PJMPS* 3 (1821): appendices I-X.

16. "Reviews," *ibid.* 7 (1824): 152–57; all emphases in original.

17. R.E. Griffith, "On Medical Jurisprudence," *ibid.* 10 (1825): 36–46.

18. See the editorial announcement in *AJMPS* n.s. 1 (1841).

19. *AJMPS* n.s. 4 (1842): 217–28, 243–47, 485–96.

20. *Ibid.* n.s. 5 (1843): 112–19, 231–42, 392–404, 484–95.

21. Orfila, *Traité des exhumations juridiques* (Paris, 1830).

22. Orfila died in 1853, making him an almost exact contemporary of the two elder Beck brothers. For an early sketch of Orfila's career and a list of his major publications see *Nouvelle Biographie Générale* (Paris, 1863) 37: 779–83. A longer treatment in the context of medical jurisprudence specifically appears in Léon Dérobert, "Histoire de la médecine légale," *Zacchia: Archivio di Medicina Legale, Sociale E Criminologica*, Series 3, vol. 9, no. 2 (1973): 167–73. Shorter summaries appear in most standard English-language collections of medical and scientific biography and in some English-language encyclopedias. Orfila's letters of faculty appointment and his papers as dean of the faculty of medicine at Paris are in a collection labeled "Doyens de la Faculté de Médecine, 1808–1937," in the Archives National, Paris. They make clear that his deanship was plagued by petty squabbling and financial bickering; deanships apparently remain an academic constant. There is still a public *place* named for Orfila in modern Paris. The Spanish also recognize him with great pride, especially since his family subsequently acquired considerable political influence in that nation. On this subject, see the notice in *Glasgow Medical Journal* 1 (1853): 260, announcing an international subscription for funds to erect a monument to Orfila in Spain. Orfila's brother was already "deputy to the Cortes" there and promised to make up any shortfall of funds for the monument. Orfila seems not to have a modern scholarly biographer in French or in English, however, even though such a biography would be of great interest to historians of social, medical, and professional development.

23. On the background and launching of this journal see William Coleman, *Death Is a Social Disease: Public Health and Political Economy in Early Industrial France* (Madison, Wisc., 1982), 18.

24. T.R. Beck, "Notes on Mr. Pickering's 'Vocabulary of Words and Phrases, Which Have Been Supposed to be Peculiar to the United States,' with Preliminary Observations," *Transactions of the Albany Institute* 1 (1830): 25–31. On Beck's preference for hiring Americans, see John McVickar to TRB, April 18, 1822, Beck Papers, NYPL. This is a letter of recommendation, and in it McVickar notes explicitly Beck's "patriotic requisite of a Native American" to fill an open professorship of mathematics and natural sciences.

25. "Reviews," *PJMPS* 7 (1824): 152–57.

26. Russell C. Maulitz, "Pathology," in Ronald L. Numbers, ed., *The Education of American Physicians* (Berkeley, 1980), 126–27; Edward Atwater, "Internal Medicine," *ibid.* 144–151; and John Duffy, *The Healers: A History of American Medicine* (Urbana, Ill., 1979), 129.

27. *PJMPS* 8 (1824): 154.

28. James H. Cassedy, *American Medicine and Statistical Thinking, 1800–1860* (Cambridge, Mass., 1984), 55–67.

29. M. Meredith to TRB (n.d.); John Patterson to TRB (n.d.); Thomas Dobson to TRB, July 10, 1817; M. La Sueiz to TRB, Jan. 14, 1820; Wm Milbert to TRB, Nov. 11, 1821; all in Beck Papers, NYPL; and TRB to JWF, Feb. 15, 1815, in JWFP. See also *Catalogue of a Part of the Library of the Late Dr. T. Romeyn Beck* (Albany [?], 1855), in Catalogues of Private Medical Libraries, Vol. 1, Rare Book Room, NYAM.

30. John B. Beck, "An Historical Sketch of the State of Medicine in the American Colonies, from their first settlement to the period of the Revolution," *Transactions of the New York State Medical Society*, published as *Assembly Document, No. 174* (Albany, 1850), 41–93; the plug for French, 91. John B. Beck's library was surveyed

in James E. Cooley, agent, *Catalogue of the entire Professional and Private Library of the Late John B. Beck* (New York, 1851), NYAM.

31. *Transactions of the New York Medical Society* (1850): 233–34. For evidence of collaboration between T.R. Beck and Amariah Bringham on cases of legal insanity, see [T.R. Beck and Amariah Bringham] "Analysis of Testimony on the Trial of Alvin Cornell for Murder, and of the Subsequent Proof which led to the Commutation of his Punishment," *ibid.* 6 (1844–46): 196–216.

32. For an excellent example of the use of French authorities in American courts, see Alonzo Clark, "Case of Supposed Murder," a lecture given to the NYAM, Dec. 18, 1861 (Bound pamphlet, Rare Books and Manuscripts Room, NYAM), in which Clark, a prominent physician, describes his testimony in a case that hinged upon whether a woman had been murdered or had commited suicide. Clark cited nine different French authorities in defense of his position in this case.

33. Coleman, *Death Is a Social Disease*, 19–20 and *passim*.

34. Some American jurisdictions do permit a technical bench expert under certain conditions, but that proceeding is unusual and quite different from what nineteenth-century medical jurisprudence writers admired in the French system.

35. *PJMPS* 11 (1825): 410–14.

36. M. Gendrin, "Du devoir des médecins experts et des limites du droit de visite dan les enquêtes médico-légales," *Annales D'Hygiène Publique et de Médecine Légale* 2 (1829): 480–81; Alfred Lechopié and Ch. Floquet, *Droit Médical ou Code de Médecins* (Paris, 1890), 5–9, 152–80.

37. A. Lacasagne, *Des Transformations du droit pénal et les progrés de la médecine légale de 1810 à 1912* (separately published from *Archives d'Anthropologie Criminelle, de Médecine légale et de Psychologie Normale et Pathologique*, no. 233 [March 15, 1913]): 6–7, in the library of the Institut de Médecine Légale, Université René Descartes, Paris.

38. This statement is impossible to document literally, but even a cursory perusal of medical journals and law reports from the first half of the nineteenth century will quickly reveal routine instances of medical practitioners actively involved in court cases of all sorts, often as the key witness. Success stories of doctors' exploits in court became a staple of the journal literature. Many flamboyant trials received extensive coverage in the public press as well. Note that the generalization advanced here refers to cases in which the physician was not a principal in the proceedings, but rather agreed voluntarily to enter the proceedings on one side or the other.

39. The basic source for this paragraph and the next several that follow is Samuel D. Gross, *Autobiography of Samuel D. Gross, M.D.* (first published Philadelphia, 1887; rpt. in facsimile, New York, 1972), vol. 1, 26–60 and *passim*. Unless otherwise cited, the material on Gross, including the direct quotations, may be found in that source.

40. Gross later published his experiments on intestinal wounds under the title "An Experimental and Critical Inquiry into the Nature and Treatment of Wounds of the Intestines," *Western Journal of Medicine and Surgery* 7 (1843): 1–50, 81–141, 161–224; and in bound book form under the same title (Louisville, 1843).

41. Gross later published the results of those experiments under the title "Observations on Manual Strangulation, illustrated by Cases and Experiments," in *ibid.* 9 (1835): 25–38. He also performed a post-mortem examination on the body of someone who had committed suicide by hanging in March of 1833, right after the Goetter trial, and included those findings as well, since they confirmed his own conclusions about the physiological signs of strangulation.

42. Beck and Beck, *Elements* (1838 edition), vol. 2, 160–161, and subsequent editions under different pagination.

43. No one could accuse Gross of winning gracefully, however, for he could not resist adding a note about Porter's subsequent career. The latter failed to be confirmed by the U. S. Senate as Secretary of War under President John Tyler and ended his professional life "in straitened circumstances," half incapacitated by apoplexy himself and "begging" Gross for a job teaching medical jurisprudence. Gross all too obviously reveled in the triple irony and sharp contrasts. Gross, *Autobiography*, 54–55.

44. Samuel D. Gross, "Address of Samuel D. Gross, M.D., LL.D., President of the Association," *TAMA* 19 (1868): 57–74.

45. Gross, *Autobiography*, 374–76. Medical jurisprudence at the centennial celebration will be discussed later in a different context.

46. T.R. Beck, "Contributions in Medical Jurisprudence, No. 1., Of Insurance upon Lives," *NYMPJ* 5 (1826): 26–27. In this context, see also John C. Greene, "Science and the Public in the Age of Jefferson," in Brooke Hindle, ed., *Early American Science* (New York, 1974), 201–13.

47. These developments are summarized in Joseph G. Richardson, "On the Detection of Red and White Corpuscles in Blood-Stains," *AJMS* n.s. 58 (1869): 50–58. Richardson, an M.D., was microscopist to the Pennsylvania Hospital. See also William H. Schneider, "Chance and Social Setting in the Application of the Discovery of Blood Groups," *BHM* 57 (Winter 1983): 545–62.

48. See the report of a San Francisco rape case in (Aug.?) 1850, contained in Pamphlet No. 7, TC.

49. For a recent discussion of anatomy instruction during the eighteenth century see Christopher Lawrence, "Alexander Monro *Primus* and the Edinburgh Manner of Anatomy," *BHM* 62 (1988): 193–214.

50. For examples of the sort of work referred to here, see the unsigned review essay discussion of Addison and Morgan, "An Essay on the Operation of Poisonous Agents upon the Living body," in *PJMPS* 11 (1832): 127–37; and John B. Beck, "On the Modus Operandi of Medicine," *AJMS* n.s. 7 (1844): 27–43.

51. On this shift generally see John Harley Warner, *The Therapeutic Perspective: Medical Practice, Knowledge, and Identity in America, 1820–1885* (Cambridge, Mass., 1986). Warner concludes that therapeutic practices changed gradually, but by the late 1860s and early 1870s began to resemble the early twentieth century more than the early nineteenth. That conclusion, though reached in an altogether different context, meshes neatly with the overall position being developed in this study: profound professional changes took place in the United States around the middle of the nineteenth century.

52. For examples, see John B. Beck's ongoing and revised sections on infanticide in successive editions of the *Elements; J.B. Beck, "An Examination of the Medico-Legal Question, whether, in Cases of Infanticide, the Floating of the Lungs in Water can be depended on as a certain test of the Child's Having Been Born Alive," *NYMPJ* 1 (1822): 441–63; J.B. Beck on the signs of stillbirth and livebirth in *AJMS* n.s. 4 (1842): 243–47; and especially J.B. Beck, "Observations on some of the signs of live and still birth, in their application to Medical Jurisprudence," *Transactions of the New York State Medical Society* 5 (1841–43): 150–57. The latter summarizes the results of ten infant autopsies.

53. See, for example, "Marks of Vitality in New-Born Infants," *NYMPJ* 5 (1826): 521–22; the piece on respiration in newborns is in the medical jurisprudence section of *NYMPJ* 5 (1826): 644–45; R.E. Griffith, "Remarks on Infanticide," *PJMPS* 13

(1826): 259–73 and *ibid.* 14 (1827): 38–60; Charles A. Lee, "Report of a Trial for Infanticide, with Remarks," *PJMPS* 12 (1835): 327–41; and J.H. Thompson, "Case of Suspected Infanticide," *AJMS* n.s. 8 (1844): 269–70.

54. The medico-legal literature on this subject is voluminous. For representative examples, see [T.R. Beck] "Contributions in Medical Jurisprudence and Police, No. IV: Duration of Human Pregnancy," *NYMPJ* 6 (1827): 224–42; T.R. Beck, "Contributions to Legal Medicine," *AJMS* n.s. 1 (1841): 55–64; Aristide Rodrigue, "Contributions to Legal Medicine," *ibid.* n.s. 10 (1845); Washington L. Atlee, "Legal Medicine," *ibid.* n.s. 12 (1846): 535–40; [T.R. Beck] "Medical Jurisprudence and Toxicology," *ibid.* n.s. 23 (1852): 548–56; *ibid.* n.s. 29 (1855): 263–68.

55. The first observation is from the notebook of George B. McKnight, "Notes of Lectures on Legal Medicine [by James S. Stringham at the College of Physicians and Surgeons, New York City]," for the date Dec. 7, 1815, TC; the second is from the same source under the heading "Concealed Pregnancy."

56. The *Maryland Medical Recorder* 3 (1832): 349, reported the use of the stethoscope to determine pregnancy and claimed that others had been doing the same since 1821. On the quickening doctrine see James C. Mohr, *Abortion in America: The Origins and Evolution of National Policy, 1800–1900* (New York, 1978), 3–6.

57. T.R. Beck, "On the Signs of Pregnancy," *AJMS* n.s. 5 (1843): 112–19, summarizes the early tests.

CHAPTER FIVE

1. A large portion of Wharton and Stillé, *A Treatise on Medical Jurisprudence* (Philadelphia, 1855) was material on insanity that Francis Wharton had previously published by himself. That work remained in print separately: Wharton, *A Treatise on Mental Unsoundness, Embracing a General View of Psychological Law* (Philadelphia, 1873). Wharton came to the subject from the perspective of the law; he was an attorney, not a physician.

2. Thanks to a burst of scholarly activity on the history of insanity and its treatment in the United States during the nineteenth century, this conclusion, and several others in this chapter, may be verified in other contexts as well. The place to start is three volumes by Gerald Grob: *The State and the Mentally Ill: A History of the Worcester State Hospital in Massachusetts, 1830–1920* (Chapel Hill, 1966); *Mental Institutions in America: Social Policy to 1875* (New York, 1973); and *Mental Illness and American Society, 1875–1940* (Princeton, N.J., 1983).

3. An especially good example is Beck, "An Account of Some of the Lunatic Asylums in the United States," *NYMPJ* 7 (1828): 186–206, 251–54, in which he presents optimistic statistics on cures. For lobbying elsewhere, see Grob, *Mental Institutions to 1875.*

4. The quote and the story are from Andrew Dickson White, *Autobiography of Andrew D. White,* vol. 1 (New York, 1905), 333. See also *Albany Evening Journal,* April 3 and 6, 1865. White, incidentally, struck a deal in the midst of this bizarre train of events that secured state support for the establishment of Cornell University. See James C. Mohr, *The Radical Republicans and Reform in New York During Reconstruction* (Ithaca, 1973), 164–66.

5. Michel Foucault, *Folie et déraison: histoire de la folie,* translated by Richard Howard as *Madness and Civilization: A History of Insanity in the Age of Reason* (New York, 1965), and Foucault, *Discipline and Punish* (New York, 1979). Foucault's perspective has continued to generate considerable intellectual debate in the United

States through the late 1980s, and his name appears frequently in essays of social criticism.

6. David Rothman, *The Discovery of the Asylum: Social Order and Disorder in the New Republic* (Boston, 1971). Rothman also assessed the later period in his *Conscience and Convenience: The Asylum and Its Alternatives in Progressive America* (Boston, 1980). For a comparison of two asylums in Beck's own New York state (Utica and Willard) and how they functioned through 1890, see Ellen Dwyer, *Homes for the Mad: Life Inside Two Nineteenth-Century Asylums* (New Brunswick, 1987).

7. See *Notes on Medical Jurisprudence*, by Andrew Duncan, Sr., taken by J. Lee, Edinburgh, 1800, Special Collections, University of Edinburgh Library.

8. "Observations on Medical Jurisprudence delivered in Lecture in the University of Edinburgh, by Andrew Duncan [Sr.], M.D. & P, Taken in Notes by David Pollock" (2 vols., 1797–98), vol. 2: 2, Special Collections, University of Edinburgh Library.

9. Francis Wharton and Moreton Stillé, *A Treatise on Medical Jurisprudence* (Philadelphia, 1855), "Book I."

10. Benjamin Rush, *Sixteen Introductory Lectures, to Courses of Lectures upon the Institutes and Practice of Medicine, with a Syllabus of the Latter* (Philadelphia, 1811), 377.

11. *Ibid.*, 391.

12. *Ibid.*, 368.

13. Rush, *Medical Inquiries and Observations, upon the Diseases of the Mind* (Philadelphia, 1812; rpt. Birmingham, Ala., 1979).

14. *Ibid.*, 59, 66, 70–71, 347, 354; quote: 71.

15. Griffith, "On Medical Jurisprudence," *PJMPS* 10 (1825): 39–40. Blackstone's opinion about wills was from the first volume of his *Commentaries*, 13. T.R. Beck, *Elements*, vol. 1: 377–78, made the same point.

16. Beck, *Elements*, vol. 1: 377–82.

17. Dunglison, *Syllabus*, 127–29.

18. Williams, *Catechism*, 41–42.

19. "Medical Jurisprudence" by Nathan Smith, lecture notes taken by A[very] J. S[kilton] at Yale (February [1827?]), 143, NLM.

20. For an excellent example of the sharp increase of attention given to such cases in medical journals, see the *AJMS* during the 1840s.

21. William Cabell Bruce, *John Randolph of Roanoke, 1773–1833* (New York, 1970), vol. 2: 49–60.

22. T.R. Beck, "Of the state of mind necessary to constitute a valid will. Case of Stewart's executors v. Lispenard, as tried and decided in the courts of the state of New York," *AJMS* n.s. 6 (1843): 507–16. Verplanck's position is summarized 515–16.

23. *Ibid.*, 515.

24. Robert B. Warden, *A Familiar Forensic View of Man and Law* (Columbus, Ohio, 1860), 505–30.

25. "Expert Testimony," an interview with Dr. W. A. Hammond in an unidentified newspaper (hand marked October 1884), in Pamphlet No. 10, TC. Hammond will be discussed further in later chapters, but he was certainly in a position to know the fee structure for experts on insanity.

26. John J. Elwell, *A Medico-Legal Treatise on Malpractice and Medical Evidence, Comprising the Elements of Medical Jurisprudence* (New York, 1866), 296.

27. *New York Times*, April 2, 18, 19, and 21, 1856; July 19, 1856.

28. *Ibid.*, May 5, 1862.

29. "Editorial: Michigan's New Will Law," *Medico-Legal Journal* 1–2 (1883–84): 97–99.

30. In the English tradition specifically, Henry VIII provides a good example. He feared poisoning, which was considered a troublesome, dangerous, and widespread crime in early modern England. But all he could do about it was declare it a form of treason. Anyone convicted of murder by poison would thereby be subject to especially ghastly forms of execution because such forms of execution were permissible in treason cases but not permissible in simple murder cases. But the decree did not make the detection of poisoning itself any easier or more likely, and the decree may reasonably be seen as a measure of Henry's frustration rather than a step in the long slow effort to reduce the threat of poisoning. See Leon Radzinowicz, *A History of English Criminal Law and Its Administration from 1750* (London, 1948), vol. 1: 146, 238–39, 629.

31. McKnight notes of Stringham lectures, TC.

32. *NYMPJ* 1 (1822): 515. Arsenic-based rat-killers, for example, were not infrequently mistaken for coarse sugar.

33. For representative comments on the continuing public fear well into the nineteenth century, see John B. Beck, "On the Deaths from Poisoning, in the City and County of New York, during the years 1841, 42, and 43; obtained from the Records of the Coroner," *Transactions of the Medical Society of the State of New York* 6 (1844–46): 66–72; Charles T. Jackson, "Statistics of Poisoning in New England," *BMSJ* 63 (1860): 389–91 (I am indebted to James Cassedy for bringing this reference to my attention); and Elwell, *Malpractice*, 440, 452, 453–54; quote: 440.

34. The story of the Kesler evidence is in *Medical Repository* (New York) 19 (1818) [n.s. Vol. 4]: 314–19.

35. [John Clarkson Jay] "Medical Jurisprudence by Dr. [John B.] Beck," 14 (a student notebook from a course that began November 17, 1829), Rare Books, NYAM. Jay clearly got the message. In his notebook he wrote "*Rule* always make your opinion not from one test, but from all of them."

36. *NYMPJ* 3 (1824): 375.

37. *Maryland Medical Recorder* 1 (1829): 90.

38. J.K. Mitchell, "Observations on Arsenic," *AJMS* 10 (1832): 121–28; quote: 128. John K. Mitchell, the father of S. Weir Mitchell, had graduated from Edinburgh and would later play a large role in the early development of physiology. See *DAMB* 2: 529.

39. On the importance of combining tests, see Benjamin S. Downing, "Lectures on the Materia Medica and Medical Jurisprudence Delivered at the College of Physicians and Surgeons at the University of the State of New-York By John B. Beck, M.D., Professor &c" (a student notebook, undated), vol. 2: 195–205, Rare Books, NYAM.

40. John B. Beck instructed his students on how to meet "objections usually raised by the Court," including apparently routine allegations that arsenic found in a corpse might have been introduced after death through the rectum or the vagina in order to frame someone. See Downing, "Lectures," 202–4.

41. In addition to his private practice, Jackson was professor at the Philadelphia College of Pharmacy at the time of this trial, and later a professor at the University of Pennsylvania Medical School. See *DAMB*, 388–89. Jackson, incidentally, and by no accident, was among the country's most fervent advocates of French medical methods.

42. Samuel Jackson, "Case of Supposed Poisoning with Arsenic," *AJMS* 5 (1829): 237–48.

43. The account in this and the following paragraphs is taken from William F. Packer and Alexander Cummings, Jr., *Report of the Trial and Conviction of John Earls for the Murder of his Wife Catharine Earls, Late of Muncy Creek Township, Lycoming County, Pennsylvania, in the Court of Oyer and Terminer held at Williamsport, for Lycoming County, February Term, 1836, Including the Arguments of Counsel, at length, together with the Confession of the Prisoner* (Williamsport, 1836). Only direct quotations will be cited.

44. *Ibid.*, 137.

45. *Ibid.*, 176.

46. *Ibid.*, 173–74.

47. W.A. Campbell, "Some Landmarks in the History of Arsenic Testing," *Chemistry in Britain* 1 (May 1965) 198–202. In 1841 the Marsh test was replaced in the United States by the even more popular and more easily performed Reinsch test. See D.P. Gardner, "On the Application of M. Reinsch's test for the detection of Arsenic to Medico-Legal Enquiries," *American Journal of Science* 44 (1842): 240.

48. These conclusions are impressions, of course, but they are based upon a perusal of hundreds of volumes of medical journals and a close reading of extant student notebooks from medical jurisprudence courses in medical schools. Many of the latter have already been cited in other specific contexts.

49. T.R. Beck, "Review," *AJMS* n.s. 2 (1841): 403–35. The essay reviewed nine recent articles from France, one from a South Carolina physician studying in Paris, and one from England.

50. T.R. Beck, "Contributions to Legal Medicine," *AJMS* n.s. 1 (1841): 55–64, Case II.

51. Lewis C. Beck, *Adulterations of Various Substances Used in Medicine and the Arts, with the means of detecting them* (New York, 1846).

52. The English treatise was Frederick Accum, *A Treatise on Adulterations of Food, and Culinary Poisons* (American edition, Philadelphia, 1820). Beck also discussed such things as the adulteration of coffee by adding chicory.

53. On this and the other nineteenth-century precursors of twentieth-century pure food and drug efforts, see Mitchell Okun, *Fair Play in the Marketplace: The First Battle for Pure Food and Drugs* (Dekalb, Ill., 1986); and James Harvey Young, *Pure Food: Securing the Federal Food and Drugs Act of 1906* (Princeton, N.J., 1989). There is a substantial literature on the milk controversies specifically.

54. T.G. Wormley, *Ohio Medical and Surgical Journal* 12 (1859): 32–39; and John J. Reese, "On Detection of Strychnia as a Poison, and the Influence of Morphia in disguising the Usual Colour-test," *AJMS* n.s. 41 (1861): 409–21.

55. Robert P. Thomas, "On the Colour Tests of Strychnia, as modified by the presence of Morphia," *AJMS* n.s. 43 (1862): 340–47.

56. Susan Brownmiller, *Against Our Will: Men, Women and Rape* (New York, 1975), 23–30. While Brownmiller and Susan Griffith, "Politics of Rape," *Ramparts* (1971), deserve credit for initiating a long-overdue modern analysis of rape, reference to their work here does not signify agreement with all of their contentions. For Brownmiller and Griffith, rape has remained a sort of unchanging cultural metaphor, a gender-based constant of oppression. While that argument may be taken seriously at a metaphorical level, the discussion here is based upon the premise (and the evidence) that rape, like other actions and other crimes, has undergone substantial change in different societies at different times for different reasons. Here the

suggestion is that Americans altered some of their attitudes and policies toward rape during the second quarter of the nineteenth century and that the new champions of medical jurisprudence played a key role in that alteration.

57. On the impact of the Scottish and French Enlightenments on modern Western concepts of rape, see the perceptive "Introduction," by Sylvana Tomaselli, in Tomaselli and Roy Porter, eds., *Rape* (Oxford and New York, 1986), esp. 6–9.

58. A[very] J. S[kilton], " 'Medical Jurisprudence' by Nathan Smith."

59. See the previous discussion in Chapter Three about Williams's *Catechism* and the review of that work by R.E. Griffith in *AJMS* 16 (1835): 159–62.

60. Beck and Beck, *Elements* (11th ed., 1860), vol. 1: 204.

61. William Coleman, *Report of the Trial of Levi Weeks, &c. taken in short-hand by the clerk of the court* (New York, 1800), cited in Beck, *Elements* (1st ed., 1823), vol. 1: 86 and vol. 2: 67–69.

62. See, for example, the editorial exhortation in *PJMPS* 9 (1824): 427–33, urging physicians to get involved in rape cases and to testify. For a good example of the way rape cases were kept before the profession see *AJMPS* n.s. 3 (1842): 490–95.

63. Beck and Beck, *Elements* (11th ed., 1860), vol. 1: 225–26.

64. S.D. Gross, "Observations and Experiments on Spermatic Stains, in their relation to Medical Jurisprudence," *Western Medical Gazette* 2 (1834): 244–49.

65. Beck, *Elements* (1st ed., 1823), vol. 1: 72–103; quote, 101. The legal opinion about female pleasure, incidentally, has intriguing implications in the debate over the nature of sexuality in the United States during the nineteenth century. See, for example, on this subject Carl N. Degler, "What Ought to Be and What Was: Women's Sexuality in the Nineteenth Century," *American Historical Review* 79 (1974): 1467–90.

66. Scholars of medical jurisprudence did, however, still debate the exact nature of the conception process. For a hypothesis based on electrical theory see James A. Harrell, "Thesis on Medical Jurisprudence" (doctoral dissertation, Washington University of Baltimore, 1842), longhand copy in TC.

67. See *AJMS* n.s. 45 (1863): 272, which comments on an article by E.S. Arnold in the *American Medical Times* of Nov. 29, 1862, defending the old British position.

68. Thomas Laqueur explores some of the key, often ironic, relationships between this shift in the understanding of conception, on the one hand, and the place of women in society, on the other, in an essay entitled "Orgasm, Generation, and the Politics of Reproductive Biology," *Representations* 14 (1986): 1–41.

69. Dunglison, *Syllabus*, 121.

70. Thomas W. Blatchford, "Observations on Equivocal Generation, prepared as evidence in a Suit for Slander," *Transactions of the Medical Society of the State of New York* 6 (1844–46): 22–33; quotes, 23.

71. Thomas W. Blatchford, *An Inaugural Dissertation on Feigned Diseases* (New York, 1817).

72. Blatchford, "Observations on Equivocal Generation," 22–33. The case appeared in *Wendell's Reports* 19: 296.

CHAPTER SIX

1. George Rosen, *From Medical Police to Social Medicine: Essays on the History of Health Care* (New York, 1974), 120–46, 246–58, argued that state-sanctioned medi-

cal jurisprudence typical of late eighteenth- and early nineteenth-century Europe had arisen from German cameralism; was overtly authoritarian and paternalistic; and was, as a consequence, the "diametrical opposite" (p. 258) of Enlightenment republicanism in general and of American Jeffersonian thought in particular. Rosen may be correct for the German tradition, but his arguments are difficult to sustain in the Anglo-American context. The surge of activity in medical jurisprudence at Edinburgh, for example, was directly associated with the Scottish Enlightenment, not its opposite. In the United States people like Thomas Cooper, whose political philosophy could hardly be characterized as cameral, not only went along with but actually took the lead in pushing a medico-legal agenda. Indeed, in almost direct rebuttal of Rosen's explicit arguments about Jeffersonianism, it was Jefferson himself who asked Dunglison, a professional trained in the German tradition, to come to the University of Virginia to build medical jurisprudence. In short, there seems to have been an altogether comfortable ideological fit between Jeffersonian republicanism and the sort of civic-minded medical jurisprudence envisioned by Beck and others like him; not the philosophical conflict that Rosen asserted. That is not to say, however, that the pervasive opposition to a powerful and paternalistic state had nothing to do with the fate of medical jurisprudence in the United States; it certainly did, as will become evident. But not for the reasons Rosen suggested.

2. For excellent data and specific examples of the way this worked in Beck's own Albany area, see Michele A. L. Aldrich, "New York Natural History Survey, 1836–1845" (Ph.D. dissertation, University of Texas, 1974), 55–56 and *passim*. Gerard W. Gawalt, *The Promise of Power: The Emergence of the Legal Profession in Massachusetts, 1760–1840* (Westport, Conn., 1979) demonstrates the way in which networking and family alliances helped solidify the position of elite lawyers in early Massachusetts.

3. There is a large and detailed literature on early American common law, legal codes, and codification. The discussion throughout this section draws most heavily upon Maurice Eugen Lang, *Codification in the British Empire and America* (Amsterdam, 1924); Roscoe Pound, *The Formative Era of American Law* (Boston, 1938); James Willard Hurst, *The Growth of American Law: The Law Makers* (Boston, 1950) and *Law and the Conditions of Freedom in Nineteenth Century America* (Madison, Wisc., 1956) and *Law and Social Order in the United States* (Ithaca, 1977); Anton-Hermann Chroust, *The Rise of the Legal Profession in America*, vol. 2, *The Revolution and the Post-Revolutionary Era* (Norman, Okla., 1965); Charles Warren, *A History of the American Bar* (New York, 1966); Lawrence M. Friedman, "Law Reform in Historical Perspective," *Saint Louis University Law Journal* 13 (1969): 351–74, and *A History of American Law* (New York, 1973); William E. Nelson, *Americanization of the Common Law: The Impact of Legal Change on Massachusetts Society, 1760–1830* (Cambridge, Mass., 1975); Morton J. Horwitz, *The Transformation of American Law, 1780–1860* (Cambridge, Mass., 1977); Charles M. Cook, *The American Codification Movement: A Study of Antebellum Legal Reform* (Westport, Conn., 1981); and Kermit L. Hall, *The Magic Mirror: Law in American History* (New York, 1989).

4. Friedman, *American Law*, 96–97.

5. New York State Constitution of 1821, Article 7, Section XIII.

6. This section follows the excellent discussion in Cook, *Codification*, 136–53; quotes: 141, 142.

7. On this chronology and on the New York codes generally, see Ernest Henry Breuer, "The New York Revised Statutes, 1829: Its Several Editions, Reports of the Revisers, Commentaries and Related Publications Up to the Consolidated Laws

of 1909," unpublished typescript and bibliography, New York State Library, Albany, Aug. 1, 1961.

8. On Spencer's dominant role in writing the 1829 code, see the preface to the 1846 edition of the *Revised Code of the State of New York* (Albany, 1846), vii.

9. *DAB* 9: 443–45.

10. *Ibid.*, 449–50; *NCAB* 6: 6–7; *Revised Statutes of the State of New York* (Albany, 1836), vol. 3: 420.

11. James M. Hobbins, "Shaping a Provincial Learned Society: The Early History of the Albany Institute," in Alexandra Oleson and Sanborn C. Brown, eds., *The Pursuit of Knowledge in the Early Republic: American Scientific and Learned Societies from Colonial Times to the Civil War* (Baltimore, 1976), 117–50.

12. See, for example, Stephen Van Rensselaer to TRB, Dec. 16, 1821, July 21, 1823, and Dec. 8, 1823; Beck Papers, NYPL. Van Rensselaer was in Congress at the time.

13. Edward Livingston to TRB, March 22, 1829; Beck Papers, NYPL. Beck and Livingston doubtless met while the latter was still a citizen of New York state. Livingston had represented New York in the national House of Representatives before moving to Louisiana. He subsequently represented his new state both in the national House and the national Senate. Livingston wrote Beck from Washington.

14. For a discussion of the legislature's reaction to this specific section, and its implications for the origins of anti-abortion legislation, see *Revised Statutes of New-York . . . 1828 to 1835 Inclusive* (Albany, 1836), vol. 1: 578, and vol. 3: 829–30; and James C. Mohr, *Abortion in America: The Origins and Evolution of National Policy, 1800–1900* (New York, 1978), 26–31; and note 19: 270–271. Discovery of Spencer's short letter to T.R. Beck, which was unknown in 1978, strengthens further the professional-based argument advanced in *Abortion in America* (since we now know exactly which medical professionals the committee of revision relied upon), and the influence of John B. Beck's ideas about abortion must now be beyond dispute.

15. [John C. Spencer] *Notes on the Revised Statutes of the State of New-York: Pointing Out the Principal Alterations Made by Them in the Common and Statute Law* (Albany, 1830), 24–27, 213–14; *Revised Statutes of the State of New York* (Albany, 1836), vol. 3: 848, and "Appendix, Containing Extracts From the Original Reports of the Revisers," *passim*.

16. Cook, *Codification*, 28. Kilty made these revisions in 1797 and more extensive compilations and revisions of different sorts in 1811: William Kilty, *A Report on All Such English Statutes* (Annapolis, 1811).

17. Jeremy Bentham himself coined the word "codification" and once offered to draft a code for New Hampshire. See Cook, *Codification*, 74–78, 102. The tendency to consider codification a failure has deep scholarly roots, which go back at least half a century and continue to the present day to inform legal history. See Lang, *Codification*, 114–86; and Friedman, *American Law*, 351–55.

18. For heuristic suggestions about the physician as modernizer on a broad scale see Christopher Lasch, "What the Doctor Ordered," *New York Review of Books* 22, no. 20 (Dec. 11, 1975): 52. For a specific example of the professions setting social policy during the nineteenth century see Mohr, *Abortion in America, passim*. In the latter are many examples of the way physicians used the process of code revision to bring about policy changes. Especially obvious ones are documented in A[lexander] J. Semmes to Horatio R. Storer, March 24, 1857, and L[evin] S. Joynes to Horatio R. Storer, May 4, 1859; Horatio R. Storer Papers, Countway Library, Harvard Medical School.

19. Beck, *Elements* (1823 edition), vol. 1: xxiii–xxiv. The previous year Beck had called for state subsidies to physicians who came up with ideas that served the public good. New York state had actually done that once in 1806, but the person who received the subsidy turned out to be a charlatan whose purported antidote to rabies proved ineffective. T. R. Beck, "A Sketch of the Legislative provision of the Colony and State of New-York, respecting the Practice of Physic and Surgery," *NYMPJ* 1 (1822): 142–51.

20. R.E. Griffith, "On Medical Jurisprudence," *PJMPS* 10 (1825): 38–39.

21. "Medical Jurisprudence," *NYMPJ* 5 (1826): 384, and the review of "A Letter to the Hon. Isaac Parker, Chief Justice of the Supreme Court of the State of Massachusetts, containing Remarks on the Dislocation of the Hip-joint, occasioned by the publication of a Trial, which took place at Machias, in the State of Maine, June, 1824," *NYMPJ* 5 (1826): 597–607; quotes: 607.

22. See John B. Beck's introductory lecture at the College of Physicians and Surgeons of New York for fall term 1829, reprinted in *NYMPJ* n.s. 2 (1830): 350–55.

23. T.R. Beck, "Annual Address," 14–15.

24. The history and eventual triumph of "regular" medicine in the United States is well known; readers may consult the previously cited works of Shryock, Kett, Rothstein, and Starr for details. "Regularism" itself, however, remains difficult to define with historical precision, in part because the line between regular practice, on the one hand, and various forms of irregular practice, on the other, was always blurry and continued to shift throughout the nineteenth century. Regulars in New York City in 1846, seeking to separate themselves from the irregulars, found it easiest to define themselves negatively. In their minds regularism excluded "all homoeopathic, hydropathic, chronothermal and botanic physicians, and also all mesmeric and clairvoyant pretenders to the healing art, and all others who at any time or on any pretext claim peculiar merits for their mixed practices not founded on the best system of physiology and pathology, as taught in the best schools in Europe and America." The quote is from Philip Van Ingen, *The New York Academy of Medicine: Its First Hundred Years* (New York, 1949), 13.

25. William G. Rothstein, *American Physicians in the Nineteenth Century: From Sects to Science* (Baltimore, 1972), 77; Joseph F. Kett, *Formation of the American Medical Profession: The Role of Institutions, 1780–1860* (New Haven, 1968), 35–46.

26. Beck, "Annual Address," 16.

27. After the Norman Conquest, these inquiries were also designed to discover incidents of Normans being murdered by Saxons. See Faruk B. Presswalla, "Historical Evolution of Medico-Legal Investigative Systems," *Medico-Legal Bulletin (of Richmond, Virginia)* 25 (1976): 1–8.

28. F. W. Maitland, *The Constitutional History of England* (1908, 1950), 534, 536, 590, 644; Austin Lane Poole, *From Domesday Book to Magna Carta, 1087–1216* (Oxford, 1951), 390–91.

29. E. Donald Shapiro and Anthony Davis, "Law and Pathology Through the Ages: The Coroner and His Descendants—Legitimate and Illegitimate," *New York State Journal of Medicine* 72 (1972): 805–9.

30. Gordon Smith, England's leading expert on medical evidence in the first decades of the nineteenth century was typical. "It is impossible to resist the wish that special qualifications were required by law on the part of medical witnesses," he wrote. "There is something of this nature on the continent; and though one of the last of my countrymen who would wish to see the customs and institutions of

Great Britain shaped according to foreign patterns, yet I think we might in some matters take a hint from and improve upon their practice." *Medical Evidence*, 103, quoted in a note of Beck's "Annual Address," 16.

31. Even Shakespeare poked fun at the way coroners conducted their investigations. See the comic dialogue between the gravediggers in *Hamlet*, Act V, Scene 1.

32. A. Keith Mant, "Milestones in the Development of the British Medicolegal System," *Medicine, Science, and the Law* 17, no. 3 (1977): 155–63; Richard Harrison, " 'How Came They By Their Death' Inquests Two Hundred Years Ago," *Lancet* (Sept. 2, 1978): 518; Dorothy L. Lansing, "The Coroner System and Some of Its Coroners in Early Pennsylvania," *Transactions and Studies of the College of Physicians of Philadelphia* 44 (Jan., 1977): 135–40.

33. New York Constitution of 1777, Arts. XXIII and XXVI, Nathaneil H. Carter and William L. Stone, reporters, *Reports of the Proceedings and Debates of the Convention of 1821, Assembled for the Purpose of Amending the Constitution of the State of New-York* (rpt., New York, 1970), 17; James A. Henretta, "The Rise and Decline of 'Democratic Republicanism': New York and the Several States, 1800–1915," an unpublished paper presented at the University of Maryland Baltimore County Faculty Seminar series, 1988.

34. Carter and Stone, *Reports of the Convention of 1821*, 161.

35. *Ibid.*, 663.

36. John B. Beck, "On the Deaths from Poisoning, in the City and County of New York, during the years 1841, 42, and 43; obtained from the Records of the Coroner," *Transactions of the Medical Society of the State of New York* 6 (1844–46): 66–67.

37. "Medical Coroners," *BMSJ* 48 (May 25, 1853): 346; *ibid.*, 49 (Oct. 19, 1853): 249.

38. Horace Binney, *Opinion of Horace Binney, Esq., Upon the Jurisdiction of the Coroner* (Philadelphia, 1853). For a brief biographical sketch of one of thousands of mid-nineteenth-century coroners, see Andrew Forest Muir, "Heinrich Thuerwaechter, Colonial German Settler," *Texana* 4 (1966): 33–40. Muir makes clear that this 1856 Harris County, Texas, coroner was a "character" and an "eccentric" politician.

39. Benjamin F. Butler, John Duer, and John C. Spencer, *Reports of the Revisers* (7 vols., Albany, 1826–28), vol. 3, part IV, chapter 2, title vii, sections 4 and 5: 65.

40. *Revised Statutes of the State of New York* (Albany, 1829), vol. 2: 742–43.

41. The best recent portrait of this world of overlapping healers in the early republic is in Laurel Thatcher Ulrich, *A Midwife's Tale: The Life of Martha Ballard, Based on Her Diary, 1785–1812* (New York, 1990), esp. chapters 3 and 7.

42. For information about irregular sects in the nineteenth century, see Norman Gevitz, ed., *Other Healers: Unorthodox Medicine in America* (Baltimore, 1988).

43. Alexander Wilder, *History of Medicine: A Brief Outline of Medical History and Sects of Physicians, from the Earliest Historic Period; with an Extended Account of the New Schools of the Healing Art in the Nineteenth Century, and Especially a History of the American Eclectic Practice of Medicine, Never before Published* (New Sharon, Me., 1901), 502, 504.

44. Charles B. Coventry, "History of Medical Legislation in the State of New York," *New York Journal of Medicine* 4 (1845): 151–61.

45. "Law in Relation to Medical Charges in Massachusetts," *BMSJ* 25 (Dec. 1, 1841): 278.

46. "Medical Miscellany," *BMSJ* 26 (March 24, 1842): 115; and "Legalized Quackery," *ibid.*, 29 (Aug. 19, 1843): 25.

47. "Physicians' and Counsels' Fees," *Pennsylvania Law Journal* 2 (1843): 126–28. Those rulings, which outraged physicians, reversed professional traditions that went back to the Romans.

48. This provision was of great interest to pharmacists as well as physicians, incidentally. See Harley R. Wiley, *A Treatise on Pharmacal Jurisprudence* (San Francisco, 1904), 102.

49. "Law of Medicine in Mississippi," *BMSJ* 32 (July 2, 1845): 447.

50. Wilder, *History of Medicine*, 510.

51. Rothstein, *American Physicians*, 39–174; Shryock, *Medical Licensing in America, 1650–1965* (Baltimore, 1967), 3–42; Edward C. Atwater, "The Medical Profession in a New Society, Rochester, New York (1811–1860)," *BHM* 47 (May-June 1973): 221–35.

52. William M. Wood, "Thoughts on Suits for Malpractice, suggested by certain Judicial Proceedings in Erie County, Pennsylvania," *AJMS* n.s. 18 (Oct. 1849): 395.

53. See *Revised Statutes of the State of New York* (Albany, 1836), vol. 2, part 3, chapter 2, title 7, article 1; *ibid.* (Albany, 1846), under the same sections; and *ibid.* (Albany, 1848), vol. 3: 782.

54. Beck and Beck, *Elements* (6th ed., 1838), vol. 2: 681.

55. Beck, "Presidential Address," 30–31.

56. Beck and Beck, *Elements* (5th ed., 1835), vol. 2: 3.

57. *Ibid.*, 639.

58. The travel and *per diem* provisions adjusted in 1840 had been in the original Spencer-Beck code of 1830. *Revised Code of the State of New York* (Albany, 1848), vol. 2: 734, 827–28, and 913. Physicians could, of course, be paid by the defense in criminal cases.

59. T.R.B[eck]., "Are medical men liable to punishment if they refuse to make a medico-legal dissection, or a chemical analysis, when called upon by the coroner?" *AJMS* n.s. 4 (1842): 224–25.

60. James Webster, *Introductory to the Course of Anatomy, in Geneva Medical College, March 7th, 1850: On the Frequency of Suits for Mal-Practice in Western New-York* (Geneva, 1850), 14–15.

61. H. John Anthon, "A Course of Lectures on Medical Jurisprudence," *New York Medical Press* 2 (1859): 461–68, 487–95, 519–25, 551–56, 583–88, 615–20, 665–70, 697–701; quote: 467.

62. See "Opinion of the Hon. Judge Ellis Lewis," *AJMS* n.s. 12 (1846): 538–40.

63. "The Right of a Physician to compensation for making a Post-mortem examination at the request of a Coroner," *AJMS* n.s. 13 (1847): 257–58.

64. Alexander H. Stevens, "Annual Address, before the Medical Society of the State of New-York and Members of the Legislature. Delivered in the Capitol at Albany, February 6, 1850," *Transactions of the Medical Society of the State of New York, 1850* (Albany, 1850), 5–23, and reprinted as *Assembly Document # 174*; and Jenks S. Sprague, "Observations on various subjects in Forensic Medicine," *ibid.*, 208–24.

65. Samuel Parkman, "On the Relations of the Medical Witness with the Law and the Lawyer," *AJMS* n.s. 23 (1852): 126–34 (Parker originally read this paper before the Boston Society for Medical Observation); and "Medical Men as Witnesses in Court," *New Orleans Medical and Surgical Journal* 8 (1852): 685.

66. *Constitution, By-Laws, and Code of Ethics of the Illinois State Medical Society,*

adopted 1850 (Chicago, 1865), 25. Illinois physicians were especially annoyed about having to perform uncompensated post-mortem examinations.

67. Beck and Beck, *Elements* (1851 ed.), vol. 2: 921.

68. *Ibid.* 921–22, and *Elements* (1860 ed.), vol. 2: 958–59.

69. Medicus, "Testimony of Experts," *New York Medical Press* 3 (1860): 350.

CHAPTER SEVEN

1. R.E. Griffith, "On Medical Jurisprudence," *PJMPS* 10 (1825): 36–46.

2. T.R. Beck, "Annual Address Delivered before the Medical Society of the State of New-York, Feb. 6, 1828," *NYMPJ* 7 (1828): 9–34, and also reprinted in *Transactions of the Medical Society of the State of New-York* (Albany, 1828), 41–63.

3. Thomas Starkie, *A Practical Treatise on the Law of Evidence, and Digest of Proofs in Civil and Criminal Proceedings, with References to American Decisions, By Theron Metcalf* (Boston and Philadelphia, 1826), vol. 1: 74–75; the same *With References to American Decisions, by Theron Metcalf and Edward D. Ingraham* (Philadelphia, 1832); and the same *With References to American Decisions, and to the English Common Law and Ecclesiastical [sic] Reports*, by Theron Metcalf, Edward D. Ingraham, and Benjamin Gerhard (Philadelphia, 1837), 68–69. Not until the second edition did the American annotators have a specific case to cite for this doctrine.

4. Beck, "Annual Address," 18.

5. Burton J. Bledstein, *The Culture of Professionalism: The Middle Class and the Development of Higher Education in America* (New York, 1976), 65–79; JoAnne Brown, "Professional Language: Words That Succeed," *Radical History Review*, 34 (1986): 33–51; Joseph Ben-David, "Roles and Innovations in Medicine," *American Journal of Sociology* 65 (1965): 557–68; Harold L. Wilensky, "The Professionalization of Everyone?," *American Journal of Sociology* 70 (1964): 137–58; S. E. D. Shortt, "Physicians, Science, and Status: Issues in the Professionalization of Anglo-American Medicine in the Nineteenth Century," *Medical History* 27 (1983): 51–68.

6. Michael Ryan, *A Manual of Medical Jurisprudence, Compiled from the Best Medical and Legal Works: Being an Analysis of a Course of Lectures on Forensic Medicine, Annually Delivered in London* (1st American ed., Philadelphia, 1832), R. Eglesfeld Griffith, ed., editor's footnote, 315.

7. Beck, "Annual Address," 19.

8. *Ibid.*, 24.

9. The Donellan case was much discussed by Americans interested in medical jurisprudence. Beck was convinced that John Hunter erred in that case and said so in the *Elements*, though he considered the evidence sufficient for the verdict. Stephen Williams at Berkshire, on the other hand, thought the evidence insufficient in his *Catechism* of 1835, 12. The quote here is from Beck, "Annual Address," 26. Hunter's testimony appears verbatim in some editions of the *Elements*. See, for example, the seventh edition (London, 1842), 1017–20.

10. Beck's own New York began to undercut the use of books and the admissibility of their contents as evidence in a major ruling in 1858. While some states, including Iowa and Alabama, continued to allow the admissibility of medical texts through the 1880s, most followed New York. At least one state, Maine, had barred texts earlier, in 1831. Later medico-legal theorists went along with this shift in the law of evidence largely on the grounds stated by a court in North Carolina in 1877: "The medical work which was a 'standard' last year becomes obsolete this year." For the situation after the Civil War, see John J. Elwell, *A Medico-Legal Treatise on*

Malpractice and Medical Evidence, Comprising the Elements of Medical Jurisprudence [new edition] (New York, 1866), 331–37. For a fine overview of this issue in the nineteenth century see Henry Wade Rogers, *The Law of Expert Testimony* (St. Louis, 1883), 234–51, from which the quotation above is taken.

11. Beck, "Annual Address," 26.

12. Beck and Beck, *Elements* (5th ed., 1835), vol. 2: 656.

13. I.R. [Isaac Ray?], "Medical Evidence," *American Jurist* 24 (1841): 294–306; quotes: 294, 295, 306.

14. Beck, "Annual Address," 14.

15. Griffith, "Medical Jurisprudence," 42–43.

16. N[athan]. S. Davis, "Medico-Legal Testimony, on the Trial of Mrs. Turpening for the Murder of Her Husband, with Observations on the Same," *Transactions of the Medical Society of the State of New-York* (Albany, 1846), 50–65.

17. "Medical Men as Witnesses in Court," *New Orleans Medical and Surgical Journal* 8 (1852): 685–86.

18. A.K. Taylor, "Law and Physic," *Memphis Medical Recorder* 3 (1854): 106–8.

19. *DAMB* 2: 722.

20. David Humphreys Storer, "Medical Jurisprudence," *Medical Communications of the Massachusetts Medical Society* 3 (1851): 131–163. This address was also reprinted separately by John Wilson and Son of Boston in 1851 and circulated under the title *An Address on Medical Jurisprudence: Its Claims to Greater Regard From the Student and the Physician*.

21. The son, Horatio Robinson Storer, would emerge by the late 1850s as the leader of America's first national anti-abortion crusade. See James C. Mohr, *Abortion in America: The Origins and Evolution of National Policy, 1800–1900* (New York, 1978), 147–70.

22. *BMSJ* 24 (1841) 92–94, 121–23.

23. *Ibid.*, 123.

24. D.H. Storer, "Medical Jurisprudence," 135.

25. *Ibid.*, 137.

26. Samuel Parkman, "On the Relations of the Medical Witness with the Law and the Lawyer," *AJMS* n.s. 23 (1852): 126–34; quote: 126–27.

27. *Ibid.*, 129–32.

28. Thomas A. Logan, "Physicians as Witnesses," *Cincinnati Lancet and Observer* 2 (1859): 149.

29. James Wynne, *Importance of the Study of Legal Medicine, A Lecture Introductory to the Course on Medical Jurisprudence, at the New York Medical College* (New York, London, and Paris, 1859), 1.

30. Parkman, "Relations of the Medical Witness," 127.

31. *DAB* 9: 515–16. Thurman, one of Ohio's leading Democrats, would remain a first-rank political figure through Reconstruction.

32. William Frederick Norwood, *Medical Education in the United States Before the Civil War* (Philadelphia, 1944), 328–29.

33. Hon. A. G. Thurman, "Annual Address, Delivered at Commencement of Starling Medical College, March 3, 1857," *Ohio Medical and Surgical Journal* 9 (1857): 347–56; quote: 349.

34. *Ibid.*, 351, 352, 353.

35. Many historians of American law have demonstrated that lawyers worked during the first half of the nineteenth century to formalize rules of procedure that would enhance both the courts and the legal professionals who controlled them. For

recent discussions of that process, see Morton Horwitz, *The Transformation of American Law, 1780–1860* (Cambridge, Mass., 1977), and the debate over his position in Wythe Holt, "Morton Horwitz and the Transformation of American Legal History," *William and Mary Law Review* 23 (1982): 663–723; Robert W. Gordon, "Historicism in Legal Scholarship," *Yale Law Journal* 90 (1981): 1017–56; and Charles J. McClain, Jr., "Legal Change and Class Interests: A Review Essay on Morton Horwitz's *The Transformation of American Law*," *California Law Review* 68 (1980): 382–97.

36. Thurman, "Annual Address," 354–55; quote: 355.

37. *Ibid.*, 356.

38. *Ibid.*

CHAPTER EIGHT

1. William Blackstone, *Commentaries on the Laws of England* (facsimile rpt. of 1st ed.), vol. 3, *Of Private Wrongs* (originally 1768), Chapter 8: 122. In various forms, of course, the concept of medical malpractice far predated Blackstone as well, though they are less germane to the situation in the United States. See, for example, Michael T. Walton, "The Advisory Jury and Malpractice in 15th Century London: The Case of William Forest," *Journal of the History of Medicine* 40 (Oct. 1983): 478–82.

2. See, for example, the first three editions of Thomas Starkie, *A Practical Treatise on the Law of Evidence, and Digest of Proofs in Civil and Criminal Proceedings, with References to American Decisions, by Theron Metcalf* (Boston and Philadelphia, 1826; slightly variant title, Philadelphia, 1832; and another slightly variant title, Philadelphia, 1837). These multi-volume standards do not address medical malpractice.

3. R.E.G[riffith]., review of Adolphe Trebuchet, *Jurisprudence de la médecine, de la chirurgie, et de la pharmacie, en France* (Paris, 1834), in *AJMS* 15 (1834–35): 168–70.

4. "Michael O'Neil vs. Gerard Bancker," *NYMPJ* 6 (1827): 145–52. Irregularities occur in the spelling of the physician's name, but it is rendered throughout the text of the story as Banker. That spelling will be used in the text.

5. *Ibid.*, 151.

6. Many of the principals in this well-known case, *Lowell v. Hawks and Faxon*, ended up publishing their own version of what they considered most important about the affair. See, for example, Charles Lowell, *An authentic report of a trial before the Supreme judicial court of Maine, for the county of Washington, June term, 1824: Charles Lowell vs. John Faxon & Micajan Hawks, surgeons and physicians, in an action of trespass on the case for ignorance and negligence* (Portland, 1825); Lowell, *Report of the trial of an action, Charles Lowell against John Faxon and Micajah Hawks, doctors of medicine, defendants, for malpractice in the capacity of physicians and surgeons, at the Supreme judicial court of Maine, holden at Machias for the county of Washington—June term, 1824. Before the Hon. Nathan Weston, Jun., Justice of the court* (Portland, 1825); and the public letter issued by John C. Warren: *A Letter to the Hon. Isaac Parker, Chief Justice of the Supreme Court of the State of Massachusetts, Containing Remarks on the Dislocation of the Hip Joint, Occasioned by the Publication of a Trial which took place at Machias, in the State of Maine, June, 1824* (Cambridge, Mass., 1826).

7. " 'Medical Jurisprudence' by Nathan Smith," 138; lecture notes by A[very]. J. S[kelton]. taken at Yale; probably in Feb. 1827; NLM. The Connecticut dislocation case involved a shoulder.

8. The standard essay on this subject for some time has been Chester R. Burns,

"Malpractice Suits in American Medicine Before the Civil War," *BHM* 43 (1969): 41–56. Burns, in turn, had benefitted from the surveys of Hubert W. Smith, "Legal Responsibility for Medical Malpractice, IV: Malpractice Claims in the United States and a Proposed Formula for Testing Their Legal Sufficiency," *JAMA* 116 (1941): 2670–79; and Andrew A. Sandor, "The History of Professional Liability Suits in the United States," *JAMA* 163 (1957): 459–66. More recently, Kenneth A. De Ville completed a monograph that has added enormously to this and related inquiries about medical malpractice in the United States during the nineteenth century. De Ville was kind enough to share his manuscript with me prior to its publication. References here are to that manuscript. The book itself, which is now available, is Kenneth Allen De Ville, *Medical Malpractice in Nineteenth-Century America: Origins and Legacy* (New York, 1990).

9. De Ville, *Origins*, 1–5. The 2.3 percent represented 5 of the 216 total cases. What percentage of all medical malpractice cases reached appellate courts, of course, is also impossible to judge. There is some reason to use a 1 percent ratio for later periods, but that seems a bit low for the early period, when malpractice cases, precisely because they were oddities, might more likely be appealed. In any event, it seems safe to state that fewer than 500 medical malpractice actions were brought in all American courts combined prior to 1835, and the total is probably much lower.

10. *Ibid.*, 4–5 and Table 1.

11. *Ibid.*, *passim*, discusses many of these and other factors. On the erosion of therapeutic differences by region, see John Harley Warner, *The Therapeutic Perspective: Medical Practice, Knowledge, and Identity in America, 1820–1885* (Cambridge, Mass., 1986).

12. De Ville, *Origins*, 45.

13. *Ibid.*, 4, Table 1.

14. "Doings of the Courtland County (N. Y.) Medical Society," *BMSJ* 26 (Feb. 16, 1842): 33–34.

15. William G. Rothstein, *American Physicians in the Nineteenth Century: From Sects to Science* (Baltimore, 1972), 324–25.

16. William Wood, "Thoughts on Suits for Malpractice, suggested by certain Judicial Proceedings in Erie County, Pennsylvania," *AJMS* n.s. 18 (1849): 400.

17. De Ville, *Origins*, 373–459, and *passim*. All of these trends are evident as well in many articles that appeared during the 1840s and 1850s in the nation's leading contemporary medical journals.

18. Walter Channing, "A Medico-Legal Treatise on Malpractice and Medical Evidence—A Review," *BMSJ* 62 (1860): 306; emphasis in original.

19. *Ibid.*, 233–41, 259–65, 300–307.

20. "Medical Miscellany," *BMSJ* 42 (Feb. 20, 1850): 67.

21. *American Law Journal* n.s. 1 (1849): 284–85.

22. *Ibid.*, 284; n.s. 2 (1849–50): 330–33. On the adoption of anesthetics, see Martin Pernick, *A Calculus of Suffering: Pain, Professionalism, and Anesthesia in Nineteenth-Century America* (New York, 1985).

23. *JAMA* (1887): 839.

24. "Medical Miscellany," *BMSJ* 35 (Oct. 7, 1846): 207.

25. "Liability of Physicians and Surgeons," *BMSJ* 48 (July 20, 1853): 506–7.

26. The quote is from "Medical Notes," *BMSJ* 100 (1878): 91. The larger report is E[ugene]. F. Sanger, "Report of the Committee on Suits for Malpractice," *Transactions of the Maine Medical Association* 6 (1878): 360–82.

27. On Geneva Medical College at this time see William Frederick Norwood, *Medical Education in the United States Before the Civil War* (Philadelphia, 1944), 155–59, 164, 411–42.

28. "Accusation of Mal-practice," *BMSJ* 31 (1844): 123.

29. This case, *Smith v. Goodyear and Hyde,* is developed at length by De Ville, *Origins,* 281–302, and may easily be tracked in detail through the medical journals and regional newspapers of the period.

30. *Ibid.,* 200–203, 277; Frank H. Hamilton, *Fracture Tables* (Buffalo, 1853); and James H. Cassedy, *American Medicine and Statistical Thinking, 1800–1860* (Cambridge, Mass., 1984), 87–88.

31. James Webster, Jr., *Medical Jurisprudence* (Philadelphia, M.D. thesis, submitted April 8, 1824; now bound with Miscellaneous Theses, College of Physicians of Philadelphia, Vol. 1), 2.

32. James Webster, *Introductory to the Course on Anatomy, in Geneva Medical College, March 7th, 1850* (Geneva, 1850), 6 (now in the pamphlet collection, College of Physicians of Philadelphia).

33. *Ibid.,* 6–7.

34. *Ibid.,* 6, 12.

35. C.R. Gilman, who was professor of medical jurisprudence at the College of Physicians and Surgeons of New York, took the editorial lead in preparation of the eleventh edition, but at least fifteen other medical scientists also contributed to the effort.

36. E [dward]. H [artshorne]., "Art. XXXII," *AJMS* n.s. 39 (1860): 211–12.

37. John J. Elwell, *A Medico-Legal Treatise on Malpractice and Medical Evidence, Comprising the Elements of Medical Jurisprudence* (New York, 1860), Preface, 7–9, 10, 12, and *passim.*

38. S [tephen]. S [mith]., "Art. XV," *AJMS* n.s. 40 (1860): 155.

39. See, for example, the resolution of the Medical Association of Southern Central New York, reprinted and endorsed in *BMSJ* 52 (July 5, 1855): 444.

40. Walter Channing to J.J. Elwell, May 16, 1860, reprinted in the front matter of the 1866 edition of Elwell's *Malpractice.* For Channing's long, favorable review of the book see *BMSJ* 62 (1860): 233–41, 259–65, 300–307.

41. Jno. Ordronaux to J.J. Elwell, March 8, 1860, reprinted in the front matter of the 1866 edition of Elwell's *Malpractice.*

42. Robley Dunglison to J.J. Elwell, n.d., reprinted *ibid.*

43. Excerpts from these reviews are reprinted *ibid.*

44. "Notice" of Elwell's *Malpractice, New York Medical Press* 3 (1860): 141–42; italics in original.

45. *BMSJ* 52 (July 5, 1855): 444.

46. For Smith's activities as a health reformer, see James C. Mohr, *The Radical Republicans and Reform in New York during Reconstruction* (Ithaca, 1973), 61–85. Smith's review of Elwell's *Malpractice* appeared as S [tephen]. S [mith]., "Art. XV," *AJMS* n.s. 40 (1860): 153–66; quote: 166.

47. On Ordronaux, see *NCAB* 12: 331–32; *DAB* 7: 50–52. Both Ordronaux and the lunacy commission are also discussed in Chapter Twelve.

48. Milo McClelland, *Civil Malpractice* (New York, 1873). This was a reprint for national publication of a report McClelland had done on malpractice for the Chicago Medical Society.

49. *NCAB* 27: 351–52. After his retirement in 1924, interestingly enough, Lewis switched sides and took "numerous malpractice actions, this time on behalf of the

plaintiff." The other two people singled out for work in the field of medical juris-prudence were James W. Putnam, the AMA president and neurologist who was considered among the nation's leading authorities on the forensic aspects of insanity, and William C. Woodward, the Washington, D.C., sanitation reformer who also taught medical jurisprudence many years at Georgetown and other universities.

50. De Ville, *Origins*, 373–78, 399–402. The Medical and Surgical Society of Baltimore was a good example of a local medical association that pledged its members to mutual defense in court: *Maryland Medical Journal* 6, no. 2 (1879): 135–36. An excellent example of a local medical society responding effectively to a malprac-tice threat in San Francisco in 1885 is chronicled in Neil Larry Shumsky, Paul Knox, and James Bohland, " 'All for One and One for All': Medical Professional-ization in San Francisco, 1850–1900," unpublished paper kindly supplied by the authors.

51. The reverse, according to Paul Starr, was also true by 1900: consolidation helped mute some of the most professionally damaging aspects of the early malprac-tice crisis. Starr, *The Social Transformation of American Medicine: The Rise of a Sovereign Profession and the Making of a Vast Industry* (New York, 1982), 111.

CHAPTER NINE

1. T.R. Beck, "Review," *AJMS* n.s. 2 (1841): 403–35. Seven of the nine pieces reviewed, incidentally, were French; one was English; and one was by a South Carolinian working in Paris. This article also takes a look at the 1840 trial of the infamous poisoner Madame Lafarge, in which Orfila was a key witness.

2. *Albany Evening Journal*, March 10, 1853.

3. This summary, as well as what follows, is taken from David M. Barnes and W[infield] S. Hevenor, reporters and compilers, *Trial of John Hendrickson, Jr., for the Murder of his Wife Maria, by Poisoning, At Bethlehem, Albany County, N. Y., March 6th, 1853. Tried in the Court of Oyer and Terminer, at Albany, N. Y., in June and July, 1853* (Albany, 1853), vii and 176 pps. Barnes was a newspaper reporter; Hevenor was assistant district attorney of Albany County. All subsequent references to the trial, unless otherwise noted, are from this book. The *Albany Evening Journal* also tracked the entire case from start to finish and beyond. References specific to the *Journal*'s account will be cited separately.

4. *Albany Evening Journal*, March 12 and 15, 1853.

5. *Ibid.*, March 16, 21, 24, 25, 28, 30, 1853; April 1, 9, 16, 1853.

6. Among the classical writers who mention aconite are Ovid, Pliny, and Theophrastus.

7. Aconite is, of course, still in the *American Pharmacopeia* and still used as a heart depressant. For the use of aconite by regular physicians at mid-century see John Harley Warner, *The Therapeutic Perspective: Medical Practice, Knowledge, and Identity in America, 1820–1885* (Cambridge, Mass., 1986), 101, 117, 119, 130, 212, 227.

8. James H. Salisbury, "An Account of Some Experiments and Observations on the Influence of Poisons and Medicinal Agents upon Plants," *New York Medical Journal* n.s. 12 (1854): 9–15.

9. Reid had emigrated to the United States from Edinburgh. His brother's book was *Reid's Elements of Practical Chemistry*.

10. Those interested in Wells's later fame as a leading political economist and governmental adviser can begin with the *DAB* 10: 637–38. Wells's papers are at LC, but do not contain anything on this incident.

11. *BMSJ* 50, no. 15 (May 10, 1854): 289–304.

12. David A. Wells, "Poisoning by Aconite: A Second Review of the Trial of John Hendrickson, Jr.," *Medical and Surgical Reporter* (Philadelphia) 8 (1862): 110–18; C[harles] A. L[ee], "Review of Barnes and Hevenor, *Trial of John Hendrickson, Jr., for the Murder of his Wife by Poisoning, at Bethlehem, Albany County, N.Y., March 6, 1853* (Albany, 1853) 8 vo. pp. 176," in *AJMS* n.s. 28 (1854): 459; *Albany Evening Journal*, May 1, 1854, 2.

13. Clark to Beck in Wells, "Interesting Case," 302–3. On Clark personally see *Appleton's Cyclopaedia of American Biography* 1: 624.

14. Clark to Beck in Wells, "Interesting Case," 302–3.

15. *Albany Evening Journal*, April 29, 1854; Wells, "Poisoning by Aconite," 117; and Lee, "Review," 453.

16. The resolution is reprinted in Wells, "Interesting Case," 303–4; and in Lee, "Review," 453–54.

17. On Lee's national reputation as a statistically minded leader of the profession see James H. Cassedy, *American Medicine and Statistical Thinking, 1800–1860* (Cambridge, Mass., 1984), 72, 117–19, 183, 200–202.

18. Lee, "Review," 466.

19. George H. Tucker, "A Contribution to our Knowledge of Poisoning by Aconite," *New York Journal of Medicine* n.s. 12 (1854): 222–39. Tucker found only 53 cases in the entire world literature.

20. Charles D. Smith, "Case IV, poisoning by aconite," *New York Medical Journal* 3 (1854): 200–201, and Oswald Warner, "Case of Poisoning by Aconite," *ibid.* 4 (1855): 242–44.

21. The Supreme Court affirmed the conviction December 8, 1853, and the Court of Appeals did the same, by a vote of 5–3, on April 4, 1854. See *New York Times*, May 8, 1854: 1–2. The legal press also followed the appeal, part of which hinged upon the issue of self-incrimination while testifying before coroners' juries prior to indictment. See *American Law Register* 2 (1853–54): 531–42.

22. *Albany Evening Journal*, April 29, 1854: 2.

23. *Ibid.*, May 1, 1854, p.2. The piece was signed only A.J.C., but is legalistic in its arguments and may confidently be attributed to the district attorney.

24. The letter is reprinted in John Swinburne, "Poisoning by Aconite: Trial of John Hendrickson, Jr., for the Poisoning of His Wife in 1853," *Medical and Surgical Reporter* (Philadelphia), n.s. 7 (1862): 369–70.

25. *Albany Evening Journal*, May 3, 1854: 2.

26. Stewart Mitchell, *Horatio Seymour of New York* (Cambridge, Mass., 1938) and *DAB* 9: 6–9.

27. Barnes and Hevenor, *Trial*, 176.

28. *New York Daily Times*, May 8, 1854: 1–2; *BMSJ* 50, no.15 (May 10, 1854): 307.

29. *Examination as to the Death of Priscilla Budge Before the Coroner and a Jury* (New York, 1860), 11–12, 114–40; the question-and-answer duel: 129. This case was also mentioned frequently in later years in medico-legal writings. Unlike the Hendrickson case, however, Swinburne had a good deal of national and international support for his position in the Budge trial, which helped rehabilitate his standing. See [Citizens' Association of New York] *A Typical American; or, Incidents in the Life of Dr. John Swinburne of Albany, the Eminent Patriot, Surgeon, and Philanthropist* (Albany, 1888), 195–211.

30. Alfred Taylor, *Medical Jurisprudence*, Edward Hartshorne, ed., 4th American from the 5th London ed. (Philadelphia, 1856), 169.

31. *Ibid.*, 5th American from the 7th London ed. (Philadelphia, 1861), 37.

32. David A. Wells, *Wells's Principles and Applications of Chemistry* (New York and Chicago, 1858), 457.

33. Swinburne, "Poisoning by Aconite," 361–76.

34. Wells, "Poisoning by Aconite: A Second Review," 110–18.

35. This request was reported in the *Albany Evening Journal*, March 16, 1853: 2.

36. J. H. Salisbury, "Some Experiments on Poisoning with the Vegetable Alkaloids," *AJMS* n.s. 44 (1862): 413, and Salisbury, "Experiments Connected with the Discovery of Cholesterine and Seroline as Secretions . . . ," *ibid.* n.s. 45 (1863): 289.

37. See, for example, Salisbury, "Physiological Observations and Experiments . . . ," *ibid.* n.s. 50 (1865): 413–16; Salisbury, "Microscopic Researches . . . ," *ibid.* n.s. 51 (1866): 307–39; Salisbury and M. W. House, "Physiological Experiments," *ibid.* n.s. 52 (1866): 92–96.

38. Salisbury, "Some Experiments on Poisoning with the Vegetable Alkaloids," 413–40.

39. *Ibid.* n.s. 54 (1867): 571, and *ibid.* n.s. Vol. 55 (1868): 17–24. Salisbury based his claims on his microscopic observations of matter taken from the sores of people suffering from the two diseases.

CHAPTER TEN

1. T. R. Beck, "Review," *AJMS* n.s. 2 (1841): 403.

2. The discussion in this chapter is entirely within the context of *public* asylums, creations of the state, since one of the key relationships involved here is that between physicians, on the one hand, and the state, including its laws and its secondary institutions, on the other. *Private* asylums for the insane, which paying customers made separate decisions to use or to avoid, continued to exist, even proliferate, through this era. But *private* asylums tended to serve particular subsets of society and would have disappeared if they ceased to perform the functions their clients desired.

3. This, ironically enough, is one of the few subjects in the entire history of legal medicine to receive anything like the serious analytical attention it deserves. Some scholars have approached the subject from the perspective of legal history, and readers should have little trouble finding numerous references to the development of the insanity defense in American law. Among studies that have integrated that legal story into larger medical, social, and political patterns, Charles E. Rosenberg's excellent monograph *The Trial of the Assassin Guiteau: Psychiatry and Law in the Gilded Age* (Chicago, 1968) still stands out and is still the place to begin.

A long bibliographical essay would be required to explain exactly why the history of insanity has received so much more attention than other aspects of medical jurisprudence; and this is really not the place for such an essay. At minimum, that essay would need to look closely at shifting concepts of consciousness in the post-Freudian West, at the profound doubts concerning individual motivation that have arisen in late twentieth-century intellectual life, at the modern resurgence of interest in the irrational, at the use of the concept of insanity for overtly political ends, at the debate over those political usages, and at the increased power of what might be called the interventionist professions.

4. Edward Jarvis, "The Influence of Distance from and Proximity to an Insane Hospital, on Its Use by Any People," *BMSJ* 42 (1850): 209–22.

5. In Massachusetts, see *Report of the Joint Committee of the Legislature of Massachusetts, Appointed April 20, 1848, on the Subject of Insanity in the State, and Directed to Sit During the Recess of the Legislature, and to Report at the Early Part of the Session of 1849, Senate Documents* (1849), No. 60; in Rhode Island, see Thomas R. Hazard, *Report of the Poor and Insane in Rhode Island; Made to the General Assembly at Its January Session, 1851* (Providence, 1851); and in New York, see *Report of the Select Committee on Report and Memorial of County Superintendents of the Poor, on Lunacy and Its Relation to Pauperism, New York Senate Documents* (1856), No. 71, and *Report of Select Committee Appointed to Visit Charitable Institutions Supported by the State, and All City and County Poor and Work Houses and Jails, New York Senate Documents* (1857), No. 8.

6. Helen E. Marshall, *Dorothea Dix: Forgotten Samaritan* (New York, 1937 [and rpt. 1967]), 148–54; Dorothy Clarke Wilson, *Stranger and Traveler: The Story of Dorothea Dix, American Reformer* (Boston, 1975), 205–12; Edith Abbott, *Some American Pioneers in Social Welfare: Select Documents with Editorial Notes* (New York, 1937 [rpt. 1965]), 124–27; *A Compilation of the Messages and Papers of the Presidents*, James D. Richardson, ed. (New York, 1897), vol. 6: 2780–89.

7. This section follows the analysis in Gerald Grob, *Mental Institutions in America: Social Policy to 1875* (New York, 1973), 115–150; quote: 150.

8. [Edward Jarvis] *Report on Insanity and Idiocy in Massachusetts, by the Commission on Lunacy, Under Resolve of the Legislature of 1854, Massachusetts House Documents* (1855), No. 144.

9. See, for example, *BMSJ* 42 (1850): 146; 42 (1851):467; 45 (1852): 537; and 46 (1852): 85.

10. Grob, *Institutions to 1875*, 84–131 and Appendix IV.

11. There are many survey overviews of the *mens rea* doctrine and the insanity defense. Readers should have no trouble documenting the points made in this paragraph. Among the most recent, many of which were triggered by the 1982 trial of would-be presidential assassin John W. Hinckley, Jr., is Thomas Maeder, *Crime and Madness: The Origins and Evolution of the Insanity Defense* (New York, 1985), 1–22. The "lucid interval" debate, which continued to rage through the nineteenth century, hinged upon the possibility that a person could be perfectly sane and reasonable some of the time but deranged and unreasonable at other times, hence responsible some of the time and not responsible at other times.

12. William E. Nelson, *Americanization of the Common Law: The Impact of Legal Change on Massachusetts Society, 1760–1830* (Cambridge, Mass., 1975) and *The Roots of American Bureaucracy, 1830–1900* (Cambridge, Mass., 1982); Lawrence M. Friedman, *A History of American Law* (New York, 1973), esp. 248–58; Kermit L. Hall, *The Magic Mirror: Law in American History* (New York, 1989).

13. On this point, see Janet Ann Tighe, *A Question of Responsibility: The Development of American Forensic Psychiatry, 1838–1930* (Ph.D. dissertation, UP, 1983; University Microfilms International, Ann Arbor, 1984), esp. 1–19.

14. Suicide appears to have been an exception to this rule. Many suicides were routinely judged (after the fact, of course) to have been temporarily insane. But that ruling constituted something of a special case, for it risked no danger to society, assuaged family images, sometimes affected the disposition of inheritance, and often preserved insurance policies. On suicide in American history see Howard I. Kushner, *Self-destruction in the Promised Land: A Psychocultural Biology of American Suicide* (New Brunswick, 1989).

15. Exactly what to do with the criminally insane remained a difficult problem for decades. In the 1820s the Chancellor of New York's equity courts had theoretical jurisdiction over insane criminals, but it was not clear where he could put them or for how long. That solution ended in any event with the subsequent elimination of the equity courts in New York. *ALJ* 7 (1873): 85, 100, 273–79, tracks a debate in the New York legislature over how to address the problem.

16. Stanley L. Block, "Daniel Drake and the Insanity Plea," *BHM* 65, no. 3 (1991): 326–39.

17. Isaac Ray, *A Treatise on the Medical Jurisprudence of Insanity* ([Boston, 1838] rpt. Cambridge, 1962), 78.

18. Rush had alluded to criminal implications in his *Inaugural Address* of 1811, but made little of them.

19. Beck, *Elements* (1832 ed.), vol. 1: 362–63.

20. *NYMPJ* 3 (1824): 250–52; quote: 252.

21. These observations are drawn primarily from the best recent study of Ray: John Starrett Hughes, *In the Law's Darkness: Insanity and the Medical-Legal Career of Isaac Ray, 1807–1881* (Ph.D. dissertation, Rice University, 1982; Ann Arbor, 1983), iii, 8–29, 77, and *passim*.

22. Ray, *Treatise*, 78. For a detailed analysis of Ray's shifting arguments over the years and of his impact on forensic psychiatry, see Tighe, *Question of Responsibility*.

23. Tighe, *Question of Responsibility*, 45–46.

24. On Ray and the editions of his book, see Isaac Ray, *A Treatise on the Medical Jurisprudence of Insanity* [Winfred Overholzer, ed.], reprint edition (Cambridge, Mass., 1962), "Editor's Introduction," vii–xvi, and "A Note on the Text," xvii.

25. See, for example, I. R. [probably Isaac Ray, this was a Boston-based journal], "Mittermaier on the Excuse of Insanity," *American Jurist* 22 (1840): 311–29.

26. The literature on the M'Naghten case and the M'Naghten Rule is extensive. Readers may wish to consult the following, all of which have proved useful in developing the discussion here: Roger Smith, *Trial by Medicine: Insanity and Responsibility in Victorian Trials* (Edinburgh, 1981); Anthony Platt and Bernard Diamond, "The Origins of the 'Right and Wrong' Test of Criminal Responsibility and Its Subsequent Development in the United States: An Historical Survey," *California Law Review* 54 (1966): 1227–60; Jacques Quen, "Anglo-American Criminal Insanity: An Historical Perspective," *Journal of the History of the Behavioral Sciences* 4 (1974): 313–23; and Quen, "An Historical View of the M'Naghten Trial," *BHM* 42 (1968): 43–51. For true aficionados, there is even a literature on the spelling of M'Naghten's name.

27. Tighe, *Question of Responsibility*; Hall, *The Magic Mirror*, 185–87; Maeder, *Crime and Madness*; Hughes, *In the Law's Darkness*; Louis E. Reik, "Doe-Ray Correspondence: A Pioneer Collaboration in the Jurisprudence of Mental Disease," *Yale Law Review* 63 (1953): 183–96.

28. Hughes, *In the Law's Darkness*, iii, 63.

29. Charles R. King, "Review of J. Ray's *A Treatise on the Medical Jurisprudence of Insanity*, 2nd ed. (Boston, 1844)," *AJMS* n.s. 9 (1845): 391–93.

30. Robley Dunglison, ed., *The Cyclopaedia of Practical Medicine* (Philadelphia, 1845), 332.

31. Samuel White, "Annual Address delivered before the Medical Society of the State of New-York, Feb. 7, 1844," *Transactions of the New-York State Medical Society, 1844–46* 6 (Albany, 1846), 1–21; quotes: 8, 9.

32. John McCall, "Annual Address, delivered before the Medical Society of the State of New-York, in the Assembly Chamber of the Capitol, at the City of Albany, February 3, 1847," *ibid.*, *1847–49* 7 (Albany, 1849), 1–13; quote: 12.

33. E[ward] H[artshorne], "Art. XVIII [a review of Wharton and Stillé, *Medical Jurisprudence*]," *AJMS* n.s. 31 (1856): 171.

34. Tighe, *Question of Responsibility*, 48–54.

35. James Wynne, *Importance of the Study of Legal Medicine; A Lecture Introductory to the Course on Medical Jurisprudence, at the New York Medical College* (New York, London, and Paris, 1859), 13.

36. "Common Pleas of the City and County of Phil'a *[sic]*," *American Law Journal* n.s. 3 (1850–51): 531.

37. C. B. Coventry, "Report on the Medical Jurisprudence of Insanity," *TAMA* 11 (1858): 471–524; and D[avid] Meredith Reese, "Report on Moral Insanity in its Relations to Medical Jurisprudence," *ibid.*, 721–46.

38. Coventry, "Insanity," 473.

39. *Ibid.*; quotes: 510, 518, 520.

40. "Medical Miscellany," *BMSJ* 26 (Aug. 3, 1842): 419 for an announcement of Reese's invitation to accept the chair of medical jurisprudence at Washington Medical College in Baltimore.

41. Reese, "Moral Insanity"; quotes: 736, 741.

42. The Sickles-Key murder case was one of the best-covered stories of the decade, and may be followed in any of several papers of the period. I tracked it in the *New York Times*, the New York *Tribune*, and the *Baltimore Sun*. The version that follows is taken from those sources collectively. Those three together provided a full view, since the first was reasonably straightforward, the second was anti-Sickles for political reasons, and the third was more sympathetic to the Key family than most American papers (because the family was so well connected in Maryland). Only direct quotations, however, will be cited hereafter, along with references from other sources. The case is also covered in a biography of Sickles: W. A. Swanberg, *Sickles the Incredible* (New York, 1956), 37–76.

43. *New York Times*, April 11, 1859; italics in original.

44. *Ibid.*, April 15, 1859.

45. *Ibid.*, April 11, 1859.

46. *Ibid.*, April 15, 1859.

47. *The Liberator* (Boston) 29, no. 18 (May 6, 1859), editorial "Acquittal of Sickles." The fact that Garrison's paper would discuss this case at all is evidence of the wide publicity it received.

48. *New York Times*, April 27, 1859, and *Supplement to the New York Times*, April 27, 1859.

49. In defense of this general reaction, it was all but universally conceded that Sickles (or anyone else for that matter) would not have been indicted in the first place under American precedent had he come upon the couple *in flagrante* and shot on the spot the man who was clearly in the act of violating his wife (with or without his wife's complicity, incidentally, which would probably not have been at issue in such a situation, though it could later become grounds for divorce). Though Sickles had learned about the adulterous relationship several days before the shooting, and of the signal Key used to summon Teresa, those who approved of the verdict reasoned implicitly that the sight of Key again offering that signal in Lafayette Park was, under the circumstances, tantamount to catching Key *in flagrante*. The lack of serious punishment for Key, if Sickles had simply confronted him with the law,

was also cited by many editorials that approved the verdict; that is, there were some circumstances in which the law did not mete out the punishment people deserved, and this was one of them. Lost, of course, was the fact that Sickles had a relatively long period to "cool off" after learning about the relationship, and the fact that Sickles's actual procedures (the taking of Teresa's statement, for example, and the nature of the fateful confrontation, during which Key pleaded for his life) resembled a deliberate assassination, however charged the circumstances, more than an act of spontaneous, reflexive emotion. Lost also was the fact that Sickles himself was a flamboyant philanderer. Not the least of the curious sequels to this strange event, however, was the reconciliation of Sickles and his wife, who continued their unhappy marriage until Teresa's relatively early death.

50. New York *Tribune*, April 27, 1859.

51. *Baltimore Sun*, April 28, 1859.

52. Leonard W. Levy, *The Law of the Commonwealth and Chief Justice Shaw* (Cambridge, Mass., 1957), 211–12, discusses *Commonwealth v. Rogers*, an 1844 case that might, depending upon interpretations of temporary insanity, stand as an earlier example of the basic tack taken by Sickles' attorneys. For a generation after the Sickles case, popular publications referred to the decision as a sort of metaphor for controversial justice, and, because the case was so well known, they could do so without explanation. See, for example, *Frank Leslie's Illustrated Newspaper*, May 28, 1870: 162.

CHAPTER ELEVEN

1. George Worthington Adams, *Doctors in Blue: The Medical History of the Union Army in the Civil War* (New York, 1952), 47, asserts that "more than 12,000 doctors had seen service in the field or in hospitals" by April 1865. Mary C. Gillett, *The Army Medical Department, 1818–1865* (Army Historical Series: Washington, D.C., 1987), 181, notes that "more than 5,500 civilian doctors assisted the Medical Department" during the Civil War. Along with Horace H. Cunningham, *Doctors in Gray: The Confederate Medical Service* (Baton Rouge, 1958), those books contain most of the information upon which the next several pages are based. Actual quotations and additional sources will be cited separately, but these studies will not be repeated in general reference.

2. On the role of physicians in support agencies see [United States Sanitary Commission], *The Sanitary Commission of the United States Army: A Succinct Narrative of Its Works and Purposes* (New York, 1864; rpt. New York, 1972); William Quentin Maxwell, *Lincoln's Fifth Wheel: The Political History of the United States Sanitary Commission* (New York, 1956); Sarah Edwards Henshaw, *Our Branch and Its Tributaries; Being a History of the Work of the Northwestern Sanitary Commission and Its Auxiliaries, During the War of the Rebellion* (Chicago, 1868); and William E. Parrish, "The Western Sanitary Commission," *Civil War History* 36, no. 1 (1990): 18–35.

3. On the Metropolitan Board of Health, see James C. Mohr, *Radical Republicans and Reform in New York during Reconstruction* (Ithaca, 1973), 61–114; on Swinburne's career see [Citizens' Association of New York] *A Typical American; or, Incidents in the Life of Dr. John Swinburne of Albany, the Eminent Patriot, Surgeon, and Philanthropist* (Albany, 1888), a campaign biography prepared for the gubernatorial race. In this biography, incidently, the Citizens' Association tried to make a virtue of Swinburne's controversial role as an expert witness and of his rivalries with some of those who attacked him in the Hendrickson and later cases. The clear intent was

to create the image of a people's expert, one who understood community realities and placed them above professional nit-picking. Swinburne never fully reconciled, however, with the Albany medical establishment. See *Report of the Special Committee of the Common Council of the City of Albany on the Affairs of the Albany Medical College and the Removal of Dr. John Swinburne* (n.p., n.d., but probably Albany, 1880).

4. Adams, *Doctors in Blue*, 49. Hammond himself had a lifelong interest in medico-legal issues, particularly in the medical jurisprudence of insanity, which will be discussed further in the next chapter.

5. Maxwell, *Lincoln's Fifth Wheel*, 293.

6. The best overview of the examining surgeons is Eugene C. Murdock, "Pity the Poor Surgeon," *Civil War History* 16 (1969–70): 18–36.

7. Peter T. Harstad, "A Civil War Medical Examiner: The Report of Dr. Horace O. Crane," *Wisconsin Magazine of History* 48 (1965): 222–31; quotes: 228, 229.

8. Hasket Derby, "The Relations of the Ophthalmoscope to Legal Medicine, Particularly as Regards the Detection of Simulated Myopia or Amaurosis in the Case of Persons Drafted for Military Service," *BMSJ* 66 (July 31, 1862): 525–28.

9. Murdock, "Surgeons," 27–29.

10. Some of the specific problems associated with the war on a large scale echoed long afterward on a smaller scale. M. A. McClelland, a close analyst of legal medicine after the war, noted in 1875 that "the medical practitioner is frequently applied to by parties seeking to evade public work such as road labor." Many of the sorts of evasions practiced by reluctant soldiers were practiced by reluctant road workers, and many of the same complications for and with physicians continued. "The Medical Expert and Medical Evidence," *Chicago Medical Journal and Examiner* 32 (1875): 102–3.

11. Murdock, "Surgeon," 26.

12. Harstad, "Civil War Medical Examiner," 227, 229.

13. John David Smith, "Kentucky Civil War Recruits: A Medical Profile," *Medical History* 24 (1980): 191.

14. Murdock, "Surgeon," 32–36.

15. [William A. Hammond] *A Statement of the Causes Which Led to the Dismissal of Surgeon-General William A. Hammond from the Army: With a Review of the Evidence Adduced Before the Court* (New York, 1864), esp. 6–8, 15, 18–19.

16. Gillett, *Medical Department*, 216, gives an excellent example of insubordination in the Sea Islands.

17. Gillett, *Military Department*, 268–69.

18. *Sanitary Commission*, 52.

19. Gillett, *Military Department*, 231.

20. A null hypothesis is inherently difficult to prove conclusively, but in over twenty years of research on this and related topics I have never seen any serious discussion in the record. Perhaps more significant, neither has Mary Gillett, the person who knows best the internal records of the Army Medical Department. Gillett to the author, May 1991.

21. Gillett, *Medical Department*, 251–52.

22. The general history of the Freedmen's Bureau is well known. On some of its specifically medical aspects see Marshall S. Legan, "Disease and the Freedmen in Mississippi During Reconstruction," *Journal of the History of Medicine and Allied Sciences* 28 (July 1973): 257–67; Todd L. Savitt, "Politics in Medicine: The Georgia Freedmen's Bureau and the Organization of Health Care," *Civil War History* 28 (March 1982): 45–64; Gaines M. Foster, "The Limitations of Federal Health Care

for Freedmen, 1862–1868," *Journal of Southern History* 48 (Aug. 1982): 349–72; and Eric Foner, *Reconstruction: America's Unfinished Revolution, 1863–1877* (New York, 1988), 151–52.

23. Foster, "Limitations of Federal Health Care," 368. The Freedmen's Hospital in the District of Columbia, which was administered directly by Congress, survived longer.

24. Paul Starr, *The Social Transformation of American Medicine: The Rise of a Sovereign Profession and the Making of a Vast Industry* (New York, 1982), 181–82, 191.

25. Henry I. Bowditch, *Public Hygiene in America: Being the Centennial Discourse Delivered Before the International Medical Congress, Philadelphia, September, 1876* (Boston, 1877); Hermann M. Biggs, "An Address: Sanitary Science, the Medical Profession, and the Public," *Medical News* 72 (1898): 44–50; John Duffy, *A History of Public Health in New York City, 1866–1966* (New York, 1974). Public opposition to public health reform showed clearly in central Wisconsin at least through the 1880s, where antipathies remained intense. See Jan Coombs, "Rural Medical Practice in the 1880s: A View from Central Wisconsin" (manuscript version of a convention paper kindly supplied by the author), 16–22.

CHAPTER TWELVE

1. Gerald Grob, *The State and the Mentally Ill: A History of the Worcester State Hospital in Massachusetts, 1830–1920* (Chapel Hill, 1966); *Mental Institutions in America: Social Policy to 1875* (New york, 1973); and *Mental Illness and American Society, 1875–1940* (Princeton, N.J., 1983); Charles E. Rosenberg, *The Trial of the Assassin Guiteau: Psychiatry and the Law in the Gilded Age* (Chicago, 1968); Janet Ann Tighe, *A Question of Responsibility: The Development of American Forensic Psychiatry, 1838–1930* (Ph.D. dissertation, UP, 1983; University Microfilms International, Ann Arbor, 1984), esp. 133–302; and John Starrett Hughes, *In the Law's Darkness: Insanity and the Medical-Legal Career of Isaac Ray, 1807–1881* (Ph.D. dissertation, Rice University, 1982; University Microfilms International, Ann Arbor, 1982), esp. 322–67. Their bibliographies, in turn, are rich sources of more detailed primary and secondary literature. Hughes subsequently published a revised version of his work: *In the Law's Darkness: Isaac Ray and the Medical Jurisprudence of Insanity in Nineteenth-Century America* (New York, 1986).

2. Tighe, *Question of Responsibility*, 63.

3. Ellen Dwyer, *Homes for the Mad: Life Inside Two Nineteenth-Century Asylums* (New Brunswick, 1987), 29–54, has a fine discussion of this process in the context of New York state.

4. Oliver Dyer and Dennis Murphy, *Speeches of Defendants' Counsel and the Charge of Judge Burnside in the Case of Hinchman vs. Richie, et al.* (Philadelphia, 1849), 87.

5. Grob, *Institutions to 1875*, p. 265, n. 8, cites two early exposes: Robert Fuller, *An Account of the Imprisonments and Sufferings of Robert Fuller, of Cambridge* (Boston, 1833), and Elizabeth T. Stone, *A Sketch of the Life of Elizabeth T. Stone, and of Her Persecutions, with an Appendix of Her Treatment and Sufferings While in the Charlestown McLean Asylum, Where She was Confined Under the Pretence of Insanity* (n.p., 1842). A somewhat later protest, which had attacked Isaac Ray personally, was Isaac Hunt, *Astounding Disclosures! Three Years in a Mad-House by a Victim. Written by Himself* (Boston[?], 1852).

6. My account of the Packard case has been drawn from the following sources: Mrs. E.P.W. Packard, *Modern Persecution, or Insane Asylums Unveiled, As Demonstrated*

by the *Report of the Investigating Committee of the Legislature of Illinois, Vol. 1* (Hartford, 1873); Packard, *Modern Persecution, or Married Woman's Liabilities, As Demonstrated by the Action of the Illinois Legislature, Vol. 2* (Hartford, 1873); Andrew McFarland, "Case History [Packard]," *American Journal of Insanity* 20 (1863): 89–94; Myra Samuels Himelhoch, with Arthur H. Shaffer, "Elizabeth Packard: Nineteenth-Century Crusader for the Rights of Mental Patients," *American Studies* 13 (1979): 343–75; and Hendrik Hartog, "Mrs. Packard on Dependency," *Working Papers of the Legal History Program* (Institute for Legal Studies, Madison, Wisconsin, 1988), Series 1, No. 9. Only where the foregoing are specifically supplemented or where individual citation seems necessary will separate footnotes be added to the paragraphs that follow.

7. Grob, *Institutions to 1875*, 265, comments on McFarland's career.

8. Community sentiment was strongly with Mrs. Packard. See the transcript of her trial in Packard, *Modern Persecution, Vol. 2*, 21–58 and the editorial of the Kankakee *Gazette*, Jan. 21, 1864, *ibid.*, 58–60.

9. Hartog, "Packard," 25, 26.

10. Mrs. Packard went so far as to blame medical attendants specifically for driving asylum patients to suicide. See the section, "Mrs. Cheneworth's Suicide—Medical Abuse," in Packard, *Modern Persecution, Vol. 1*, 231–39.

11. Hughes, *In the Law's Darkness*, 184–85.

12. Dwyer, *Homes for the Mad*, 111–13.

13. This generalization is made for clarity and emphasis, and is not intended as a blanket statement or exclusive conclusion. In actual practice, of course, Americans of the late nineteenth century took many different views of asylums. See Constance M. McGovern, "The Myths of Social Control and Custodial Oppression: Patterns of Psychiatric Medicine in Late Nineteenth-Century Institutions," *Journal of Social Medicine* 20 (1986): 3–23. The point here is that the negative aspects of asylums were receiving unprecedented attention.

14. [Isaac Ray], "Confinement of the Insane," *American Law Review* 3 (1869): 193–217; quote: 193–94.

15. *ALJ* 12 (1875–76): 385.

16. *First Annual Dinner of the Medico-Legal Society of the City of New York*, Clark Bell, compiler (New York, 1873), 18.

17. Emotional insanity, like moral insanity thirty years earlier, became the focal point of protest. See the attack upon emotional insanity by the prominent legal scholar David Dudley Field in a formal paper before the Medico-Legal Society, April, 24, 1873. The *ALJ* 7 (1873): 273–79, which reprinted and discussed Field's paper, also thought that emotional insanity pushed the whole concept of responsibility too far.

18. *Annual Banquet*, 32. On Reid, see *DAB* 8: 482–86.

19. *Annual Banquet*, 42–43.

20. The McMaster article appeared Sept. 13, 1873. For the debate among lawyers, see S.D.K., "James A. McMaster on the Bench, Bar, Press, and Medical Faculty of New York," *ibid.* 8 (1873): 242–45.

21. *Frank Leslie's Illustrated Newspaper*, July 19, 1876.

22. *ALJ* 23 (1881): 501.

23. James C. Mohr, *The Radical Republicans and Reform in New York during Reconstruction* (Ithaca, 1973), 61–114.

24. James C. Mohr, "New York: The De-politicization of Reform," in James C. Mohr, ed., *Radical Republicans in the North: State Politics during Reconstruction* (Baltimore, 1976), 66–81.

25. Isaac Ray, *A Treatise on the Medical Jurisprudence of Insanity* (Boston, 1838), section 29.

26. Wharton later changed his mind. The best discussion of his thinking is in Tighe, *Question of Responsibility*, 110–11, 133–73.

27. D. Meredith Reese, "Report on Moral Insanity," *TAMA* 11 (1858): 723–46; C.B. Coventry, "Report on Medical Jurisprudence of Insanity," *TAMA* 11 (1858): 473–524.

28. *ALJ* 9 (1874): 153, 268–69.

29. For an excellent example see John Ordronaux, "In re William Winter (The Value of Expert Testimony)," *American Journal of Insanity* 27 (1870–71): 47–80.

30. *ALJ* 7 (1873): 54, 273–79; 9 (1874): 153; Tighe, *Question of Responsibility*, 198–200.

31. *ALJ* 11 (1875): 105–7, 176–77; Dwyer, *Homes for the Mad*, 186–93.

32. Dwyer, *Homes for the Mad*, 188–208; Bonnie Blustein " 'A Hollow Square of Psychological Science': American Neurologists and Psychiatrists in Conflict," in Andrew Scull, ed., *Madhouses, Mad-Doctors and Madmen* (Philadelphia, 1981), 241–70.

33. *ALJ* 11 (1875): 54–55.

34. Tighe, *Question of Responsibility*, 121–123, 199–202.

35. *ALJ* 11 (1875): 176–77; Dwyer, *Homes for the Mad*, 188–208.

36. William J. Mann, "Insanity Considered As A Defense in Criminal Cases," *ALJ* 13 (1876): 210–12, 225–27; see also 33, 52.

37. See his letter in *ibid.* 15 (1877): 27–29.

38. *ALJ* 19 (1879): 205, 305–06, 385; 20 (1879–80): 501.

39. *Ibid.* 21 (1880): 121–22.

40. The best work on Hammond is Bonnie Ellen Blustein, *A New York Medical Man: William Alexander Hammond, M.D. (1828–1900), Neurologist* (University Microfilms, Ann Arbor, 1979), a dissertation done at the University of Pennsylvania. Readers who wish to learn more about Hammond and gain full citation to his many works should consult Blustein's study. I am grateful to Professor Blustein, who shared additional insights about Hammond.

41. Eugene Grissom, "True and False Experts," *American Journal of Insanity* 35 (1878): 1–36; quotes: 33, 35.

42. Quoted in *Philadelphia Medical Times* 9 (1878): 62.

43. *American Journal of Insanity* 35 (1878): 163–67, and *Philadelphia Medical Times* 9 (1878): 62.

44. "Expert Testimony," an interview with Dr. W. A. Hammond from an unidentified newspaper (hand marked Oct. 1884). Clipping in pamphlet No. 10, TC.

45. John B. Chapin, "Experts and Expert Testimony," *Alienist and Neurologist* 1 (1880): 521.

46. For a copy of one of those bills and a medical discussion of it, see J. Marcus Rise, "Medical Expert Testimony," *BMSJ* 107 (1882): 27.

47. Rosenberg, *Trial of the Assassin Guiteau.* See also Tighe, *Question of Responsibility*, esp. 181–233; and Blustein, *Hammond*, esp. 282–94.

48. See, for example, Louis E. Reik, "The Doe-Ray Correspondence: A Pioneer Collaboration in the Jurisprudence of Mental Disease," *Yale Law Journal* 63 (1953): 183–96, and John P. Reid, "A Speculative Novelty: Judge Doe's Search for Reason in the Law of Evidence," *Boston University Law Review* 39 (1959): 321–48.

49. See Tighe, *Question of Responsibility*, 198–226.

CHAPTER THIRTEEN

1. Robert Christison, *A Dispensary; Or Commentary on the Pharmacopoenias of Great Britain (and the United States)*, second revised and improved American edition with a supplement, R. E. Griffith, ed. (Philadelphia, 1848); John James Reese, *Chemistry: Its Importance to the Physician* (Philadelphia, 1852); Reese, *Syllabus of the Course of Lectures on Medical Chemistry, Delivered in the Medical Department of Pennsylvania College* (Philadelphia, 1857); Reese, *On the Detection of Strychnia as a Poison, and the Influence of Morphine in Disguising the Usual Colons-test* (Philadelphia, 1861); William Thomas Brande and Alfred Swaine Taylor, *Chemistry* (Philadelphia, 1863); T[heodore]. G[eorge]. Wormley, *Micro-Chemistry of Poisons, Including their Physiological, Pathological, and Legal Relations, Adapted to the Use of the Medical Jurist, Physician, and General Chemist* (New York, 1867 and 1869); Alfred Swaine Taylor, *A Manual of Medical Jurisprudence*, sixth American from eighth revised London edition with notes and references to American decisions, Clement B. Penrose, ed. (Philadelphia, 1866); S.W.M., "Forensic Medicine: Observations on the Tests for Arsenic," *American Law Register* 1 (1852–53): 11–15. On the dominance of these texts in courses on medical chemistry and toxicology through 1900, see Patricia German, "Textbooks in American Medical Schools, 1860–1900," M.A. thesis, History Department, University of Maryland Baltimore County, 1991. *Taylor's Principles and Practice of Medical Jurisprudence*, A. Keith Mant, ed., went to its thirteenth edition in 1984. According to the Preface, that 1984 edition was the first to discard much of Taylor's own original historical material.

2. Two commercial printers published transcripts and accounts of this trial. The story that follows draws from both: *The Schoeppe Murder Trial: The Trial of Dr. Paul Schoeppe, in the Court of Oyer and Terminer of Cumberland County, Pa., charged with the murder of Miss Maria M. Stennecke, by poison. Hon. James H. Graham, president judge, Hugh Stuart and T. F. Blair, associate judges. The court convened on Monday, May 24th, 1869* (Philadelphia, 1869); and *The Schoeppe Tragedy, Entire: Trial of Dr. Paul Schoeppe for the murder of Miss Maria Steinnecke [sic] by poison* (Carlisle, 1869). These two sources will not be repeatedly cited, but other sources will be cited separately. As is common in virtually all nineteenth-century accounts of this sort, the spelling of names varied greatly. Stennecke, for example, was rendered Stineke, Steinecke, Stinnecke, and Stinecke in various newspapers and court documents. The first "e" in Schoeppe sometimes disappeared. I have used the spellings of the Cumberland County court documents. Other details varied as well, including such things as Stennecke's age and the monetary value of her estate, though they varied within consistent orders of magnitude and do not affect the point of this story in the present context.

3. For a glimpse at Aiken's undistinguished background, see Michele A. L. Aldrich, "New York Natural History Survey, 1836–1845" (Ph.D. dissertation, University of Texas, 1974), 96, 388. T.R. Beck had once rejected Aiken's application to work on the New York State natural history survey, and Amos Eaton had characterized the young Aiken as a poorly trained "itinerating lecturer."

4. Geary is one of those nineteenth-century figures who turn up in a host of intriguing contexts. For an analysis of the Pennsylvania political situation at this point, and Geary's place in it, see David Montgomery, "Radical Republicanism in Pennsylvania, 1866–1873," *Pennsylvania Magazine of History and Biography* 85 (1961): 439–57, and reprinted as "Pennsylvania: An Eclipse of Ideology," in James C. Mohr, ed., *Radical Republicans in the North: State Politics during Reconstruction* (Baltimore,

1976), 50–65. The standard biography of Geary remains Harry M. Tinkcom, *John White Geary: Soldier-Statesman, 1819–1873* (Philadelphia, 1940).

5. More than forty years ago Whitfield Bell, Jr., made this same surmise about physicians' motives in the Schoeppe case. See his manuscript, "Prussic Acid in Pomfret Street," 26, typescript dated March 20, 1947 in Cumberland County Historical Society. I am indebted to Evelyn Kassouf for this and related local references.

6. Reese published his statement in the *Philadelphia Age*, and it was reprinted in *Schoeppe Murder Trial*, 71–73.

7. Baltimore *Sun*, Aug. 21, 1869: 1.

8. *Philadelphia Inquirer*, Nov. 12, 1869: 2.

9. "Medico-Legal Report on the Medical Testimony of the Schoeppe Murder Trial Presented to the College of Physicians of Philadelphia, and Unanimously Adopted, November 3, 1869," reprinted in *Schoeppe Murder Trial*, 75–91.

10. *Philadelphia Inquirer*, Nov. 12, 1869: 2.

11. Baltimore *Sun*, Aug. 21, 1869: 1. The New York Medico-Legal Society's piece appeared in the New York *Medical Review* in August, 1869, and was reprinted in *Schoeppe Murder Trial*, 68–70.

12. "From the New Haven Medical Association," in *Schoeppe Murder Trial*, 92–96; *Philadelphia Inquirer*, Nov. 12, 1869: 2.

13. *Philadelphia Inquirer*, Dec. 4, 1869: 1.

14. *Ibid.*, Nov. 12, 1869: 2.

15. *Ibid.*, Dec. 14, 1869: 2. The Baltimore *Sun*, Dec. 6, 1869, suggested that these Baltimore efforts were organized by the city's German doctors.

16. Baltimore *Sun*, Aug. 21, 1869 1.

17. *Ibid.*, Aug. 23, 1869: 1; *Philadelphia Inquirer*, Nov. 12, 1869: 1.

18. Schoeppe to Governor Geary, Nov. 29, 1869, reprinted in the Baltimore *Sun*, Dec. 3, 1869: 1.

19. The Baltimore *Sun* later summarized the efforts of the German press. See Jan. 10, 24, Feb. 9, 15, 1870. Events in Germany itself eventually proved chilling for Schoeppe's supporters in the United States, however, since the authorities in Berlin, while disagreeing with the medico-legal evidence that convicted him, also suspected Schoeppe of being the same man who tried a similar scheme in the old country before emigrating to America. The historian George Bancroft was United States ambassador in Berlin at the time of the Schoeppe affair. He worked to calm the volatile situation, and the Prussian government finally decided to sit out the whole business rather than press it as an international incident. I am indebted for a number of these *Sun* references to my friend Joseph Arnold, whose own close survey of the Baltimore press has uncovered material of interest to his colleagues as well as to himself.

20. *Philadelphia Inquirer*, Nov. 12, 1869 1; Baltimore *Sun*, Dec. 14, 1869: 1.

21. *Philadelphia Inquirer*, Nov. 12, 1869: 2.

22. *Schoeppe Murder Trial*, 97.

23. *Philadelphia Inquirer*, Nov. 12, 1869: 1, 2.

24. Bell, "Prussic Acid," 26; Baltimore *Sun*, Feb. 15, 1870; *New York Times*, June 20, 1875.

25. Interview reported in the Baltimore *Sun*, Dec. 14, 1869: 1.

26. The retrial may be followed in detail in the Baltimore *Sun*. See especially the stories for Aug. 29, 30, 31 and Sept. 1, 3, 6, 7, 9, 1872. The quote is from

Aug. 30, 1872. Many other papers carried extensive trial reports as well, of course, especially the German-language papers.

27. Baltimore *Sun*, Nov. 28, 1872: 1. The *Sun* disapproved of Schoeppe trying to capitalize upon his notoriety and considered his attack on the American justice system offensive.

28. Baltimore *Sun*, Aug. 8, 9, 20, and March 19, 20, 21, 23, 1874; *New York Times*, Oct. 12, 1872: 4–5; and June 6, 1875: 7; *Philadelphia Inquirer*, June 21, 1875: 1.

29. My sketch of this case is drawn primarily from the *Baltimore Gazette*'s separately published, book-length account: *Trial of Mrs. Elizabeth G. Wharton, on the Charge of Poisoning General W. S. Ketchum, Tried at Annapolis, Md. December, 1871–January, 1872* (Baltimore, 1872). That account has been supplemented by stories in the *New York Times*, the *Baltimore Sun*, the *Baltimore American and Commercial Advertiser*, the *American Law Review*, the *New York Herald*, and a large number of medical articles. The last will be cited separately. In the interim, only direct quotes of significance will be cited in order to avoid pointless multiple footnoting of this composite account. As usual, various versions of this twisted story disagree on peripheral details. Some have Henry Wharton dying in 1863, for example, and others have Dr. Nugent's chief practice in Pittstown, Pennsylvania. There is substantial agreement, however, on the points germane to the analysis here.

30. Both direct quotes are from the *Gazette, Trial*, 153.

31. *Ibid.*, 112.

32. Steele must have had little other reason for these witnesses, however, since one of them, Dr. Abram Claude, professor of natural science at St. John's, was so marginal that the bench denied him formal status as an expert in analytical chemistry. That sort of denial was most unusual, especially for a local professor. See *Gazette, Trial*, 132.

33. The illustrations appeared in *Frank Leslie's Illustrated Newspaper*, Dec. 23, 1871: 236; Feb. 3, 1872: 333; and Feb. 10, 1872: 345; quote: Feb. 10, 1872: 347.

34. All of the foregoing newspaper comments are quoted from the *Baltimore American and Commercial Advertiser*, Jan. 26, 1872, which carried columns of editorial excerpts from all over the nation upon the conclusion of the Wharton trial.

35. John J. Reese, "A Review of the Recent Trial of Mrs. Elizabeth G. Wharton on the Charge of Poisoning General W. S. Ketchum," *AJMS* (April, 1872): 329–55; quote: 329.

36. Horatio C. Wood, "Review of the Medical Testimony in the Trial of Mrs. E. G. Wharton, for the Alleged Attempt to Poison Mr. Eugene Van Ness," *Medical Record* (New York) 8 (1873): 169–73.

37. *ALJ* 7 (1873): 258–60.

38. S[amuel]. C[laggett]. Chew, "A Medical Survey of the Trial of Mrs. E. G. Wharton on the Charge of Poisoning Gen. W. S. Ketchum," a 23–page pamphlet printed separately as a reprint from the *Richmond and Louisville Medical Journal* (July 1872); and Chew, "An Examination of the Medical Evidence in the Trial of Mrs. E. G. Wharton, on the Charge of Attempting to Poison Eugene Van Ness, Esq.," *Medical Record* 8 (1873): 332–338. The latter was also republished separately in pamphlet form by W. Wood of New York in 1873. Philip C. Williams, "A Correct Statement of the Medical and Chemical Facts Developed During the Trials of Mrs. Wharton, for the Alleged Murder of Gen. Ketchum, and the Alleged Attempt to Murder Mr. Van Ness," a 31–page pamphlet reprinted separately from the *Richmond and Louisville Medical Journal* (Lexington, Ky., 1873); and Williams, "An Ex-

amination of Dr. Reese's Review of the Trial of Mrs. Wharton," pamphlet reprint from the *Medical and Surgical Reporter*. In a preface to the last, Williams claimed that the *AJMS* would not publish his reply to Reese, so he approached the rival Philadelphia journal, which agreed to carry his essay.

39. John J. Reese, "Card from Dr. Reese, of Philadelphia," *Medical Record* 8 (1873): 439–40.

40. William E.A. Aiken, *A Review of "Prof. Reese's Review" of the Wharton Trial, with a Brief Notice of the Schoeppe Trial* (New York, 1873), 3.

41. "Expert Testimony," *Indiana Journal of Medicine* 4 (1873–74): 264–75; esp. 265–66 and 269–73.

42. John Thomas, "Notice of John H. Thomas, one of the Counsel for the Defence in the Cases against Mrs. E.G. Wharton, of Attacks Made on Him and His Colleagues, by Drs. S.C. Chew and P.C. Williams and Prof. Wm.E.A. Aikin" (n.p., n.d.), now bound with other pamphlets related to the Wharton case in the collection of the Peabody Library, Baltimore; quotes: 3, 10.

43. Thomas, "Notice," 13.

44. Scores of examples could be cited. Two of the best are Jacob F. Miller, "Expert Testimony—Its Nature and Value," *Sanitarian* 6 (1878): 67, and H. N. Sheldon, "Medical Testimony From a Legal Standpoint," *Transactions of the Massachusetts Medico-Legal Society* 2 (1888–1898): 82. The language in the former, written by a lawyer, was typical: ". . . within the last ten years trials have taken place in this and neighboring States in which the medical witnesses did more harm than good—did more to mislead the jury than to instruct them. I need not speak of Scheppe's [sic] case, the Wharton case, and others a little nearer home. They are familiar to you."

45. *Baltimore American*, Jan 25, 1872.

46. See letter of Jan. 8, 1872, from J. W. Mallet of the University of Virginia to the Baltimore *Sun*, published in the Baltimore *Sun*, Jan. 18, 1872; and the *Sun*'s editorial comment of Jan. 25, 1872.

CHAPTER FOURTEEN

1. Stanford E. Chaillé, *Origin and Progress of Medical Jurisprudence, 1776–1876: A Centennial Address* (Philadelphia, 1876), 9–10. This essay was reprinted separately from *Transactions of the International Medical Congress, 1876*.

2. W. F. Sanford, "Medical Testimony in Courts of Law," *Proceedings of the Medical Society of Kings County* 4 (1879–80): 254. As was the case for this Brooklyn doctor, discussions of the subject generally began with this premise, which was never challenged and never needed defending.

3. M. G. Ellzey, "Application of Chemistry in Medico-Legal Science," *Maryland Medical Journal* 2, no. 6 (1878): 527.

4. S. H. Tewksbury, "Medico-Legal Evidence," *Transactions of the Maine Medical Association* (1869–70): 97–114; quotes: 97, 107.

5. Alexander Young, "Medical Evidence," *BMSJ* n.s. 3 (1869): 461.

6. "Expert Testimony," *BMSJ* 87 (Sept. 26, 1872): 219.

7. Quoted in *BMJS* n.s. 3 (1869): 356. Chapman's charge later appeared in somewhat different words and phrasings both in the *BMSJ* itself and in the writings of other medico-legal experts, but the sentiments remained unmistakably the same.

8. See Young, "Medical Evidence," 465.

9. Clemens Herschel, *On the Best Manner of Making Use of the Services of Experts in the Conduct of Judicial Inquiries* (Boston, 1886), 14.

10. J[oseph]. Snowden Bell, *The Use and Abuse of Expert Testimony* (Philadelphia, 1879), 8.

11. For a good example involving a prominent medico-legalist see M. A. McClelland, "The Medical Expert and Medical Evidence," *Chicago Medical Journal and Examiner* 32 (1875): 249–50. McClelland was double-crossed by lawyers who had used his library and solicited his opinions on the express promise that he would not be called to the stand.

12. In one of the worst examples, physicians from New York City had been summoned to a court in Buffalo, at the standard witness compensation rate of a dollar a day, and made to testify against their wills in a malpractice matter. See Medicus, "Testimony of Experts," *New York Medical Press* 3 (1860): 349–50.

13. *BMSJ* n.s. 2 (1868): 160.

14. "Rights of Medical Experts as Witnesses," *BMSJ* n.s. 2 (1868): 224.

15. *Ibid.*

16. "Report of the Committee Appointed to Memorialize the Legislature of the State of Massachusetts on the Subject of Expert Testimony," *Proceedings of the American Academy of Arts and Sciences* (Boston, 1873–74) n.s. 1: 31–34. Washburn had written and lectured often on the problems of the medical witness. The National Union catalogue contains several pages of citations of his works, many of which touch upon that subject directly.

17. "Medical Testimony and Experts: A Report to the Suffolk District Medical Society," *BMSJ* 82 (1870): 119–23; quote: 123. The efforts described here and below may be tracked in great detail through the decade of the 1870s in the *BMSJ*; only direct quotes will be footnoted.

18. Washburn had first made his points in *American Law Review* 1 (1866): 61, but they resurfaced nationally in the debates of the mid-70s. See M.A. McClelland, "The Medical Expert and Medical Evidence," *Chicago Medical Journal and Examiner* 32 (1875): 85–86.

19. For a draft of the bill proposed in Massachusetts in 1874 see "An Act Concerning the Testimony of Experts," *BMSJ* 90 (1874): 387–88. Washburn is quoted on its ultimate fate, after repeated failure, in C.H. Boardman, "Report of the Committee on Medical Jurisprudence," *Transactions of the Minnesota State Medical Society* (St. Paul, 1882): 199–201.

20. See "Medical Expert Testimony: What It Is and What It Should Be," *Transactions of the Massachusetts Medico-Legal Society* 1 (1878–1887): 134. This article also contained the report of a committee that Marston chaired.

21. Letter from Attorney General Marston, *ibid.*, Appendix: x–xi.

22. Thomas Kennard, "Medical Experts: Their Duties and Relations to Courts of Justice and to Their Profession," *Medical Archives* n.s. 8 (1872): 65–74; quotes: 65, 66, 67.

23. *ALJ* 7 (1873): 258–60.

24. *American Journal of Insanity* (Jan., 1874).

25. C. Goepp, "Experts in Judicial Proceedings," *ALJ* 9 (1874): 146–47.

26. "Expert Testimony in Judicial Proceedings," *ibid.*, 122, 153.

27. *Ibid.*, Vol. 12 (1875–76): 399–400.

28. Doremus also taught chemistry at City College and was internationally known as a scientific inventor. During the Civil War he had perfected a form of compressed gunpowder that greatly facilitated the muzzle-loading of field artillery.

Emperor Napoleon III had invited Doremus to France to help the French armies gain the benefit of that breakthrough. See *DAB* 3: 376–77.

29. *ALJ* 12 (1875–76): 2.

30. For a summary, see Boardman, "Report of the Committee on Medical Jurisprudence," 189–204.

31. Christopher Johnston, "Opening Address," *Transactions of the Medical and Chirurgical Faculty of Maryland at Its Seventy-ninth Annual Session, 1877* (Baltimore, 1877), 37–50. Johnson deserves credit for coming up with one of the most inventive reasons for reform: the best physicians were always being dragged into court as experts, which left the public in the hands of lesser doctors.

32. "Reports of Societies," *Maryland Medical Journal* 1 (1877): 54.

33. D.A. Morris, "The Duties of the Medical Witness, and His Privileges," *Cincinnati Lancet and Observer* 13 (1870): 129–50; esp. 147.

34. "Expert Testimony," *Indiana Journal of Medicine* 4 (1873–74): 264–75.

35. Wilson Hobbs, "The Medical Witness," *Transactions of the Indiana State Medical Society, 1877* (Indianapolis, 1877), 33–49; quote 47.

36. R.W. Hazlett to Wilson Hobbs, in Hobbs, "The Medical Witness," *Transactions of the Indiana State Medical Society, 1878* (Indianapolis, 1878), 15–16.

37. Decision quoted in *ibid.*, 16–24; quote: 20; italics in original.

38. Proceedings, *State of Indiana v. Thomas J. Dills*, quoted in *ibid.*, 26.

39. *Buchman v. Indiana*, opinion of Worden, J., *ibid.*, 37–47; quotes: 45, 45–46.

40. For a representative editorial and confirmation of Hobbs's statement, see *Maryland Medical Journal* 2, no. 6 (1877): 535.

41. Hobbs, "Expert Witness [1878]," 51, 52.

42. *Ibid.*, 51.

43. J.W. Gordon, "True and False Experts," *American Practitioner* 18 (1878): 133–41, 197–206, 278–89.

44. William Protzman, "Should Experts Speak in Our Courts Without Extra Remuneration? Were Drs. Dills and Buchman, of Ft. Wayne, Rightfully Treated?" *Ohio Medical Recorder* 2 (1877–78): 446–50; quotes: 449, 450.

45. [Editorial] *ibid.*, 326–32.

46. W.H. Philips, "The Testimony of Medical Experts," *Transactions of the Ohio State Medical Society* 33 (1878): 43–61; quotes: 44, 48, 49.

47. Philips recognized that the French system, hailed in theory for so long by American physicians, did not work well in France in actual practice. Individual judges were too susceptible to favoritism and political pressure to guarantee selection of the best available experts in every case.

48. Philips, "Testimony," 57–61; "Report of Committee Upon Compensation of Medical Experts," *Transactions of the Ohio State Medical Society* 33 (1878): 62–64; quotes: 63.

49. W.J. Conklin, "The Medical Expert," *Ohio Medical and Surgical Journal* 3 (1878): 127–46; quotes: 127, 139; italics in original.

50. [Editorial] "Expert Testimony in Toledo," *Toledo Medical and Surgical Journal* 4 (1880): 457–59; quote: 459.

51. Francis B. James, *The Ohio Law of Opinion Evidence, Expert and Non-Expert* (Cincinnati, 1889), 18–19, citing *State v. Darby*, 17 Bull. (Warren Co. Com. Pleas) 62 (1887).

52. Edward Cox, "Our Relations to Jurisprudence," *Detroit Lancet* 2 (1879): 273.

53. *Ibid.*, 267–74.

54. John J. Reese, "Medical Expert Testimony," *Medical and Surgical Reporter* (Philadelphia) 38 (1878): 301–6; quote: 305.

55. "The Payment of Medical Experts" [editorial], *Philadelphia Medical Times* 8 (1878): 227–28; quotes: 227.

56. E. Bowyer, "Compensation of Expert Witnesses," *Transactions of the Twenty-ninth Anniversary Meeting of the Illinois State Medical Society* (Chicago, 1879), 248–57; quotes: 248, 249.

57. F.T. Ledergerber, "Medical Experts as Witnesses in Courts of Justice," *St. Louis Medical and Surgical Journal* 34 (1878): 47–50, 119–24, 207–10, 365–66; L.B. Valliant, "Doctors as Ministers of Law," *Saint Louis Courier of Medicine and Collateral Sciences* 1 (1879): 271–80; H.C. Baker, "Professional Witnesses: The Law as to Compensation," *Louisville Medical News* 7 (1879): 208–9.

58. W.S. Thorne, "Medical Experts and Insanity," *Transactions of the Santa Clara Medical Society for 1877, 1878 and 1879* (San Jose, 1879), 26–40.

59. A.W. Saxe, "Criticism on Medical Experts and Insanity," *ibid.*, 41–52; quotes: 42, 47; italics in original.

60. J. Bradford Cox, "Scientific Witnesses Before Courts of Justice," *ibid.*, 52–61; quote: 52.

61. *Ibid.*, 4.

62. Henry Wade Rogers, *The Law of Expert Testimony* (St. Louis, 1883), 260–61.

63. George W. Cothan, "Practical Suggestions to Physicians as Witnesses," *Physicians and Surgeons' Investigator* (Buffalo) 1 (1880): 97–103; quote: 99.

64. George W. Cothan, "Compensation of Medical Experts," *ibid.*, 161–67.

65. Charles Beckwith, "Testimony of Medical Experts," *Buffalo Medical and Surgical Journal* 19 (1880): 421–28, 469–75; quotes: 426, 474, 475; italics in original.

66. F.W. Draper, "Medical Expert Testimony," *BMSJ* 103 (1880): 442–46; quote: 442.

67. Matthew P. Deady, *Proceedings of the Eighth Annual Meeting of the Oregon State Medical Society, Held at Portland, June 14 and 15, 1881* (Portland, 1881), 55–59.

68. C.H. Boardman, "Report of the Committee on Medical Jurisprudence: Medical Expert Testimony," *Transactions of the Minnesota State Medical Society* (St. Paul, 1882), 189–204; quote: 195.

69. For a summary, see Rogers, *Expert Testimony*, 252–53.

CHAPTER FIFTEEN

1. For typical articles in the *BMSJ* alone, see "Medical Men as Coroners," 42 (1850): 298; "Coroners' Inquests," 44 (1851): 206; "Medical Coroners," 45 (1851): 106; "Medical Coroners," 48 (1853): 346–47; "Medical Coroners," 49 (1853): 249; "Coroners' Bills and Medical Coroners," 55 (1857): 534–35; "Notices," 57 (1857): 430; "Medical Coroners for Suffolk County," 57 (1858): 474–75; "A Homoeopathic Coroner," 58 (1858): 386–87; "The Boston Courier and the Coroner," 59 (1858): 47; "Coroners' Inquests and the Boston Courier," 59 (1858): 27–28; and "The Malden Murder and Coroners," 69 (1864): 503–4. I would like to acknowledge the efforts of a graduate assistant, Patricia German, who helped run down these and related references in the *BMSJ*.

2. "Coroners," *BMSJ* 85 (1871): 138–40.

3. "The Office of Coroner," *BMSJ* 86 (1872): 94–95. This article stated that New York City had eight coroners, but it probably had only four. The author may

have been combining New York City with Brooklyn and surrounding jurisdictions. See "The Reform of the Coroner System," *BMSJ* 95 (1876): 768. In "Coroners," 96: 387–88, the *BMSJ* retroactively admitted failure to overcome the initial resistance of the coroners.

4. "How Coroners Are Appointed," *BMJS* 93 (1875): 337–39.

5. See "About Coroners," *BMJS* 94 (1876): 53–54; and "The Office of Coroner," *BMSJ* 94 (1876): 229–30; quote: 229.

6. For representative expressions, see "English Coroners," *BMSJ* 95 (1876): 622–24; "The Reform of the Coroner System," *BMSJ* 95 (1876), 767–69; and "Coroners in Philadelphia," *BMSJ* 96 (1877): 91–92.

7. For the outcome see "Coroner A. W. K. Newton," *BMSJ* 96 (1877): 295–96. A number of Boston's most eminent regulars, including D.H. Storer and Henry I. Bowditch, signed a formal petition to the Massachusetts House of Representatives alleging Newton's corruption and unfitness for office.

8. For more on this group, what it represented, and why this context was so apt, see Thomas L. Haskell, *The Emergence of Professional Social Science: The American Social Science Association and the Nineteenth-Century Crisis of Authority* (Urbana, Ill., 1977).

9. Theodore H. Tyndale, "The Law of Coroners," *BMSJ* 96 (1877): 243–58.

10. *Guide to U.S. Elections* (Washington, D.C., 1975), 379.

11. The *BMSJ* felt confident enough to run the story of this bill's passage before it passed. See "The Fall of Coroners," *BMSJ* 96 (May 3, 1877): 537–38.

12. "The Medical Examiners," *BMSJ* 96 (1877): 775.

13. "Coroners," *BMSJ* 96 (1877): 387–88; "The Coroner Bill," *BMSJ* 96 (1877): 443–44; "The Fall of the Coroners," *BMSJ* 96 (1877): 537–38; "The Fall of the Coroners, II" *BMSJ* 96 (1877): 561–62.

14. "The Coroners Must Go," *BMSJ* 109 (1883): 280–81.

15. A copy of the law, from which this quote is taken, may be found in *TMMLS* 1 (1878–1887) [Boston, 1888]: vii–x.

16. W. H. Taylor, "Meeting of the Massachusetts Medico-Legal Society," *BMJS* 118 (March 22, 1888): 299–300, and *BMSJ* 119 (July 19, 1888): 65; J. A. Mead, "What Cases Shall the Medical Examiner 'View'?" *BMSJ* 131 (Oct. 11, 1894): 362–63; and 369–371; Sherman Boar, "On the Duties of a Medical Examiner as a Witness," *BMSJ* 136 (April 8, 1897): 330; and 335–37.

17. "The Work and Duties of the Medical Examiner," *BMSJ* 99 (1878): 337.

18. See, for example, "Medical Expert Testimony: What It Is and What It Should Be," *TMMLS* 1 (1878–87): 124–34; H. N. Sheldon, "Medical Testimony From a Legal Standpoint," *TMMLS* 2 (1888–1898): 74–84; and John C. Irish, "Medical Expert Testimony," *TMMLS* 3 (1899–1904): 25–33, including discussion.

19. "The Medico-Legal Society," *BMSJ* 97 (Oct. 18, 1877): 455.

20. Alfred Hosmer, "Address Delivered June 11, 1878," *BMSJ* 99 (1878): 33–40.

21. See their annual reports in *TMMLS*.

22. For additional evidence of interest see "The Coroners Must Go," *BMSJ* 109 (1883): 280; and H. O. Marcy, "Report of the Committee upon the Coroner System of the United States," *JAMA* 11 (1889): 167–69.

23. *New York Times*, May 13, 1869; May 27, 1875; May 28, 1875.

24. *Ibid.*, Feb. 11, 1877; Jan. 12, 1878. Raymond Rooks, "The Abolition of the Coroner's Office in Massachusetts and New York," senior honors paper, Department of History, University of Maryland Baltimore County, 1990.

25. *New York Times*, June 19, 1880; Jan. 6, 1881; Sept. 9, 1882. Clark Bell,

"The Coroner's Office: Should It Be Abolished?" *Bulletin of the Medico-Legal Society of New York* 4 (1880–81): 64–118.

26. The office of coroner was removed as a constitutional post in 1894, though retained as a regular position. See *New York Times*, Sept. 12, 1894; Nov. 9, 1894.

27. Julie Johnson, "The Politics of Death: The Philadelphia Coroner's Office, 1900–1956," unpublished paper presented at the 1990 annual meeting of the American Association for the History of Medicine. I am indebted to Ms. Johnson, who is completing a Ph.D. dissertation on forensic pathology in the twentieth century, for providing a fuller version of that paper. Her findings for the first half of the twentieth century mesh extremely well with the argument advanced here, and readers who would like to follow what eventually happened to coroners would do well to consult her work.

28. Gustavus Eliot, "Coroners and Medical Examiners in Connecticut," *JAMA* 1 (1883): 556–57; quote 557. See also Henry. O. Marcy, J. H. Hobart Burge, and W. W. Dawson, "Report of the Committee upon the Coroner System of the United States," *JAMA* 11 (1889): 167–69.

29. "The Coroners Must Go," *BMSJ* 109 (1883): 280–81; "An Act Relating to Medical Examiners and Coroners," *BMSJ* 111 (1884): 43; quote from latter.

30. Remarks of T.C. Finnell, in *First Annual Dinner of the Medico-Legal Society of the City of New York*, Clark Bell, compiler (New York, 1873), 7–9.

31. Charles E. Rosenberg, "The Practice of Medicine in New York a Century Ago," *BHM* 41 (1967): 223–53.

32. Frontispiece, bound with *Annual Dinner*, 1.

33. The only other non-American honorary member was Alfred Vogel, listed as a professor at Dorpat University in Russia. See frontispiece, *Annual Dinner*, 4.

34. Léon Dérobert, "Histoire de la médecine légale," *Zacchia: Archivis di Medicina Legale, Sociale E Criminologica*, Anno 48 (1973): 1–37, 161–92, 341–82, 533–47; Léon Dérobert, "Historique de la société de médecine légale et de criminologie de France," *Société de médecine légale* (Dec. 1968): 410–13; A. Lacassagne, "Des transformations du droit penal et les progrès de la médecine légale de 1810 à 1912," *Archives d'Anthropologie Criminelle, de Médecine Légale et de Psychologie Normale et Pathologique* no. 233 (1913); *Annales d'Hygiène Publique de Médecine Légale* 2nd series, 29 (1868): 415–16; 32 (1869): 447–48.

35. The inscription reads: "Aux Membres de la Société de Médecine Légale de Paris—Jno. Ordronaux New York le 5 Nov. 1869," in the library of the Société Médecine Légale, Paris.

36. For difficulties on the French side see Alfred Lechopié and Ch. Floquet, *Droit Médical ou Code de Médecins* (Paris, 1890), and Lacassagne, "Transformations." As William Coleman made clear in *Death Is a Social Disease: Public Health and Political Economy in Early Industrial France* (Madison, 1982), *passim*, the inherent tension between state medicine and liberal republicanism, the same tension that was so crucial in the United States from the beginning, began to cripple medical jurisprudence in France as well by the time of the Empire under Napoleon III. For American comments tied to the French situation, see Clark Bell, *Third Inaugural Address* (New York, 1875), separately printed edition of his 1874 speech, pamphlet collection, NLM.

37. Remarks of John C. Peters, *First Annual Dinner*, 23.

38. Clark Bell, *Third Inaugural Address*, 10.

39. Clark Bell to John Shaw Billings, Jan. 22, 1875, NLM.

40. Clark Bell, "Fifth Inaugural Address," *Medico-Legal Journal* 1 (1884): 1.

41. *First Annual Dinner*, frontispiece bound with the NLM's copy of the pamphlet: 2–4 and [7].

42. *ALJ* 10 (1874–75): 363–65.

43. Janet Ann Tighe, *A Question of Responsibility: The Development of American Forensic Psychiatry, 1838–1930* (Ph.D. dissertation, UP, 1983; University Microfilms International, Ann Arbor, 1984), 181–302, is excellent on Bell's role in the NYMLS and his forty-year effort to effect a medico-legal solution to the problems of legal insanity.

44. *BMSJ* 108 (Jan. 25, 1883): 93.

45. Tighe, *Question of Responsibility*, 181–302; Blustein, *Hammond, passim*; Bell, "Fifth Annual Address," pps. 1, 3, *passim*; James J. O'Dea, "Progress of Medico-legal Science in America," *Papers Read Before the New York Medico-Legal Society* 3 (1886): 286–314. The so-called international congresses (held respectively in New York, Chicago, and New York) are well documented.

46. Luke Tedeschi, "The Massachusetts Medico-Legal Society: The Early Years," *American Journal of Forensic Medicine and Pathology* 2, no. 3 (Sept. 1981): 257–60.

47. W. H. Taylor, "Massachusetts Medico-Legal Society" *BMSJ* 119 (July 19, 1888): 65.

48. Tighe, *Question of Responsibility*, 183.

49. Over more than a decade of reading nineteenth-century articles about medical jurisprudence, I have seen phrases suggesting the existence of medico-legal groups, probably informal discussion groups or *ad hoc* associations put together to address a single issue, in St. Louis and Detroit. But the historical record of such groups, even if the groups existed as more than the overly grand characterization of single writers, is too fleeting to merit serious consideration or additional research.

50. *Constitution and By-Laws of the Medical Jurisprudence Society of Philadelphia* (Philadelphia, 1884), 7; *Constitution and By-Laws of the Medical Jurisprudence Society of Philadelphia* (Philadelphia, 1889), 5. Both in Special Collections, College of Physicians and Surgeons of Philadelphia.

51. U. S. *Census* (1880), Population, Vol. 1, p. 894; *ibid.*, (1890), Population, Part II, p. 710.

52. *Constitution and By-Laws . . . Philadelphia* (1884), 4–5.

53. The lunacy commission has been discussed. For the abortion legislation see James C. Mohr, *Abortion in America: The Origins and Evolution of National Policy, 1800–1900* (New York, 1978), 217–19. For the school legislation see Bell, "Fifth Inaugural Address," 7.

54. Remarks of David Dudley Field, *Annual Dinner*, 16.

55. Remarks of Major-General William W. Averell, *ibid.*, 19.

56. James J. O'Dea, "Medico-Legal Science: A Sketch of Its Progress, Especially in the United States," *Sanitarian* (New York) 4 (1876): 449–57, 493–503.

57. Andrew Abbott, *The System of Professions: An Essay on the Division of Expert Labor* (Chicago, 1988), 165, has argued that the medico-legal societies of this period brought physicians and lawyers "together in forums where their boundary disputes could be recognized and decided." The argument here is that the professional boundaries were well defined and well accepted in the United States by 1870. The medico-legal societies took that as a given and functioned as tiny cells, where those few who retained cross-professional interests could talk to one another.

58. Remarks of Major-General William W. Averell, *Annual Dinner*, 19.

CHAPTER SIXTEEN

1. N[athan]. S. Davis, *History of the American Medical Association* (Philadelphia, 1855), 40–41, 46, 92, 187, and *passim*.

2. William Frederick Norwood, *Medical Education in the United States Before the Civil War* (Philadelphia, 1944), 426–27.

3. Davis, *AMA*, 71.

4. *Ibid.*, 104.

5. The quote is from *BMSJ* 57 (Dec. 24, 1857): 430, which was, in turn, citing and discussing *TAMA* 10 (1857).

6. Cited in Norwood, *Medical Education*, 428.

7. Samuel D. Gross, "Address of Samuel D. Gross, M.D., LL.D., President of the Association," *TAMA* 19 (1868): 57–74; quotes: 58, 62–63.

8. *Ibid.*, 77–79.

9. *Ibid.*, 108.

10. "Report of Committee on the Subject of 'The Appointment of a Commissioner in Each Judicial District or Circuit to Aid in the Examination of Witnesses in Every Trial Involving Medico-legal Testimony,'" *TAMA* 20 (1869): 575–78.

11. The governmental reforms associated with the Reconstruction period in the South are, of course, well known. For those in the North see James C. Mohr, ed., *Radical Republicans in the North: State Politics During Reconstruction* (Baltimore, 1976).

12. Edward C. Atwater, "The Medical Profession in a New Society, Rochester, New York (1811–1860)," *BHM* 48 (1973): 221–35.

13. Charles E. Rosenberg, "The Practice of Medicine in New York a Century Ago," *BHM* 41 (1967): 223–53.

14. See reports in *BMSJ* 72 (June 15, 1865): 413; and *ibid* 73 (June 7, 1866): 378–80.

15. Morris Fishbein, *A History of the American Medical Association, 1847–1947* (Philadelphia, 1947), 1095–96.

16. *TAMA* 21–26 (1870–1875).

17. *TAMA* 25 (1874): 42–43.

18. *TAMA* 26 (1875): 41–43.

19. *Medical and Surgical Reporter* (Philadelphia) 32 (1875): 339.

20. Stanford E. Chaillé, *Origin and Progress of Medical Jurisprudence, 1776–1876* (Philadelphia, 1876),3. This citation is a separate publication of Chaillé's paper in pamphlet form, "For the benefit of the Legal and Medical Professions of the United States." It may also be consulted in the *Transactions of the International Medical Congress, Philadelphia, September, 1876* (Philadelphia, 1876).

21. Chaillé, *Medical Jurisprudence*, 8.

22. *Ibid.*, 9, 5.

23. *Ibid.*, 9–11.

24. *Ibid.*, 25–27.

25. On the German influence in New York, see Rosenberg, "Medicine in New York." The growing influence of German medicine in this period is well documented in most of the standard surveys of American medical history. There is a large literature on the rise of German-model universities in the United States during the last quarter of the nineteenth century and the first two decades of the twentieth century.

26. Chaillé, *Medical Jurisprudence*, 27.

27. Fishbein, *American Medical Association*, 1095–96.

28. *JAMA* 2 (1884): 712. The other two sections of this article on duties to the public stated that physicians should, in essence, cut back on their "eleemosynary services" (i.e. make everybody pay) and root out quackery.

29. Henry F. Campbell, "The President's Address," *JAMA* 4 (1885): 477–86.

30. *Ibid.*, 481, 485; emphasis in original.

31. *JAMA* 5 (1885): 557.

32. *JAMA* 6 (1886): 604, 608.

33. Isaac N. Quimby, "Introduction to Medical Jurisprudence," *JAMA* 9 (1887): 161–67; quote: 161.

34. *JAMA* 8 (1887): 722.

35. *JAMA* 8 (1887): 717. Reid's secretary was C.B. Bell of Massachusetts.

36. Eugene Fauntleroy Cordell, *The Medical Annals of Maryland, 1799–1899* (Baltimore, 1903), 546.

37. E.M. Reid, "Address in Medical Jurisprudence," *JAMA* 10 (1888): 701.

38. Editorial from the Philadelphia *Medical Register*, quoted in Reid, "Medical Jurisprudence," 701.

39. See *JAMA* 11–18, for examples. An excellent specific instance occurred in 14 (1890): 804–5.

40. See the report of the Chicago Medico-Legal Society reported in *JAMA* 10 (1888): 566–71, 599–600.

CHAPTER SEVENTEEN

1. Stanford Chaillé, *Origin and Progress of Medical Jurisprudence, 1776–1876: A Centennial Address* (Philadelphia, 1876), 12–14; emphases in original.

2. M.G. Ellzey, "Application of Chemistry in Medico-Legal Science," *Maryland Medical Journal* 2, no. 6 (1878): 526–31; quote: 530.

3. R.H. Philips, "The Testimony of Medical Experts," *Transactions of the Ohio State Medical Society* 33 (1878): 46–47.

4. Edward Cox (committee chair), "Our Relations to Jurisprudence," *Detroit Lancet* 2 (April 1879): 269.

5. Information on Reese's career is in the John James Reese folder, "AR" or Alumni Record files, University Archives, UP. I would like to acknowledge the assistance of Mark Lloyd, archivist, and Hamilton Elliot, assistant archivist.

6. Medical catalogues, UP, 1867–1900.

7. Reese folder, University Archives, UP.

8. Reese to Cadwalader Biddle, Esq., Secretary of the Board of Trustees, Law Files, University Archives, UP.

9. A few law schools existed in the United States much earlier than this, of course, and some of them were associated with universities. Despite those exceptions, however, the generalization is essentially correct. The subject of legal education is well researched and references many be obtained in any of the general histories of law cited throughout this book.

10. Reese to the Board of Trustees, June 10, 1875, Archives General, UP; emphasis in original.

11. Minutes of the Trustees, July 6, 1875, Archives General, UP.

12. Reese to the Board of Trustees, April 26, 1876, Archives General, UP; emphasis in original.

13. Minutes of the Trustees, May 2, 1876, Archives General, UP.

14. Brainerd Currie, "The Materials of Law Study: Part One," *Journal of Legal Education* 3, no. 3 (Spring 1951): 331–83; esp. 359–74.

15. "Communication from Com– on Law Dept, in re, Resignation of Prof. Reese, submitted and acted upon Oct 3, 1876"; Minutes of the Trustees, Oct. 3, 1876, UP.

16. Reese to the Board of Trustees, May 9, 1887; Minutes of the Trustees, June 7, 1887; Files of the Dean of Law, 1887, UP.

17. The reluctance of the law school to appropriate medical jurisprudence, a reluctance shared by other law schools all around the country, raises serious questions about the applicability in this context of the model of professional development outlined in Andrew Abbott, *The System of Professions: An Essay on the Division of Expert Labor* (Chicago, 1988). By the end of the nineteenth century there was no real "boundary dispute" between medicine and law over medical jurisprudence, which had become, as it were, ground not worth contesting. In a literal sense, the field did not pay, and neither profession staked a claim to it by insisting upon its incorporation in their required curricula, then or since.

18. Minutes of the Trustees, Oct. 6, 1891, UP. The board thanked Reese for "his long and faithful service" and moved to afford him emeritus status.

19. Medical catalogues, UP, 1890–1900.

20. A chair of medical jurisprudence was re-created in 1904 at the University of Pennsylvania Medical School, but it was pretty clearly a ceremonial post for Daniel J. McCarthy, a wealthy friend of S. Weir Mitchell. Though McCarthy served as adviser to the Municipal Court of Philadelphia, he never made any scientific contributions of substance. When he retired in 1939, the chair was not continued. Young instructors occasionally organized lectures in the field after World War II, and Lawrence H. Eldridge, a lawyer, gave lectures to medical students into the 1960s on the legal aspects of medicine. But the statement that medical jurisprudence barely existed at Penn during the first two-thirds of the twentieth century is accurate. George W. Corner, *Two Centuries of Medicine: A History of the School of Medicine, University of Pennsylvania* (Philadelphia, 1965), 213, 291.

21. *Jefferson Medical College Catalogue*, 1868–69; 1880–81; 1891–92; 1898–99.

22. *NCAB* 12: 331.

23. *Albany Medical College Catalogue*, 1853, 1859, 1866–72, 1883, 1890, 1914–15; Surgeon General's collection, NLM.

24. *University of Missouri Medical School Catalogue*, 1886–1900; NLM.

25. Connecticut Medical Society, *Proceedings*, 1868: pamphlet in Yale University Archives.

26. *Annual Announcement . . . Medical Department of Yale College, 1862–63* through *1868–69*.

27. *Ibid., 1880–81*, 6.

28. *Ibid., 1885–86* through *1888–89*.

29. *Ibid., 1890*.

30. *Ibid., 1895*.

31. *Ibid., 1899*.

32. Henry K. Beecher and Mark D. Altschule, *Medicine at Harvard: The First Three Hundred Years* (Hanover, N.H., 1977), 121.

33. *Ibid.*, 290. The 1968 committee wanted to restore a broad version of medical jurisprudence to the curriculum. Their report was strikingly reminiscent of the professional vision of the 1820s. See the Ad Hoc Committee on the Lee Professorship in *ibid.*

34. *Catalogue of Starling Medical College,* 1867–1907, NLM.

35. *Catalogue of the Medical College of Ohio,* 1850, 1855–56, 1869, 1885–86, 1886–87, 1893–94, and *University of Cincinnati Medical School, Catalogue,* 1896–97 through 1907–08, NLM.

36. See the *Western Homoeopathic Medical College, Catalogue,* 1887–88: 9; NLM.

37. *Ibid., 1890–91* through *1901–02.*

38. Phinizy Spalding, *The History of the Medical College of Georgia* (Athens, 1987), 83–86. Spalding is candid about the nepotism and "mediocrity" that characterized MCG's treatment of several subjects during the 1880s.

39. My discussion of the situation at JHU is drawn primarily from Alan M. Chesney, *The Johns Hopkins Hospital and the Johns Hopkins University School of Medicine: A Chronicle, Volume 1: Early Years, 1867–1893* (Baltimore, 1943).

40. "Editorial," *Maryland Medical Journal* 2, no. 6 (1878): 403.

41. Ellzey, "Application of Chemistry," 530. Ellzey, a Virginian, also rued the fact that his own state's medical school failed to appreciate the importance of the subject, and he hoped that some benefactor would invigorate medical jurisprudence at the University of Virginia Medical School with a donation for that specific purpose.

42. Elizabeth Fee, *Disease and Discovery: A History of the Johns Hopkins School of Hygiene and Public Health, 1916–1939* (Baltimore, 1987), esp. 1–25; Donald Fleming, *William H. Welch and the Rise of Modern Medicine* (Baltimore [1954], 1987), 181–84.

43. Thomas Turner, *Heritage of Excellence: The Johns Hopkins Medical Institutions, 1914–1947* (Baltimore, 1974), 44–71, 169; quote: 169.

44. In addition to the schools already mentioned in this chapter, surveys were conducted for the University of Maryland Medical School and the Baltimore Medical College by a graduate student, Patricia German. The patterns were consistent, right to the adoption of defensive medical jurisprudence. The Baltimore Medical College, which had long before gone to a revolving door of local lawyers and judges lecturing irregularly, described its 1896–97 course in medical jurisprudence as one in which the students would be "taught rules of evidence, liabilities and duties of physicians, legal status of insanity, and how to testify in court, how to conduct themselves when under cross-examination on the witness stand, and to answer hypothetical questions in giving expert testimony." Examination of the advertisements for medical schools, which routinely appeared in medical journals like the *BMSJ,* also revealed fewer and fewer schools listing either professors of medical jurisprudence or courses in the subject after 1880.

45. Missouri was a case in point; see *Missouri Medical Catalogue, 1899–1900.* Western Homoeopathic, another case in point, actually announced a new professorship of life insurance in 1901; see *Western Homoeopathic Medical College, 1900–1901.*

46. Thomas Hall Shastid, "A History of Medical Jurisprudence in America," in Howard A. Kelly, ed., *A Cyclopedia of American Medical Biography,* Vol. 1 (Philadelphia, 1912), lxxv–lxxxv.

47. William G. Rothstein, *American Medical Schools and the Practice of Medicine: A History* (New York, 1987); Kenneth M. Ludmerer, *Learning to Heal: The Development of American Medical Education* (New York, 1985).

AFTERWORD

1. William J. Curran, "Medical-Examiner-System Reorganization in Massachusetts," *New England Journal of Medicine* 299, no. 6 (Aug. 10, 1978): 295. In the

law of 1978, even the newly created Chief Medical Examiner of the state was given a salary "clearly unrealistic and uncompetitive" by the standards of the day, and the act contained a number of steps that Massachusetts medical examiners considered backward rather than forward.

2. For modern examples of nationally publicized difficulties, see the *Washington Post*, July 23, 1984: A1; and the *New York Times*, July 28, 1990: 1. The latter summarizes a dispute that had dragged on for more than five years.

3. On the general process of authority-building by the medical profession, especially in the last decades of the nineteenth century and the early decades of the twentieth century, see Paul Starr, *The Social Transformation of American Medicine: The Rise of a Sovereign Profession and the Making of a Vast Industry* (New York, 1982), esp. 127–144.

4. *JAMA* 252 (1984): 251.

5. *New York Times*, June 23, 1982: A-1 and A-26.

6. *JAMA* 251 (1984): 2967–81; quote: 2981.

7. Wallace D. Riley and B. J. George, Jr., "Reform Not Abolition," *JAMA* 251 (1984): 2947–48; and Loren H. Roth, "Tighten but Do No Discard," *ibid.*, 2949–50. The AMA vote took place in Los Angeles in December 1983, and may be followed in any of the nation's major newspapers of that period.

8. David Faust and Jay Ziskin, "The Expert Witness in Psychology and Psychiatry," *Science* 241 (July 1988): 31–35; *New York Times*, "Psychologists' Expert Testimony Called Unscientific," Oct. 11, 1988: C-1.

9. Typical was an effort in 1964 in Los Angeles, where a special joint committee of the County Bar Association and the County Medical Association floated a series of procedures designed "to assist physicians and attorneys in their mutual professional contacts in the hope that misunderstandings leading to discord may be minimized and more meaningful interprofessional relationships, based on mutual respect, may be engendered." The report explored new rules for decorum in court, a "professional liability panel" to settle malpractice claims, the elimination of contingent fees, paid expert medical testimony at fixed rates, and the like; all to no real purpose. See "Interprofessional Code of the Los Angeles County Bar Association and the Los Angeles County Medical Association" (xerox of typescript, Los Angeles, 1964), Library of the Medical and Chirurgical Society of Maryland, Baltimore.

10. Losses paid by a major insurer in New York rose from less than half a million dollars in 1976 to more than $35.5 million in 1981. *New York Times*, Feb. 21, 1983, II, 4:1.

11. *Ibid.*, Aug. 31, 1983, I, 27:5.

Index